Gender-Critical Feminism

Gender-Critical Feminism

HOLLY LAWFORD-SMITH

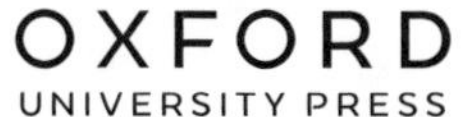

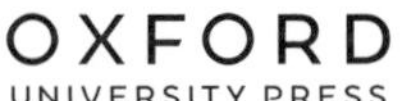

Great Clarendon Street, Oxford, OX2 6DP,
United Kingdom

Oxford University Press is a department of the University of Oxford.
It furthers the University's objective of excellence in research, scholarship,
and education by publishing worldwide. Oxford is a registered trade mark of
Oxford University Press in the UK and in certain other countries

First Edition published in 2022

Impression: 2

Published in the United States of America by Oxford University Press
198 Madison Avenue, New York, NY 10016, United States of America

British Library Cataloguing in Publication Data
Data available

Library of Congress Control Number: 2021940430

ISBN 978–0–19–886388–5

DOI: 10.1093/oso/9780198863885.001.0001

Printed and bound by
CPI Group (UK) Ltd, Croydon, CR0 4YY

For Elisa and Coda.
May you grow up in a world that has real feminism in it;
and grow old in a world that no longer needs it.

Contents

Preface

There have been countless moments throughout history when momentous social shifts occurred. We've shifted from thinking the earth was at the centre of the universe to realizing it's just one more planet to orbit the sun. We've shifted from feudal societies where accidents of birth determine who lives in luxury and who works to pay for that luxury, to societies governed by the principle of equal opportunity. We've stopped believing in 'humours', four fluids that make up the body in different proportions and determine people's mental and physical capacities. Many of us have shifted from belief in a god or gods creating life, to having an evolutionary understanding of the origins of life. We've stopped thinking it's acceptable to own people, or to keep people in conditions of slavery or servitude.

We could zoom in on any one of these moments in history and find our protagonists, people courageously challenging the prevailing orthodoxy, or working underground to help those harmed the most by that orthodoxy. Our narrative for these historical moments is often binary: the resisters, the rebels, the misfits, and the visionaries, versus everyone else. The people in the mainstream who go along with the status quo, and the people who see the problem and start to do something about it. The orthodox, and the heterodox.

There was a binary narrative like this for feminism, once: feminists were the rebels, the women who first started to ask questions about whether woman was really destined to be merely the wife and helpmate of man. Feminism was simple then. It was a single heterodoxy fighting for women's rights and opportunities. It challenged the perception that what woman appeared to be, itself a product of rigid social conditioning, was all she was capable of being. The orthodoxy it worked against, in place in many conservative countries and in many segments of progressive countries even today, was a set of ideas according to which men were meant to be masculine, women were meant to be feminine, and women were *for* the servicing of men and men's needs. Men and women were considered to be very different, and women were considered to be inferior. Feminism was *the* sex/gender heterodoxy then. This isn't *ancient* history, it was true as recently as the 1970s, but it's history nonetheless.

The moment we're in right now, when it comes to sex and gender, does not fit this binary structure. Now the heterodoxy is plural, and its factions are in fierce disagreement with each other. Here are two—very different—heterodox accounts of sex and gender:

Gender as identity. There is no sex/gender distinction, there is only gender.[1] Sex, the idea that humans can be sorted into two biological types, male and female, is an outdated concept. Sex is a spectrum; or there are many different sexes; or there is really no such thing as sex, just a set of bad ideas imposed onto arbitrary features of bodies.[2] Whatever sex is or was, it doesn't matter anymore. What matters is gender, in particular, gender understood as *identity.* Every human person has a gender identity, at minimum 'man', 'woman', or 'nonbinary'. This new way of sorting people into categories supersedes sex, but takes over the role that sex used to play, for example as the basis of romantic and sexual attractions between people, or as the trait determining which social spaces can be appropriately used. According to this view, transwomen are women, transmen are men, and nonbinary people are neither women nor men. A transwoman belongs on a women's sports team, or in a women's prison, or in a women's domestic violence refuge. Same-sex attractions are 'transphobic'.[3] Women-centred language is 'exclusionary' if it refers to biological traits.[4] Wearing pussy hats and t-shirts with uteruses printed on them to the women's march is bad; it suggests a connection between women and vulvas, women and uteruses.[5] But some men have vulvas and uteruses (transmen), and some women don't (transwomen).

Gender as social norms and expectations. There is a sex/gender distinction, and sex is indispensable to it. There are two sexes, male and female, and intersex conditions do not undermine this. Gender is a set of social norms and expectations imposed on the basis of sex. There is no understanding gender without sex. Women are subject to the expectation that they be feminine, men that they be masculine. Men are valued more highly than women. Understanding gender as norms imposed on the basis of sex allows us to make predictions, for example about who will be subject to social sanctions (masculine and other gender norm non-conforming women, feminine and other gender norm non-conforming men). And it allows us to think about the social construction of femininity, the ways that women have been 'made' to be feminine, both throughout history, and within an individual woman's lifetime. This understanding allows us to critique a range of social practices, for example the standards of beauty by which women are assessed. These may require women to spend more time and money, and accept more pain and discomfort, than men (for example, to purchase skincare regimens, makeup, hair products, clothing and shoes; to take the extra time needed to apply makeup and style hair; to have body hair plucked, waxed, or lasered; to undergo cosmetic surgeries like breast implants, nose jobs, or labiaplasties).[6] It is the social construction of womanhood that causes some women to dis-identify with womanhood and in some cases attempt to disaffiliate from womanhood ('I am not like that, so I must not be a woman'). And conversely, it is the social construction of womanhood that attracts some people who are not female to identify with womanhood and in some cases affiliate with womanhood ('I am like that, so I must be a woman').

It is not uncommon that competing heterodoxies lose sight of the common enemy they have in the orthodoxy, and focus their opposition upon each other. For example in the documentary *Rebel Dykes* (2019), women involved in lesbian feminism in London in the 1980s describe a social landscape in which homophobia was rife, and there was a lack of legal rights and protections for gay and lesbian people. The second wave feminist movement, starting in the late 1960s and taking off in the early 1970s, had created a flourishing underground scene of lesbians, many of whom were separatists (refusing the company of men entirely). But the radical feminists and the lesbian separatists were critical of lesbian romance and lesbian sex that imitated heterosexuality, and they were vehemently opposed to male violence against women, which they saw lesbian sadomasochism as imitating. This created a conflict at the time, with the lesbians who wanted to explore and enjoy all forms of sexuality, including those which could be argued to be imitating heterosexuality or male violence. The 'rebel dykes' were leather-wearing, motorbike-riding, 'sex positive' lesbians, many involved in underground clubs where there were live lesbian sex shows, including performances of sadomasochistic sex. It is clear from the documentary that the opposition between the 'rebel dykes' and the other lesbian feminists was fierce, with some of the women interviewed in the film describing a raid by the radical feminists and lesbian separatists on one of their sex clubs, where the furniture was smashed with crow bars and women were threatened.

A similar opposition has emerged within the sex/gender heterodoxy today. In the place of crow bars there is excessive social sanctioning. From both sides there is social media dogpiling, and unpleasant, *ad hominem* attacks. From the gender-as-identity crowd against the gender-as-norms crowd there are open letters, campus protests, campaigns to get women fired (some of which have been successful), malicious accusations made in the media and on social media, campaigns to get women banned from online platforms (often successful), deplatformings, taking women to court, forcing women out of political parties, the occasional physical assault, and more. The gender-as-norms crowd are diverted into expending enormous energy in defending themselves, and their views, rather than simply getting on with the work of feminism as they understand it.

Disagreement with gender as identity is taken to mean agreement with conservative or traditionalist views about gender. This is a failure to see 'beyond the binary' of disagreement about sex and gender. In this case there is not just the rebels and everyone else. There are two very different groups of rebels, who have very different ideas about what is wrong with the status quo, and what the best methods are for changing it. This is a book about one group of rebels under siege today, those resisting the political erasure of sex, and fighting to maintain the understanding of gender as norms, because of its immense utility in describing, understanding, and challenging sexist socialization. These rebels call themselves gender-critical feminists, referring to the idea that gender is something we should be critical of. I am one of them.

I wrote this book because I think gender-critical feminism presents the greatest challenge to conservative or traditionalist views about gender and has the best chance of overturning it. I think it is more ambitious, and significantly more appealing and coherent, than the alternative heterodox view of sex/gender. I worry about the future of feminism, because I do not see how we can fight for women's liberation when we have ceded any understanding of the trait on which women's oppression is based (namely sex) and the system which helps to perpetuate it (gender norms). Contemporary feminism is kind, inclusive, and affirming of women's choices, whatever they happen to be. Those traits have value, but they will not overturn thousands of years of oppression on the basis of sex, or earn women their liberation. I hope to persuade you that gender-critical feminism is the theory and movement that we need.

Acknowledgements

The period in which I wrote this book was not an easy one, which is why I am even more grateful to the people who have helped me with it. From comments on my original proposal through conversations about issues arising in specific chapters through reading groups on background material to feedback on the final chapter drafts, many people have been generous with their time and expertise. There are some people that I cannot name—such is the political landscape this book will become a part of, that doing so would create a risk to them. But they know who they are; I am grateful to them for their time and support and many interesting conversations.

To those I can name. Kathleen Stock, Sophie Allen, Nin Kirkham, Caroline Norma, Stephanie Collins, Alex Byrne, Frank Hindriks, David Schweikard, Katie Steele, Christian Barry, Dana Goswick, Luara Ferracioli, Kate Phelan, Jess Megarry, Cordelia Fine, Wolfgang Schwarz, John Matthewson, Howard Sankey, Rosa Freedman, Karen Riley, Rachael Hadoux, Tegan Larin, Bernard Lane, J. Michael Bailey, Komarine Romdenh-Romluc, Meghan Murphy, Ani O'Brien, Axel Gosseries, Anca Gheaus, Siba Harb, Marie Bastin, Eric Boot, John Thrasher, Dan Halliday, Callie Burt, Adi James, Colin Klein, Zakiya Deliefde, Lilian Gonzalez, Evie, Ole Koksvik, Sun Liu, Rene Rejon, Will Tuckwell, and Ryan Cox. Thank you so much.

Kate Phelan, especially, has been immeasurably helpful, and I am hugely grateful to her for the probably hundreds of conversations we have had about the topics in this book over the last few years.

I owe a particular thanks to Luara Ferracioli, Stephanie Collins, Ryan Cox, Alex Byrne, Rene Rejon, and Kate Phelan, as well as to my editor Peter Momtchiloff and three anonymous reviewers for Oxford University Press, who all read the whole book and made a ton of helpful suggestions for improvement. I'm also grateful to multiple reviewers, both of the initial proposal for this book and for comments on the full manuscript, many of which helped me to sharpen my ideas and my arguments. Thank you.

Thanks also to audiences at the Australian National University, University of Melbourne, Australian Catholic University, Université catholique de Louvain, York University, University of Manchester, University of Western Australia, Murdoch University, Victoria University of Wellington, University of Sydney, University of Auckland, Universität Flensburg, and University of Reading.

There are also some people I'd like to thank for something broader than the book. First, the philosophers who spoke up early, often at personal cost, about some of the issues I discuss here: Rebecca Reilly-Cooper, Jane Clare Jones, Kathleen Stock, Sophie Allen, Mary Leng, Elizabeth Finneron-Burns, Molly Gardner, Teresa Marques, Emily Vicendese, Alex Byrne, Tomas Bogardus, John Schwenkler, Daniel Kaufman, and Spencer Case. Second, the philosophers who spoke out in support of my and other gender-critical feminist philosophers' academic freedom to pursue these issues: Brian Leiter, José Bermudez, Clare Chambers, Cordelia Fine, Edward Hall, Benj Hellie, Thomas Kelly, Jeff McMahan, Francesca Minerva, John Schwenkler, Peter Singer, Nicole Vincent, and Jessica Wilson.

Epigraphs Permissions

In the radical feminist view, the new feminism is not just the revival of a serious political movement for social equality. It is the second wave of the most important revolution in history. Its aim: overthrow of the oldest, most rigid class/caste system in existence, the class system based on sex—a system consolidated over thousands of years, lending the archetypal male and female roles an undeserved legitimacy and seeming permanence.

Shulamith Firestone, *The Dialectic of Sex.*[7]

1
Introduction

Something strange has happened to feminism in the last forty years. What was once a thriving social justice movement, led by women and for the political advancement of women's interests, has today morphed into something else entirely. For one thing, it doesn't seem to be particularly *for* women anymore. It's about a lot of different issues, some of which involve women and some of which don't. For another, it doesn't seem to be particularly *by* women anymore. Increasingly, men claim the authority to tell women who must be included in feminism, or what feminism must be like. There were always divisions and often factions, but today there are tribes and they are so polarized that there seems to be little chance of reconciling differences. Below I'll give two examples of how feminism has changed. Then I'll spend a little time emphasizing the points of agreement between different types of feminists, before explaining what I'm trying to do in this book, and how I've organized it.

A brief note on terminology, before we get started. I'll use 'male' and 'female' in the standard way, to refer to the two biological sexes. The former is the sex that all going well produces small mobile gametes (sperm), the latter is the sex that all going well produces large immobile gametes (eggs).[1] The meanings of these terms are contested, with some preferring to use them synonymously with 'man' and 'woman' with both referring exclusively to gender identity. But there are no other terms available to refer to sex, and the ability to refer to sex is indispensable to my project in this book. So that is how I will proceed.

1.1 Women's Issues, from Centre to Margin

Two examples help to illustrate the shift in what is considered to be the subject matter or concern of feminism.[2] The first is about activism, the second about academia.

Gender-Critical Feminism: Holly Lawford-Smith, Oxford University Press. © Holly Lawford-Smith 2022.
DOI: 10.1093/oso/9780198863885.003.0001

Women's day march. According to the International Women's Day (IWD) website, the 8th of March 'is a global day celebrating the social, economic, cultural and political achievements of women', which 'marks a call to action for accelerating women's equality'. The first IWD gathering was in 1911, which makes the day more than a hundred years old. The image on their website linking through to the themes for IWD 2020 included posters saying 'I will challenge gender stereotypes and bias', and 'I will call out gendered actions or assumptions'.[3] The website is full of photographs of strong, empowered women: women of colour standing making the 'equals' sign with their arms; women working in technology, business, and health; women in sports and the arts. So far so good—all of this seems like a fairly standard approach to feminist activism.

And yet, the IWD Melbourne Collective, the group who organize the march for the city of Australia where I live, issued a list of demands in advance of IWD 2019 which were puzzlingly distant from this kind of feminism. This was their full list of demands:

1. Justice for First Nations peoples, Indigenous workers' rights, and land rights
2. An end to all forms of violence against women and children
3. An end to all imperialist wars
4. An end to racism
5. Access to permanent residence and citizenship rights for all refugees and migrant workers
6. Secure and decent employment for all, and equal pay for equal work
7. A living wage for all women in all industries
8. The right to organize unions and take collective action, including industrial action and solidarity action, free from violence, intimidation, and legal harassment
9. Health and safety at work, just compensation, and rehabilitation
10. Paid parental leave and affordable childcare
11. Full rights and freedom from violence for people of all sexual orientations
12. Full rights and freedom from violence for intersex people
13. Listen to sex worker peer organizations, and support the rights, health, and safety of sex workers, including the full decriminalisation of all forms of sex work
14. Justice for people with disabilities—freedom from violence, full access to public spaces, and an end to all forms of discrimination

15. Full reproductive rights for all women
16. Free and accessible healthcare for all
17. Affordable housing for all
18. Social security and a just welfare system
19. Free and accessible education for all
20. An end to environmental destruction, and compensation for all victims worldwide.[4]

Note the language here. First Nations *peoples*, Indigenous *workers*, *refugees*, migrant *workers*, employment for *all*, *parental* leave, *people* of all sexual orientations, intersex *people*, sex *workers*, *people* with disabilities, healthcare for *all*, housing for *all*, education for *all*, compensation for *victims* of environmental destruction. Out of twenty demands, the word 'women' appears only three times: 'an end to all forms of violence against women and children', 'a living wage for all women in all industries', and 'full reproductive rights for all women'. One might have expected the one day a year that is about women to have a list of demands relating exclusively to women's interests.

My point is not that feminist collectives should limit themselves to making demands that are good *only* for women. One of the IWD Melbourne Collective's demands was 'paid parental leave and affordable childcare'. This is a demand that will benefit both men and women. But it will *largely* benefit women, because in most countries—including Australia—workplaces grant more paid maternity leave than paternity leave, and in many countries there is not adequate affordable childcare, which creates a structure of economic incentives that encourage women to spend more time out of work, sometimes giving up their careers entirely. Some things that are good for women will have incidental benefits for men, and *that* they will have these benefits is no reason at all for feminists not to want them.

But consider another of the collective's demands, namely 'justice for people with disabilities—freedom from violence, full access to public spaces, and an end to all forms of discrimination'. This will benefit women, because some people with disabilities are women. But women are not disproportionately represented among the community of people with disabilities (in Australia it is 17.8 per cent females and 17.6 per cent males).[5] This is not a feminist demand; it's a demand that could be made by anyone interested in justice and equality. Most of the collective's list is like that.

When the list of demands issued by a women's collective are general demands for justice and equality, feminism is in trouble. Demands for justice and equality are no bad things, but doing global justice and calling it feminism *is* a bad thing, because it suggests to the world that there is a lot of feminism going on, when there is really much less than there appears to be. Radical and gender-critical feminists on social media frequently ask, 'why are women the only people who aren't allowed to centre themselves in their own liberation movement?'[6]

It's important to distinguish two questions. One is *what is feminism*, what does a theory and movement that deserves the name look like? The other is *whether we should be feminists*, which is the same as asking what social causes we should each choose to fight for. In this book I'll be talking only about the former. Women are a little more than half the global population, and some of the obstacles they face are extremely serious. Whether or not this is *the most important* social cause and thus has a claim to everyone's time and energy, it's *an important* social cause and thus has a claim to at least some people's time and energy.

I'm not interested in persuading you that you should abandon disability justice movements in favour of feminism. We need both. I'm interested in persuading you that *if* feminism is the social cause you choose, that cause might not be what you think it is (and what influential organizations and self-styled spokeswomen represent it as being). As radical feminist Julia Beck has said, 'if feminism was reduced to one word, it would be "no!"'[7] In this case, the 'no' is an answer to the question 'would you mind just taking care of these other 6,789 social justice issues while you're at it?'.

Women's studies. The University of Sydney was one of the first universities in the world to offer a course in women's studies, taught by Australian feminist Madge Dawson in 1956.[8] The course was called 'Women in a Changing World', which focused on the social, economic, and political situation of women in the liberal democracies of western Europe. Sydney's *Arts and Social Sciences Undergraduate Handbook 2020* lists no subject areas under either women's studies or feminism, but does list gender studies. From its description it is clear that this is not a shift in name only, but in content:

> Gender studies challenges and enriches our understanding of masculinity, femininity, transgender, sexuality and identity, and provides a framework for considering social and cultural issues gender impacts, ranging from debates about marriage equality and new forms of intimacy to gendered forms of labour, violence and representational practices; and how gender relates to other salient experiences such as race, coloniality, sexuality, class, and ability.[9]

Women's studies is about women; gender studies is about everyone.

Of the top five universities in Australia,[10] four don't have women's studies courses anymore (University of Melbourne, Australian National University, University of Sydney, and University of Queensland) but they do have gender studies (Queensland only as a minor, the others as a major); only the University of New South Wales, Sydney, has a course that tries to combine the two, namely 'Women's and Gender Studies'. They describe it as being about 'women, feminism, gender, sex, and sexualities'.[11]

During the school year 1969–70, Phyllis Chesler—one of the most prominent feminists of the second wave[12]—taught one of the first classes in women's studies in the United States (US), at what was then Richmond College in New York City. The class become a minor and then a major. In her memoir, *A Politically Incorrect Feminist*, Chesler talks about how she and five students went and sat in the office of the head of department and refused to leave until he approved the funding to cover her other teaching, so that she could teach the class (which she had completed all the paperwork and had initial approval for, but which at the last minute had been refused on grounds of insufficient funding).[13]

Marilyn Boxer said of the time that 'merely to assert that women should be studied was a radical act'.[14] According to Alice Ginsberg, editor of *The Evolution of American Women's Studies*, women's studies was political, functioning as 'the "academic arm" of the women's movement', 'restoring lost histories', and 'allowing silenced voices to be heard'.[15] In 2009, there were over 800 women's studies programmes in the US. Ginsberg said 'we can't overlook the significance of the apostrophe in the name women's studies. Born from the women's movement, women are finally claiming *their own* lost histories and taking the lead in challenging the social construction of knowledge'.[16]

While the first class happened in 1956 (and perhaps even earlier elsewhere), women's studies programmes weren't commonplace until the 1970s, and they were already starting to be broadened out and renamed in 2009. Even assuming they became commonplace in the early 1970s, which is probably a generous assumption, that's still less than forty years before they were massively diluted. Not a very long period for women to restore their lost histories, recover silenced voices, and teach young women about the history of women's rights struggles and women's oppression.

Compare it to classes and courses dedicated to histories of racial oppression. Universities in New Zealand offer courses in Maori studies, teaching Maori language, history, politics, and performing arts.[17] Imagine if after roughly forty years of this it was decided that those courses should be broadened out to include all minority ethnic and new immigrant groups in New Zealand, and after a while we renamed all the courses 'minority ethnic studies' and spent most of the time in them talking about Tuvaluan and Maldivian climate refugees. Or worse: at least that might plausibly be justified as a 'focusing on the least well-off' in some possible future state of New Zealand. Imagine instead all the time is spent talking about economic migrants from wealthy European countries.

There's nothing wrong with courses being replaced in principle. Maybe they're about technologies that become obsolete, or science that goes out of date. But these are not good parallels for women's history. The thousands of years' long history of women's oppression, and the struggle for women's rights starting in the United Kingdom (UK) in 1832,[18] and still in progress, would be important even if women had achieved full social justice—it's unlikely that we'll stop teaching civil rights history when we achieve racial justice. The way people are capable of treating one another is an important part of human history and something we should all remain aware of, lest history repeat. But it's not only history. Women have not achieved full social justice yet. Women's studies matters.

This doesn't mean gender studies programmes shouldn't exist. There are different phenomena we may be interested in. One is women's oppression, another is the many social groups that have suffered collateral damage in the oppression of women. For example, as femininity was imposed onto women and then women were disparaged, femininity came to be disparaged independently, and this had negative effects on anyone who was feminine whether they were a woman or not. As superiority was claimed for men, masculinity was imposed and while this came with benefits it also came with some harms. We might want to talk about this wider phenomenon, which would mean talking about all of the social groups—including, but not limited to, women—that have been impacted by women's oppression, looking for common causes and common impacts. But we might just as well want to focus on the narrower phenomenon, the original victims of sexism, the group that remains the largest constituency of those harmed by sexism, namely women. Women's studies did that; gender studies does not.

1.2 What Feminists Can Agree About

In writing a book about feminism, explaining disagreements and defending a particular position, it is easy to give the impression that *everything* is a disagreement. But that just isn't the case. Feminists of very different types can want the same outcomes for different reasons, or the same outcomes for the same reasons—it's just that once they've secured them, some will stop and others will carry on. Visions for a feminist future can have different levels of ambition, so that they overlap in part. One perspective within feminism has become dominant (on the left at least) and crowded out alternative perspectives, which has increased the toxicity of disagreements between its position on particular issues and that of other types of feminism. I'll be defending a feminism that has disagreements with the dominant perspective in three particularly charged areas (the sex industry, trans/gender, and intersectionality). But that shouldn't be taken to suggest that there isn't, nonetheless, a lot of common ground, at least when it comes to outcomes. Below are some examples.

Male violence against women and girls. Feminists of all types can agree that male violence against women and girls is a problem and needs to be addressed. It is uncontroversial that this includes phenomena like trafficking into sexual slavery, acid attacks, honour killings, domestic violence, rape, sexual assault, child abuse, and child marriage (which, when between a girl child and an adult man, will generally also involve rape).[19] Even those who disagree about the status of 'sex work' and how the sex industry should be regulated (if at all) can agree that the violence within the industry is a problem, including the murder, trafficking, rape, sexual assault, child abuse, and physical assault that go on across it.

Full control of reproduction. Feminists of most types (the exception being some religious feminists) can agree that a woman must have the right to choose when and whether to have a family. This means having control over her sexuality (when and whether she has sex, and whether that sex will risk pregnancy—so she needs sexual autonomy and access to contraceptives), and *both* being able to have an abortion if she decides that is what she wants, *and* being able to *not have* an abortion if she decides that is what she wants. This means she needs it not to be the case that a controlling state, or controlling individual, can force her to do one thing or the other (a one-child state policy, or a husband, may force her to abort; a state where abortion is illegal, or a religious husband, may force her to carry a pregnancy to term).

Feminists of many, or at least most, types can agree that there are good reasons why women need to have abortions, regardless of whether they have further opinions about this. Chesler writes for example, in criticizing people who protest outside abortion clinics, of

> A woman who requires a medical abortion; a woman who chooses not to carry a seriously ill fetus to term; a mother of five who cannot afford another child; a woman who needs radiation for cancer and whose physician has advised her to have an abortion; a rape-impregnated victim; a young woman who cannot afford to raise a child and also work a full-time job so she can attend college.[20]

Sexual objectification and beauty standards. Lisa Taddeo writes in her book *Three Women* (2019) 'One inheritance of living under the male gaze for centuries is that heterosexual women often look at other women the way a man would'.[21] Feminists of all types can agree on the negative impacts on women that our culture of sexual and aesthetic objectification of women has had, and be interested in finding ways to disrupt this objectification and see women represented as, and understood to be, full human persons. This is likely to mean changes to public spaces (billboards and posters), the media (particularly advertising), and film and television (how female characters are depicted). This may also have knock-on effects for other feminist issues, like increasing equality of sexual pleasure (women will get more if men don't think women are *for* the sexual pleasure of men), reducing rape and sexual assault (at least where this is caused by sexual entitlement), and increasing the representation of women in politics, leadership, and industries where they have been underrepresented (by impacting stereotypes and expectations).

Women at work. Feminists since long before the second wave have been concerned about women's access to work, whether about their being permitted to work (or work in particular industries), or about their pay and benefits in comparison to men, or about their underrepresentation within specific industries and in leadership positions across all industries.[22] Most types of feminists can agree that equal opportunity is important, so that at the very least we should be working to get rid of direct and indirect discrimination. They can also probably agree that it is likely that serious differences in the numbers of men and women in particular industries suggest that *either* there has been discrimination *or* there is a 'pipeline problem', which means that at some earlier point in time, perhaps even in early childhood, there have been influences that have steered some towards, and others away from, those industries.[23]

It is likely that feminists can agree on early childhood interventions, and educational campaigns, designed to tackle these inequalities, such as programmes to get girls interested in science, technology, engineering, and maths (STEM). None of this requires signing on to preferential hiring (where of two equally qualified candidates, preference is given to the woman), or affirmative action (where preference is given to the woman even if she is worse-qualified, so long as she is sufficiently qualified), about which there is likely to be more disagreement tracking different fundamental commitments.[24] Neither does it require settling *why* it is important for women to work, or even saying *that* they should necessarily work.

Equality of sexual pleasure. Feminists of all different types, even those at war over the sex industry, can also agree that the sheer quantity of bad and unwanted sex women are having all around the world is a serious feminist issue.[25] While feminists have long since agreed that rape and sexual assault are feminist issues, there is not as much attention given to bad and unwanted sex. This includes sex women have as a matter of duty, perhaps to preserve relationships; the casual sex women sign up for in the hopes of mutual satisfaction, but which ends up being unsatisfying; the sex which women end up having because the ways that they signal its being unwanted are not heeded by men. Feminists of different types can agree that it would be better if there were more equality in sexual pleasure, and focus on ways to make this happen—from more emphasis on consent as a clear and effective signal,[26] through to campus programmes in self-defence and assertiveness,[27] through to programmes in sex education and sexual equality[28] (particularly for boys).

1.3 Leftist Mansplaining of Feminism

'You should be able to rely on the Left to be on the side of feminists', wrote Julie Bindel in 2018. 'And yet, in recent years, I have experienced far more direct sexism from these so-called feminist "socialist" men than Tory ones.'[29] She criticizes leftist men for defending men's consumption of pornography, including Owen Jones who defended a politician's consumption of pornography at work;[30] and for supporting a decriminalized sex industry, which is exploitative of women. She also complains that these men lecture women about their understandings of what a woman is, as though they have superior knowledge about that. She writes:

> [Owen] Jones is also notorious for lecturing women about who actually has the right to decide who is female or not; he regularly berates anyone who dares suggest that people with penises are not actually women. In one

> of his articles, he declared that the group of people he terms 'transphobes' (who refuse to accept men as women) will be consigned to the 'wrong side of history' for their views.[31]

It's not surprising that someone like Owen Jones, a leftist journalist who writes frequently for *The Guardian*, thinks he gets a say in the question of what a woman/female is, because the dominant form of feminism has encouraged this by declaring that 'feminism is for everybody'.[32] Jane Mansbridge, a second-wave feminist and Harvard professor, says that feminists in the 1960s and 1970s saw their collectives as 'pre-figuring change in the society', which means, testing out the changes they desired for wider society on a smaller scale. She said, 'I consider the women's movement the least hierarchical, the most open and the most inclusive social movement that I have ever come across', but worried that the way the movement handled conflict was 'adversarial' and that this didn't bode well for wider social transformation.[33] On this way of thinking about the feminist movement, as a precursor to a wider transformation that is something like *justice for everyone*, gatekeeping membership doesn't make a lot of sense.

It might seem appealing to be so warm and inclusive, but here is an alternative view. Declaring that feminism is for everybody, and welcoming men into feminism not merely as allies but as people who can *be* feminist thinkers, leaders, and activists if they so desire, guts feminism of one of its most important accomplishments, which is the self-determination of women.[34] Women, as an oppressed class/caste,[35] have the right to form political associations to fight sex-based injustice and to advance their political interests. Women have the right to figure out, separately from men, what exactly they think it means to be a woman, *if it means anything at all.* Men, throughout history, have created and imposed femininity onto women. In order to achieve liberation, women must escape from men's ideas about women. From this it follows that *men do not get any say in what a woman is, and men cannot be feminists.*[36]

For those who like the idea that feminism is evolving from a movement for women into a movement for social justice more generally, it's worth asking why it's *women* who are being asked to (or are asking themselves to) take on this enormous project. It's perfectly conceivable that a division of labour between groups focused on specific constituencies' issues would be more effective, and that all of these groups could link up as allies at some point—when they have made sufficient gains—in order to form a broader base for a more general social justice movement. But it's hardly the case that women's issues, globally, have been resolved and we've now got some time on our hands to take on a bit more work. These issues are far from solved. And I don't see anyone telling Black Lives Matter, or Extinction Rebellion, that they should adopt a broader agenda, and stop being so narrowly focused on a 'single issue'.

This question of men's place in feminism has become particularly fraught when it comes to transgender issues. It is one thing to say that men like Owen Jones should be quiet about what a woman is because that's not a question *he* gets to have a say in. It's another to say that the increasing numbers of male people who 'identify as women' *also* simply don't get a say. Where leftist feminists may disagree over the question of whether men can be feminists, and that disagreement has practical implications such as whether it's permissible for feminists to bring boyfriends to the 'Reclaim the Night' march,[37] this doesn't generally cause a schism where those who disagree will end friendships and working relationships.

But disagreement *does* cause this schism when it comes to transgender issues. Many feminists today tend to use self-identification as the sole criterion for being a woman. For them, what it means to be a woman is to be a person of either sex who identifies as a woman. Identifying as a woman has no specific content, for example relating to appearance, behaviour, or character. To identify as something sounds like a mental state, one that manifests solely in a person's declaration that they are, in fact, a woman. When some women refuse to include male people with this mental state as feminist thinkers, leaders, and activists, those feminists see them as *discriminating against women*. And of course, all feminists can agree that feminism is for all women, whether or not it is also for all men. So this becomes a very serious, and highly moralized, point of disagreement.

1.4 The Great Gulf of Feminism

Reading through accounts of the second wave in the US, it is clear that there has always been in-fighting within feminist collectives.[38] Phyllis Chesler's colourful description of the movement gives a sense of this: 'In our midst was the usual assortment of scoundrels, sadists, bullies, con artists, liars, loners, and incompetents, not to mention the high-functioning psychopaths, schizophrenics, manic depressives, and suicide artists. I loved them all'.[39] Jo Freeman wrote in 1976 about 'trashing', the phenomenon of feminist women attacking and undermining one another. She says 'It took three trashings to convince me to drop out...I felt psychologically mangled to the point where I knew I couldn't go on.'[40]

Still, *being together* inside feminist collectives where there were issues between some individuals and others, and between some individuals and all the rest, is something very different to *not being together at all.* We've gone from fallouts and factions within a somewhat cohesive feminist movement to tribalism of the most extravagant kind, where feminists of different types are quite literally protected from hearing each other's criticisms and alternative viewpoints. These protections come in the form of social media mechanisms allowing blocking (including, on Twitter, the option to subscribe to large blocklists, the most notorious of which inside radical and gender-critical feminist circles is 'TERFblocker'), and muting; and in real life, cutting ties with people and refusing to participate in the same events or be on the same platforms.

For example, five days before the conference 'Historical Materialism' was scheduled to begin at the University of Sydney in 2018, the organizers emailed Caroline Norma—a radical feminist academic—to tell her she'd been removed from the conference programme and her registration fee had been refunded. Their reason was that comments made by Norma in an earlier media piece about the left driving women out were inconsistent with the conference's commitment to 'an inclusive space for people with diverse gender identities.'[41] In the earlier piece, she had argued that transgenderism was 'wedge politics', a way for leftists to purge feminists from their ranks.[42] Apparently academics, not usually expected to mindlessly agree with one another, had decided that women with the 'wrong' views on gender must be excised from a conference programme in the name of diversity. A quick glance through the conference programme suggests that most of the speakers were men.[43] Norma was eventually reinstated to the programme, but ended up presenting without the other panellists and to a largely empty audience, which she speculates was due to an open letter encouraging conference attendees to boycott.[44]

Why are we excising our dissidents rather than celebrating them for the role they play in forcing us all to defend our ideas and think more clearly? Why has feminism become a matter of tribes, rather than a matter of issues? In principle, it should be possible to be a feminist who thinks that sex work is work but transwomen are not women, or transwomen are women but sex work is institutionalized violence against women.[45] But in practice, it is very difficult to hold this combination of views, because having the 'wrong' views on sex work or trans issues makes you an enemy to the relevant tribe.

Feminism today is more polarized than ever before, which leads to each side misunderstanding the other, and sometimes demonizing the other, rather than having the kind of open dialogue that leads to mutual understanding, constructive (rather than destructive) disagreement, and the finding of common ground. This is just as disastrous inside the feminist movement as it is in democratic politics more broadly.

1.5 Gender-Critical Feminism

The remedy for the version of feminism that has become about everything and for everyone is gender-critical feminism. This is a feminism that has its roots in radical feminism, influential during the second wave, before the various cultural influences that broadened out the scope and constituency of feminism came along. But it won't do to simply rewind the clock sixty years. Radical feminists themselves got many things right, but some things wrong.[46] And they couldn't speak to social conditions that hadn't yet arisen, like the massive expansion of the pornography industry, or the institutional adoption of the ideology of gender identity.

Gender-critical feminism is both a continuation of radical feminism and distinct from it. There are many women who describe themselves as gender-critical feminists, who are talking and writing and doing activism and together slowly building a shared idea of what gender-critical feminism is. Some think of it as a new name for an old position, while others see it as a new position. Many perceive it as being focused on a single issue, namely the social uptake of gender identity. One of the arguments I will make in this book is that this is a mistake. Gender-critical feminism is a general feminist theory (albeit one that is still a work in progress). The fact that it currently gives the bulk of its attention to a single issue is explained by the urgency of that issue, and not anything more fundamental to the theory of gender-critical feminism itself. It is about being critical of gender, and this has implications for a wide range of feminist issues, not just gender identity.[47]

Philip Pettit made the following observation in a 1993 paper when he talked about trying to distinguish the political theories of liberalism and republicanism:

> there is a problem facing anyone who tries to describe the intellectual profile of a tradition like liberalism or republicanism. This is that traditions

> of this kind do not come with their intellectual profile already well defined. The traditions are identified and unified, individuals are selected as representatives and exemplars of the traditions, on a variety of intellectually incidental bases…One basis may be the figures acknowledged as heroes or anti-heroes, another texts taken as authoritative or heretical, yet another the events depicted as glorious or tragic, and so on across a range of possibilities.[48]

The same is true for gender-critical feminism. There is disparate theory and activism being produced across multiple countries. (The Women's Human Rights Campaign, which is gender-critical, has country contacts in Argentina, Australia, Brazil, Canada, Croatia, Denmark, France, Germany, India, Ireland, Italy, The Netherlands, Portugal, Serbia, Singapore, Slovakia, South Korea, Spain, Sweden, Ukraine, UK, and the US).[49] I will make decisions about how to unify that theory and activism that may not be to the liking of everyone who thinks of themselves as a gender-critical feminist. My heroes may not be the same as those of another gender-critical feminist; the work I take as authoritative may not be the same as what some other gender-critical feminists do; I may see particular events in a different light to other gender-critical feminists.

We will inevitably end up with something that is covered in my fingerprints. In talking with other gender-critical feminists, I have found my conclusions on the sex industry and trans/gender to be widely shared, even if not all the ideas that take me to them are. But I have taken particular liberties with intersectionality. On that topic I am arguing with everyone—radical, gender-critical, and liberal alike.

I have three aims in this book. First, I want to convince you that the version of feminism that gets the most airtime today barely deserves the name. I don't mean this in the petty way where we sneer across our differences of opinion muttering *that's not real feminism*.[50] Rather I mean, the socially dominant form of feminism—which is a distorted version of liberal intersectional feminism—has literally left a gap where a women-centred social justice movement used to be. This is an attempt to describe a theory that fills that gap.

Second, I want to show you how helpful philosophical ideas can be in diagnosing mistakes in arguments about feminism, explaining disagreements between feminists, and in articulating a clear vision of a feminism that has re-centred women. Theory—philosophical and otherwise—sometimes gets a bad reputation inside social justice movements. As one author puts it,

'For many, academic feminism is a contradiction in terms, an oxymoron, selling out feminism's commitment to everyday [practice]'.[51] There seems to be a sense, from at least some quarters, that feminist theory is elitist and unnecessary. There are real problems to be solved, on the ground, after all.

In anticipating objections to her radical proposal for women's liberation,[52] Shulamith Firestone considers what 'operates to destroy serious consideration of feminism: the failure of past social experiments'.[53] One reason she gives for such failures is 'lack of theory', commenting 'one senses the immense frustration of people trying to liberate themselves without having a well-thought-out ideology to guide them'.[54] She goes through a number of partially successful and failed feminist social experiments too, diagnosing the reasons for failure as including 'There was no development of a feminist consciousness and analysis prior to the initiation of the experiment'.[55] Theory is crucial, and philosophy is a great tool for both creating it and critiquing it.

Third, I want to reintroduce you to radical feminism, through some of the ideas of the most interesting and influential figures of the second wave, women many of whose ideas are lost to feminists today. As Louise Perry described them in an article for *Quillette* in 2019, these are 'women who produced influential work that is now often forgotten, or else misremembered by Third Wave feminists keen to distance themselves from their feminist foremothers'.[56] In revisiting their ideas we will be in a better position to articulate a version of feminism that is both *by* and *for* women.

Finally, a note on the organization of the book, and where to look if you're after something in particular. I have divided it into two parts, the first focused on explaining what gender-critical feminism is, and the second more reflective, raising further questions for gender-critical feminism. The core of the book is the first part, Chapters 2–6. It introduces gender-critical feminism and explains that it has its roots in radical feminism, which in turn warrants a fuller presentation of radical feminist theory and radical feminists' ideas (Chapter 2). It then moves back to gender-critical feminism and explains some differences between the two (Chapter 3). Having established that gender-critical feminism is a new iteration of radical feminism, it then picks up on two issues that have been important to each—the sex industry (Chapter 4) as being central to radical feminist concerns, and trans/gender (Chapter 5) as being central to gender-critical feminist concerns.

I'll argue for the abolition of the sex industry in its entirety (which means pornography as well as prostitution); and the continued protection of women's sex-based rights in the face of attempts by some feminists to replace sex with gender identity, as well as the regulation of access to medical and surgical transition for children and adolescents. There are many issues of concern to radical and gender-critical feminists, so these chapters are far from exhaustive; but they are intended to be representative, to get to the heart of a feminism concerned with sex and sex-based rights. (Further elaboration of the gender-critical feminist agenda is given in the Coda.) In the final chapter of the core (Chapter 6), I turn to the question of why gender-critical feminism has been so vilified, offering a number of different explanations. If you just want to get a good sense of what gender-critical feminism is and what its main disagreements are with other types of feminism, then you might read just the chapters in Part I.

In Part II of the book, I ask three further questions about gender-critical feminism. First, is it intersectional (Chapter 7)? It is more or less taken for granted in feminism today that feminism *ought* to be intersectional, so the extent to which it is, and whether that is defensible, needs to be worked out. I'll defend a feminism for female people concerned with a single axis of oppression, namely the oppression of women as women, meaning, on the basis of their sex. Second, is gender-critical feminism feasible? The *abolition* of gender norms and the *liberation* of women are hefty goals; gender-critical feminism is vulnerable to the accusation that those goals cannot be realized (Chapter 8). I'll argue that gender-critical feminism is not infeasible, but that differing assumptions about feasibility—left implicit rather than made explicit—might be behind some of the apparent disagreement between gender-critical and other types of feminists. Finally, is gender-critical feminism liberal? The socially dominant form of feminism is arguably a version of liberal feminism, and gender-critical feminism opposes several elements of that feminism. Does that mean gender-critical feminism is not liberal? And if so, is *that* defensible (Chapter 9)? I'll argue that gender-critical feminism is liberal, but that there remain open questions about how deep women's lack of freedom goes. If you are already familiar with the history of liberalism and have thought about the relation between liberalism and liberal feminism and criticisms of liberal feminism then you might skip Sections 9.1–9.3. There are some new ideas in Section 9.4, so you could go straight there.

At the end of the book, added as a coda, there is also a gender-critical manifesto, a list of issues designed to be the focus of a feminist movement that is about *all* women and *only* women.

My target in this book is the type of feminism you generally see represented in the media, in popular books about feminism, across social media, and inside feminist activist communities. There is a loose connection between this type of feminism and the feminist theory worked out by feminist academics. The connection is strongest to postmodern feminism, but there is also some connection to liberal feminism and intersectional feminism, albeit with some serious distortions. Gender-critical feminism is in disagreement with academic liberal and intersectional feminism *to the extent that* proponents of the latter share the commitments of popular feminism when it comes to the questions of what feminism is, who it is for, whether it may permissibly be concerned with a single axis of oppression, whether the sex industry should be abolished, whether gender is (only) identity, and whether transition should be regulated to prevent harm to girls.

PART I

WHAT IS GENDER-CRITICAL FEMINISM?

2
Gender-Critical Feminism's Radical Roots

In its insistence upon the importance of sex, gender-critical feminism is continuous with radical feminism. Radical feminism is a theory and movement that started in the United States in 1967 with women like Ti-Grace Atkinson, Shulamith Firestone, and groups like New York Radical Women (est. 1967), Redstockings (est. 1969), New York Radical Feminists (est. 1969), and The Feminists (est. 1968).[1] The Feminists, for example, split from the National Organization for Women (NOW) claiming that it was not radical enough.[2] Here's Germaine Greer in *The Female Eunuch*, describing The Feminists:

> It was not long before intelligent members of NOW realized that their aims were too limited and their tactics too genteel. One of the more interesting women to emerge in the movement is Ti-Grace Atkinson, a leader of the most radical and elite women's group, The Feminists—A Political Organization to Annihilate Sex Roles. This is a closed group of propaganda-makers who are trying to develop the notion of a leaderless society in which the convention of Love ('the response of the victim to the rapist'), the proprietary relationship of marriage, and even uterine pregnancy will no longer prevail. Their pronouncements are characteristically gnomic and rigorous; to the average confused female they must seem terrifying. They have characterised men as the enemy, and, as long as men continue to enact their roles as misconceived and perpetuated by themselves and women, they are undoubtedly right.[3]

Prior feminist theory had been trying to theorize women's situation *through* existing theory. Atkinson—an analytic philosopher and arguably the first radical feminist[4]—wrote 'Radical feminism is a new political concept. It evolved in response to the concern of many feminists that there has never been even the beginnings of a feminist analysis of the persecution of women'.[5] Many of the first-wave feminists, for example, oriented themselves

Gender-Critical Feminism: Holly Lawford-Smith, Oxford University Press. © Holly Lawford-Smith 2022.
DOI: 10.1093/oso/9780198863885.003.0002

around classical liberalism,[6] and argued for women's empowerment through education and the vote *as* equality according to liberal values. Some of the second-wave feminists were committed socialists and tried to fit feminism into Marxism. But neither of these went far enough, according to the radicals. The problem with liberal feminism was that equality with men on men's terms was thought to be under-ambitious. Gerda Lerner in *The Creation of Patriarchy* made this point with a metaphor of a stage, saying that men had written the play, made the props and costumes, cast all the roles, and were directing the play, so that even if women were on the stage, and even if they fought for equal opportunity in getting the better roles, for liberation the whole stage needed to be dismantled and something genuinely co-constructed put back in its place.[7] The problem with socialist feminism was that it ultimately subsumed sex to class as the fundamental axis of oppression. The radicals did not believe that abolishing class oppression would be sufficient to abolish sex oppression. Audre Lorde, for example, wrote 'in no socialist country that I have visited have I found an absence of racism or of sexism, so the eradication of both of these diseases seems to involve more than the abolition of capitalism as an institution'.[8] Catharine MacKinnon described radical feminism as 'feminism unmodified', saying 'just as socialist feminism has often amounted to [M]arxism applied to women, liberal feminism has often amounted to liberalism applied to women. Radical feminism is feminism'.[9]

Feminist women wanted a theory and movement in which *sex* took centre stage. Hence, the invention of radical feminism: a theory *by* women *for* women and *about* women, understood as a sex caste/class. Atkinson proclaimed in 1969 'The [radical feminist] analysis begins with the feminist *raison d'être* that women are a class, that this class is political in nature, and that this political class is oppressed'.[10] She described women as 'a political class characterized by a sexual function'.[11] Shulamith Firestone in 1970 declared 'sex class is so deep as to be invisible'.[12] Kate Millett in the same year described 'the situation between the sexes' as 'a relationship of dominance and subordinance', 'in our social order, [it] is the birthright priority where males rule females'.[13] Later, MacKinnon would take a further step from sex to sexuality, writing in 1982 'sexuality is to feminism what work is to [M]arxism: that which is most one's own, yet most taken away'.[14]

This radical feminist isolation of and assertion of the importance of sex is crucially important. The radical feminists pushed sex forward as a major axis of oppression just like class and just like race. They showed that sex caste could be theorized independently of either, even if it could *also* be theorized together with either or both. This made it possible to consider the structure of each of race, sex, and class as major systems of oppression, and draw on both similarities and differences for mutual illumination. It made it possible to ask about the *origins* of sex oppression: was it always the case? If not, when did it start, and how, and why? It made it possible to ask about the *mechanisms* by which sex oppression had been sustained throughout history, and through which it may still be sustained today. It made it possible to ask *who* or *what* is 'the oppressor'. Once we understand the origins and the mechanisms, we are then in a better position to understand how to challenge and ultimately dismantle that system, and achieve women's liberation (which, as mentioned already, is not necessarily the same thing as achieving sex equality).

Radical feminists, during the second wave, worked on all of these projects. Here is a brief overview—there is more detail in Section 2.2 below. Gerda Lerner in *The Creation of Patriarchy* (1986) and Riane Eisler in *The Chalice and the Blade* (1987) focused on the historical origins of sex oppression. Lerner, for example, pieced together a case based on archeological evidence and argued that patriarchy began around 3100 BCE—so about 5,000 years ago. She argued that women were the first slaves, and created the template for future relations of domination/subordination.[15] Andrea Dworkin gave women as a caste a history, or 'herstory' as feminists said at the time, outlining atrocities against women such as the 1,000-year period of footbinding of women in China, the estimated 500-year period of burning at the stake women accused of witchcraft,[16] and women's death and disease from illegal abortions. She also identified propaganda about women's inferiority, such as that built into the fairy tales taught to children.[17] Arguably, this makes it possible to claim historical injustice against women as a caste.

Multiple institutions were identified as helping to achieve the oppression of women, including marriage, the family, sexual intercourse, love, religion, rape, and prostitution. Different radical feminists focused their work on one or more of these institutions, trying to gain a better understanding of how they functioned. For example, Susan Brownmiller wrote about rape;[18] Firestone wrote about love and the family,[19] Atkinson wrote about love and sexual intercourse;[20] Millet wrote about sexual intercourse;[21] Dworkin and MacKinnon wrote about prostitution and pornography;[22] and there were many more radical feminists writing about these topics in various combinations. Some, like Atkinson and Marilyn Frye, wrote more broadly about the concept of oppression and how it works in the case of women.[23]

MacKinnon in particular advanced a more general theory, mentioned already, that men's control of women's sexuality was what united the many different harms against women and explained women's oppression—including rape, incest, pornography, prostitution, discrimination against lesbians, sexual harassment, and control of abortion and contraception.[24]

There was fairly widespread agreement at the time on the following cluster of views. Sex division was the 'difference' at the basis of women's oppression. Women's oppression consisted in women being pressed into the service of men, whether this was primarily sexual or more broadly about personal service, sexual service, and ego/emotional service. Women's oppression ran extremely deep, with many women having fully internalized men's views of women, and exacerbated by the fact that women were distributed among men, unlike pretty much any other minority group in relation to its oppressor.[25] Men were the oppressor (either because men were directly implicated, or because they maintained the institutions that worked to oppress women). Heterosexual love and sexual intercourse were deeply compromised in light of sex hierarchy. Prostitution was institutionalized rape.

There was also a broad range of solutions, and some of these were highly experimental, aimed at 'doing things differently' outside of male power structures. The radical feminists invented separatism, at its limit the idea of women living independently of men and avoiding contact with men. They invented political lesbianism, which on one understanding is simply separatism with added emphasis on no longer having sex with men,[26] and on another is the rejection of the idea that sexual orientation is necessarily innate, and the embracing of the idea that lesbianism can be a positive choice made by women to love women.[27] They revived women's spirituality from pagan times, focused on celebrating women's supposed difference from men and emphasizing women's closeness to nature. They developed 'difference feminism', which focused on articulating and revaluing women's supposed difference from men. They engaged in linguistic activism/conceptual engineering, by reclaiming terms of abuse and inventing new concepts. They introduced the methodology of consciousness-raising, where women would come together to talk, to begin realizing the shape of their common oppression, to work through the experience of living in male-dominated societies, and start questioning male power structures. They advocated for the end of 'sex roles', some of them by advocating for the end of sex-marking altogether. And they established services for women like domestic violence and rape shelters.

I see gender-critical feminism as the *revival* of radical feminism. I think it didn't start out intending to be that. Women were just reacting against what they saw as unsatisfactory feminist takes on issues like prostitution, pornography, surrogacy, sexual and beauty objectification, gender identity ideology, and more. But as more women gathered together under the label 'gender-critical', they discovered, or were pointed towards, continuities with the earlier radical feminist theory. This in turn made the connection stronger as people began revisiting that work. Gender-critical feminists have *the same project* that the radical feminists had, in that they are committed to the idea that women are a sex caste, and to sex oppression as a distinct and important axis of oppression.

Within that very broad project, women made many different contributions, some of which have come to be associated more strongly with the idea of radical feminism than others. In my view, virtually none of these are essential to radical feminism; we could be radical feminists and disagree with most of the ideas put forward by a particular radical feminist about the origins of patriarchy, the mechanisms by which patriarchy (or something like it)[28] is sustained, and what the feminist future looks like. Each of these thinkers' contributions is a small potential piece of a very large puzzle, which remains to be solved. Although I think they got many things right, in principle the radical feminists of the second wave could have gotten almost everything wrong about how women's oppression works and what it would take to dissolve it, and yet the core insight of radical feminism would remain untouched—that women are a sex caste/class, and that this fact opens up urgent social, political, legal, and economic questions. The core questions are why and how women are oppressed, and what women's liberation consists in. The answers are likely to change through time as women's situation changes, not least as a result of feminism itself. The answer that I think distinguishes the radical feminist from other types of feminists, and therefore *is* necessary, has to do with how deep feminine socialization goes. For the radical feminist, it goes very deep (on which more soon). In the remainder of this chapter, I'll describe some of the radical feminists' contributions in more detail, to provide a sense of the magnitude of the undertaking that radical feminism was,[29] and in order to be able to clarify in the next chapter which specific ideas gender-critical feminism leaves behind.

2.1 Pre-radical: Female Socialization

Long before the second wave kicked off, Mary Wollstonecraft[30] had made the case that women's situation was a result of social causes rather than anything innate to her 'soul' or person.[31] At the time of her writing, women (of her class) must have looked nearly like another species than men (of her class):[32] their central aspiration to be beautiful and to secure good prospects for their future by getting the right husband; their daily pursuits of pleasures like needlework and socializing; their opportunities limited to a narrow range of roles—resentful domestic drudge, coquettish mistress, or bitter economically dependent relative—relying on their beauty, their social status, their charm, and a lot of luck. A woman did not receive a meaningful education, and she depended financially on male relatives (with some exceptions when it came to inheritance). Most women at this time did not rail against their inequality with men. Wollstonecraft comments 'they have…chosen rather to be short-lived queens than labour to achieve the sober pleasures that arise from equality'.[33]

She asks her reader to imagine how different things might be were a woman at the time encouraged to engage in physical exercise rather than being confined to her rooms;[34] were she parented to stamp out her silly fears in childhood; were she to receive an education; were she to have the solitude necessary to pursue knowledge. On the last point, Wollstonecraft comments on the accomplishments of 'unmarried or childless men'[35] and speculates on how the constraints of marriage and children might similarly hinder women's accomplishments, and also on how women are often surrounded by others in their daily lives, for example in the company of other women discussing clothing.[36] Her conclusion was that 'men of genius and talents have started out of a class, in which women have never yet been placed'.[37]

Wollstonecraft's drawing attention to the numerous differences in boys' and girls'—and later men's and women's—social treatment would have been sufficient to inspire agnosticism about whether the social differences between men and women were the result of biological differences[38] between them. But she went a step further and made an innovative comparison that suggested socialization was in fact the direct cause of the differences in men's and women's situations, in particular in the number and magnitude of their accomplishments.

She drew on Adam Smith's work in *A Theory of Moral Sentiments* to compare women's situation with that of the nobility, commenting 'if…no great men, of any denomination, have ever appeared amongst the nobility, may it not be fairly inferred that their local situation swallowed up the man, and produced a character similar to that of woman?'.[39] Her suggestion was that wealth and status similarly doom members of the nobility to a life of trivial pleasures and pull them away from knowledge and substantial accomplishments. Because the nobility includes men, this is a direct demonstration of the difference that different circumstances and opportunities can make to people's—*men's*—accomplishments. It is harder to explain these differences away as a fact of biology or different 'souls',[40] and indeed it would have been uncomfortable to do so given the prevailing norms about the higher social status of members of the nobility.

The idea that women's situation is explained by social causes was picked up and developed in much more detail some 150 years later with French existentialist feminist Simone de Beauvoir's canonical and best-selling book *The Second Sex*.[41] Beauvoir compared the idea of the 'eternal feminine' to the ideas of a 'black soul' or a 'Jewish character', dismissing them all as stereotypes. She emphasized the invisibility and depth of social and cultural discrimination against women, 'whose moral and intellectual repercussions are so deep in woman that they appear to spring from an original nature'.[42] Like Wollstonecraft before her, she accepted that women were in fact at that time inferior to men, but asked whether that was necessary: 'their situation provides them with fewer possibilities: the question is whether this state of affairs must be perpetuated'.[43] She establishes that biology is not destiny,[44] and neither is [Freudian] psychology.[45] She surveys the subordination of women across different times, cultures, and mythologies.[46] And she explains in great detail the process of a woman's socialization from girlhood through sexual initiation into marriage, drawing on women's testimony throughout.[47]

Beauvoir's driving point is that 'Woman feels undermined because in fact the restrictions of femininity have undermined her'.[48] Female people are inculcated into a social system in which they have fewer opportunities, and they are made complicit in their own subordination by the fact that they accept the rewards designed to obscure the extent of that subordination from their full view (for example, the fact that women with class privilege are often 'put on pedestals' by men, and shielded from even minor physical discomforts).[49] This was the point of the soundbite that Beauvoir has been ground down into,[50] namely that 'one is not born, but rather becomes, woman',[51] which is so often misunderstood and misused by those concerned to advance a conception of gender as identity today.[52]

Many of the ideas in *The Second Sex* were taken up and developed by radical feminists, for example ideas about the male gaze and women's sexual objectification,[53] the role of the 'Prince Charming' myth and the way that women end up making themselves into what they think men want in order to secure marriage,[54] and the extent to which sex between men and women is coercive—which led some radical feminists to advocate lesbianism and separatism.[55]

These early feminist writers were advancing the idea that there is nothing about being female that *necessitates* the differences in behaviour and interests we might have seen between men and women in 1792, when Wollstonecraft was writing, or in 1949, when Beauvoir was writing, or indeed in the late 1960s, when radical feminists started writing. Throughout history and across time and place women have been subordinated, considered both 'different from' and 'inferior to' men. But the content of this difference has been entirely dependent on time and place. Feminists like Wollstonecraft and Beauvoir were suggesting that if women were socialized in the same way as men were, and given the same opportunities, we might expect to see them accomplish the same things.

What distinguishes Wollstonecraft from Beauvoir is what distinguishes the liberal feminist from the radical feminist. For the liberal, with Wollstonecraft as foremother, the main problem is that women are not treated as equals to men—they are denied crucial rights and opportunities. The differences between women and men are likely to disappear when their opportunities are equalized. For the radical, with Beauvoir as foremother, even if women were suddenly to be *treated* as equals to men, they are likely to still be very different, because they have been *shaped* to be different. The disagreement between the two is over the question of how deep feminine socialization goes. For the radical it goes very deep, and compromises women's autonomy more than in the case of perhaps any other oppressed social group.[56] Thus a feminist might be committed to the idea of women as an oppressed caste/class without being a radical feminist, because she thinks women's oppression is largely a matter of particular laws and practices which, once reformed, would largely transform her situation. According to the radical feminist, the struggle for women's liberation is both political and personal.

2.2 The Radical Feminists of the Second Wave

Ti-Grace Atkinson. Shulamith Firestone. Kate Millett. Germaine Greer. Mary Daly. Susan Griffin. Christine Delphy. Monique Wittig. Kathleen

Barry. Robin Morgan. Andrea Dworkin. Adrienne Rich. Marilyn Frye. Catharine MacKinnon. Audre Lorde. Sheila Jeffreys. Janice Raymond. Phyllis Chesler.[57] These are some of the most prominent radical feminists. Radical feminism came to prominence in the late 1960s and early 1970s, with Ti-Grace Atkinson as its earliest proponent.[58] It was a grassroots movement and, importantly and partly for that reason, not especially unified, although it is possible to find commonalities.[59] Within the movement there were many disagreements; Phyllis Chesler wrote 'we were champion hair-splitters and disagreed with each other with searing passion'.[60]

When we ask, 'why are women oppressed?', two broad types of answer are possible. The first is to give an origin story. This interprets the question as 'how did women come to be oppressed?' We suppose a time prior to women's oppression,[61] and then we try to explain what happened in order that women's oppression was produced. These stories all presuppose contingency, because if women's oppression was necessary in virtue of something essential to womanhood, then there could not have been any time prior when women were not oppressed. The second is to give an explanation of the mechanisms by which women are kept oppressed. These explanations can be agnostic about the origins, and might even suppose that the mechanisms themselves have changed a great deal over time. Identifying mechanisms may or may not involve identifying perpetrators. I'll take each of these types of answer in turn in what follows, starting with origin stories and moving on to mechanisms. Finally, I'll survey the range of solutions that radical feminists have given to the problem of women's oppression.

2.2.1 Origin Stories

All of the explanations that radical feminists gave for how women's subordination got started were oriented around female-specific biology or physiology, in one way or another.

Mary Jane Sherfey saw women as naturally having an insatiable sexual appetite, related to her capacity for multiple orgasm. This drive would disrupt the family unit and leave men uncertain of their paternity if not subdued.[62] Susan Brownmiller saw the root of women's oppression in the differences in human anatomy: the penis can be used as a weapon of rape, the vagina can be a site of rape. Brownmiller describes the possibility of rape as 'a conscious process of intimidation by which *all men* keep *all women* in a state of fear'.[63] Fear leads to domination. Shulamith Firestone explained women's oppression as stemming from her role in reproduction. This made her physically weaker—because more encumbered—during pregnancy and breastfeeding, and so generated a sex-based division of labour in which women were dependent on and thus inferior to men.[64] Mary Daly saw women's power to create life as giving her distinctive capacities that were then devalued by men.[65] Susan Griffin saw women as closer to nature, similarly creating a difference from men that was then devalued by men.[66]

Alison Jaggar criticizes radical feminism for this tendency towards the biology of femaleness as an explanation for women's oppression.[67] She says this focus can be dangerous insofar as it naturalizes and hence may seem to justify women's oppression, particularly if proposed solutions can be shown not to succeed. But her criticism is too strong, because she fails to distinguish biological *determinism*, biological *essentialism*, and biological *explanation*. Biological determinism is something feminists reasonably object to, because it holds that biological features of female persons determine their status as socially inferior (and similarly, that biological features of male persons determine their status as socially superior). There's a kind of fatalism or necessity here: the fact that a group of human persons has these particular biological features makes it inescapably the case that they will end up worse off. If the question is 'how did women come to be oppressed?' and the answer is 'in virtue of their reproductive organs', it's easy to end up thinking that women would have been oppressed in any possible world, that there's something about women's reproductive capacities that goes hand-in-hand with oppression.

But there's not necessarily anything wrong with biological essentialism—the idea that biological organisms have essential (necessary) properties—and there's certainly nothing wrong with mere biological explanation. Natalie Stoljar has shown that accusations of 'essentialism' (biological or otherwise) are often overblown in feminist theory, that 'essentialism' has long since become a 'term of abuse'.[68] Single necessary and sufficient conditions for class membership can be glossed as 'essential properties' of members of classes, but that need not involve any claim about the normative properties of those members. It does not follow from a mere definition of a thing that it is *good* to be that thing, or *bad* to be it, or that being it is better or worse than being some other thing.

A radical feminist might say that it is a necessary and sufficient condition for being oppressed as a woman in the actual history of our world that one had a female sexual appetite (Sherfey), a vagina (Brownmiller), a likelihood of becoming pregnant (Firestone, Daly), or an embodied experience that was more 'animalistic' (Griffin). Another way to put each of these claims is to say that the relevant property is an essential property of being oppressed as a woman. This is 'essentialist' in a descriptive sense, but it's not clear why this should be a term of abuse. So long as we think there are classes of things and we don't think they all have vague boundaries, we'll be interested in giving definitions.

When feminists object to essentialism because it attributes a fixed and unchanging nature to women, they conflate biological essentialism and biological determinism. When they object to essentialism because it will inevitably exclude some people—namely those without the essential property—they assume that 'inclusion' is so valuable as to require giving up on biological definitions altogether.[69] This is far from obvious.

Finally, it is hard to see any good reason for objecting to mere biological explanation. Beauvoir, for example, gave an explanation of woman's subjugation in terms of her biology, but it was a contingent explanation. On her account, it happened that at a particular time in early hunter-gatherer history, the tools that humans used to defend themselves against predation were heavy enough that the men in the groups could use them effectively but the women in the groups generally couldn't.[70] This led to a sex-based division of labour where the males defended the group and hunted large animals, and the females cared for the young and gathered plants and berries. The explanation depends on biology, in that the relative strength of male and female people was the difference-maker in who was able to use the existing tools effectively. But the explanation is also contingent, because *had* the tools been smaller and lighter, everyone could have used them effectively, and the group might not have ended up with a sex-based division of labour.

As Caroline Criado-Perez discusses in *Invisible Women*,[71] we know that the decisions that go into the design of tools and technologies are not always innocent; we might also want to ask who was making the tools in Beauvoir's imagined history, and why they weren't made in a way that everyone could use. If it was because they wouldn't have been effective in actually killing the animals being hunted, then this explanation of the origin of women's oppression has no real culpability in it. It *just so happens* that tools needed to be this size and weight to do their job, and it *just so happens* that men could use tools of that size and weight well while women couldn't, and *for that reason* men and women ended up separating into different roles, and *from there* a lot more got packed into sex roles until we got to where we were at Beauvoir's time of writing. Whether or not it's the right explanation of our actual history, it's a good example of an explanation of women's oppression that is both biological and contingent.[72]

Having set aside the worry that explanations of women's oppression in terms of their distinctive physiology or biology naturalize and therefore may seem to justify women's oppression, we can turn to what seems to be the most plausible explanation of the origins of women's subordination that has been offered by radical feminists. This came from Gerda Lerner in her book *The Creation of Patriarchy*.[73] Before her book came out, the most widely accepted account of patriarchy was that offered by Friedrich Engels in *The Origin of the Family, Private Property, and the State*.[74] On Engels' account, prior to the advent of agriculture men and women had a division of labour, but equal social status. After it, intensive labour was needed, which led to men appropriating the labour of others. This in turn lead to the creation of private property: men owned slaves, and animals, and land, and so came to own women.[75] Beauvoir criticizes Engels for offering no real explanation of *how* these developments lead to women's oppression. She says '[t]he whole account pivots around the transition from a communitarian regime to one of private property: there is absolutely no indication of how it was able to occur... Similarly, it is unclear if private property necessarily led to the enslavement of women'.[76]

Lerner's account improves on Engels' and answers Beauvoir's criticism, by offering a fuller explanation of one process by which patriarchy came to be established. (She says that patriarchy is likely to have emerged in different places at different times and in different ways; she focused on the evidence available about ancient Mesopotamia, drawing on the laws of archaic states, remnants of stone tablets, sealed tombs, and other archaeological evidence.) She argued that patriarchy became established over a process of roughly 2,500 years, between 3100 BC and 600 BC. She puts the origins at 'the development of intertribal warfare during periods of economic scarcity', which 'fostered the rise to power of men of military achievement'.[77] Groups coming out of the hunter/gatherer period began to roam and conquer. Men from the conquered tribes would not have been easy to enslave; it would take a lot of labour power to oversee them and guard against insurrection. But women could be enslaved more easily. Their will could be broken through rape, and more importantly, through rape they could be impregnated, and after giving birth their desire to protect their children would ensure loyalty to the conquering tribe. Lerner describes this as 'submission for the sake of their children'.[78] For these reasons, when one tribe conquered another, the conquered men were murdered, the conquered women enslaved.

A further explanation, which entrenches women's situation, relates to the shift to agricultural societies, because it became advantageous to groups to have more children, thereby more *labour* power. This led to men with military power exchanging women, in order to furnish more labour power by furnishing more reproductive power. Lerner writes that 'the first appropriation of private property consists of the appropriation of the labour of women as *reproducers*'.[79] On this view, women were the first slaves, and men's capacity to subdue and control women became the template for future enslavements. There was a shift from the sexual exploitation of women in the early period of agricultural revolution to the more general exploitation of human labour after it. The nails in the coffin for women's equal treatment, Lerner argued, were the later emergence of organized monotheistic religion, which reduced women's position even further through an attack on the pagan cults worshipping fertility goddesses, along with ancient philosophical ideas about women's substandard humanity that would become 'the founding metaphors of Western civilization'.[80]

Can Lerner's historical explanation of how men ended up gaining power over women, which makes reference to woman's biology (at first, that she was rapeable/impregnable; later, that her reproductive labour could be co-opted to meet a demand for productive labour power) be considered biologically determinist? Only if we think what happened according to this explanation would have happened in any merely *possible* history too. But as Beauvoir pointed out, there are possible histories of the world where men saw women as friends rather than slaves:

> Woman's powerlessness brought about her ruin because man apprehended her through a project of enrichment and expansion. And this project is still not enough to explain her oppression: the division of labour by sex might have been a friendly association. If the original relation between man and his peers had been exclusively one of friendship, one could not account for any kind of enslavement.[81]

Such an origin story is essentialist in the way discussed above, though, in that it excludes from the history of women's oppression anyone who didn't have the underlying biological feature. But it's not clear why an explanation of how women's oppression got started, which may be crucial in working out remedies to that oppression, should be interested in inclusion. How sex hierarchy got started, and what the physical basis for it was, are explanatory questions that have answers that can be assessed according to a range of criteria for theories in science and social science, like coherence, simplicity, and explanatory power. Inclusiveness is not one of those criteria. Woe be to science if it ever becomes one.

Does it matter that we figure out what the *specific* biological feature of female people was that sex roles were formed on the basis of? Maybe it was nothing more than the fact that female people were visibly detectable as *different* from male people, creating two 'types' of humans that could be used to solve complementary coordination problems (problems that require a division of different labour).[82] Skin pigmentation doesn't make a difference to a person's capacities, but it was still used at various historical junctures as a biological marker onto which the social meaning of race was piled in order to justify segregated social roles and social hierarchy. The fact that female bodies are observably different from male bodies in normal cases is enough. There is ample documentation throughout feminist literature since the first wave of the ways in which members of the female sex caste have been treated as inferior, and socialized to act out exactly the limitations that men have imposed upon them.[83]

2.2.2 Sustaining Mechanisms

Other feminist writing focuses less on how the oppression of women got started, and more on what it is that keeps it in place. For Atkinson it is *men* as the oppressor; for Frye it is a broader system of threats and sanctions; for MacKinnon it is men's control of women's sexuality; for Firestone and Atkinson it is (heterosexual) love; for Wittig, Dworkin, and Atkinson it is the social construction (and social sustaining) of sex; for Millett, Frye, Firestone, and others it is the social construction (and sustaining) of gender.

Atkinson argued in her essay 'Declaration of War' that the women's movement at the time—1969—was being avoidant in the naming of its enemy. It pointed to 'society', meaning something like the social institutions through which women's oppression was implemented. But, she asks, who maintains those institutions? Her answer is men. She says that 'Women have been massacred as human beings over history', and that they must take the first step, together, from '*being* massacred to *engaging in* battle (resistance)'.[84] Feminism is the war between women and men, oppressed and oppressor. Women remain oppressed because men oppress them (and because women do not resist).

Frye described women's oppression as being *kept down* or *caged in*.[85] Frye wrote about the way that women's oppression involved them being pressed into the service of men, including men's personal service (e.g. housework, cooking, running errands), sexual service (e.g. providing him with sex, bearing him children, looking attractive for him), and what Frye called 'ego service' (e.g. giving him support, encouragement, attention, and praise).[86] For Frye, the 'women's sphere' was the service sector.[87] But *why* do women end up servicing men? Frye thought others' threats and sanctions create our masculine or feminine (and not both) behaviour. She says, 'The fact that there are such penalties threatened for deviations from these patterns strongly suggests that the patterns would not be there but for the threats'.[88] She talks about the way in which a 'double bind'—a conflicting set of standards—is imposed upon women in a way that makes them damned whatever they do. On this account, what keeps women's oppression in place is the threats, or actual implementation, of social penalties. It is not only men that make these threats, it is everyone. (Although Frye does not put things in terms of 'norms', this is a way to understand what she was pointing to. Certain norms about male and female behaviour exist, and individuals reinforce and uphold those norms by sanctioning departures or violations. I'll develop this idea further in Chapter 3, Section 3.2.)

MacKinnon identifies the 'male pursuit of control over women's sexuality' as the key issue.[89] For MacKinnon, this male control of female bodies is not 'about' biology, but about the way that maleness and femaleness have been socially constructed, which makes this control of the latter by the former *constitutive* of maleness. On her view 'it is sexuality that determines gender'.[90] This may be realized through rape, (denial of / insistence upon) abortion, sexual objectification, or sexual use; and it explains why incest, contraception, abortion, sexual harassment, the treatment of lesbians, pornography, prostitution, and rape are all feminist political issues.[91]

There are clear perpetrators on MacKinnon's account, namely the men who commit sexual crimes against women. But there is also something more amorphous, namely the social construction of sex/gender categories. Social meaning can build up over time without anyone much intending it; individuals who make culpable contributions, as undoubtedly many influential men throughout history have done, may be long dead; and even those who are victims of constructions that position them as inferior can help to sustain those constructions. I'll say more about the social construction of sex below in talking about Wittig, Dworkin, and Atkinson; and I'll say more about the social construction of gender below in talking about Kreps, Millett, Frye, Firestone, and others.

Firestone and Atkinson both pointed to *love* as a mechanism of patriarchal control. (Atkinson also points to other institutions, including marriage, the family, sexual intercourse, religion, and prostitution).[92] Atkinson thought that 'uniting' with the oppressed was a clever strategy by men to keep women from organizing.[93] Firestone thought women exchanged love for economic and emotional security and emotional identity (the latter men can get through work, but women at the time largely could not).[94] She thought that genuine love required mutual exchange, and that this was not possible when there was an unequal balance of power, which there always was between men and women.[95] This kind of thought is likely what lead some radical feminist women to advocate separatism from men.

Monique Wittig wrote in her 1976 essay 'The Category of Sex' that 'there is no sex', and that 'oppression creates sex and not the contrary'.[96] She insists that 'the category of sex does not exist a priori, before all society'.[97] Andrea Dworkin says similarly that not only are masculinity and femininity culturally constructed, but so too are the biological categories of man and woman 'fictions, caricatures, cultural constructs'.[98] Atkinson suggests the same: 'Traditional feminism is caught in the dilemma of demanding equal treatment for unequal functions, because it is unwilling to challenge political (functional) classification by sex'. She continues,

> The feminist dilemma is that it is as women—or 'females'—that women are persecuted, just as it was as slaves—or 'blacks'—that slaves were persecuted in America. In order to improve their condition, those individuals who are today defined as women must eradicate their own definition. Women must, in a sense, commit suicide.[99]

On this view, what sustains women's oppression is the fact that we sustain and reproduce sex categories. If we didn't, there would be no *difference* that we could attach differential treatment or socialization to. Everyone who participates in the 'social construction' of sex, which is basically everyone in the society, would be complicit. (The related solution, which I will discuss in more detail below, is that we stop constructing sex.)

Instead of identifying the social construction (and sustaining) of *sex* as the mechanism by which women are oppressed, other radical feminists identified the social construction (and sustaining) of *gender* as the mechanism. Bonnie Kreps, for example, identified as the 'crux of the problem' that 'man has consistently defined woman not in terms of herself but in relation to him'.[100] Like Atkinson, she thought there were a number of institutions that perpetuated social roles for the sexes (what she called 'sex roles'), including 'love, marriage, sex, masculinity, and femininity'.[101] Dismantling the socialization of women into these social roles would go a long way to liberating women. Others who took roughly this view included Kate Millett;[102] Marilyn Frye;[103] Firestone;[104] Atkinson;[105] and two radical feminist collectives based in New York, 'The Feminists',[106] and the 'New York Radical Feminists'.[107]

On this view, there is a complex network of social ideas about what female people *should be like* and what male people *should be like*, and those ideas include value judgements that allow the positioning of male people as superior to female people. It is something physical, namely male and female biological difference, that these ideas are applied to, but it is the ideas themselves, and the social incentives (threats and sanctions) that create women's oppression. This broad picture allows us to capture the basic points that many feminists have made, including that gender is a role hierarchy, or that gender is a system of dominance and subordination; it allows us to say more about how these ideas are socially and culturally transmitted (e.g. through the family unit, through the media); and it allows us to ask questions about whose interests this system serves (e.g. men's, because it positions men as superior and it secures women's service for them). It also allows us to make predictions, for example about how women who are not feminine and men who are not masculine will be treated by others. All of these are routes into *dismantling* the system and therefore relieving women's oppression.

2.2.3 Utopias and Solutions

As we have seen, different radical feminists had different solutions to the problem of women's oppression. It is possible to discern at least six broad categories, although probably there were more: valuing women's difference; women's religion; technological advances; changes to language; consciousness-raising; the end of sex differentiation; and the end of the social construction of gender categories (gender abolitionism). Let's take these in turn.

Valuing women's difference. Some radical feminists saw a solution in the celebration of women's difference. Bracket what *makes* men and women different (biology, culture, or a combination of the two), and just notice that they *are* different. On this view, the problem is not necessarily with the difference, but with how it is treated. Women are perceived as inferior, when actually their unique traits are complementary to men's (and so equal), or superior to men's (and so unequal, but in a way that flips the hierarchy). A 'maternalist' position sees women as more altruistic because they have maternal instincts, and more virtuous because they have lower sex drives; women can rescue society from the 'destruction, competition, and violence' of men (this position was developed in the first wave).[108] Carol Gilligan, working with prominent male psychologists through the 1970s, noticed that they focused on separation, autonomy, and independence, while the women she interviewed all talked about relationships and interdependence. This lead her to argue that women think differently about moral problems, and further to conclude that something had gone wrong with men's moral development to lead to non-relational thinking (initiation into maleness being the likely culprit).[109] Women applied her ideas to ethics and developed a feminist 'ethics of care'.[110]

There's something important here. Women pursuing this solution, who have come to be known as 'difference feminists', were attempting to undercut the subordination of women by revaluing women's differences, not as making them inferior to men, but as making them either equal, or superior, to men.[111] We need not deny the difference; as MacKinnon said, 'can you imagine elevating one half of a population and denigrating the other half and producing a population in which everyone is the same?'.[112] But there is a worry that in celebrating difference we reinforce or perpetuate it, making it harder for both men and women to act in ways that do not conform to the supposed differences between them. Stephanie Collins, writing in *The Core of Care Ethics*, argues that an ethics of care can (and should) be completely detached from women, and treated as an ethical system in its own right which *everyone* can make use of.[113]

Women's religion. In 1971, a small group of women in Malibu started the Susan B. Anthony Coven No. 1, an experiment at the time which turned into a group of between twenty and 120 women who met twenty-one times a year to observe solstices, equinoxes, and full moons. They took as their starting point Florence Nightingale's question 'Do you think it is possible for there to be a religion whose essence is common sense?', and answered it with 'a common sense that glorifies practical things and the improvement of our lives right now, not later, after death, which is absurd'.[114] They thought of themselves as feminist witches, practicing a Dianic religion. 'Diana' is the

European name for the Goddess of the Moon; their witchcraft included worship of this Goddess but also 'a women-centred, female-only worship of women's mysteries'.[115] But the 'Goddess' is really nature: 'each time we talk about the Goddess what we really mean is Life—life on this earth. We always recognize, when we say "Goddess," that she is the life-giver, the life-sustainer. She is Mother Nature'.[116]

The women ran a candle shop and practiced stargazing astrology.[117] There were priestesses and teachers, psychics, and tarot card readers. For these women, a 'witch' was a woman with spiritual power, and they were witches.[118] They named their coven after Susan B. Anthony because of a remark she made to a reporter when asked mockingly about what she was going to do in the afterlife, and she replied 'I shall go neither to heaven nor to hell, but stay right here and finish the women's revolution'.[119] Within the manifesto of the Susan B. Anthony coven we can find commitments to women's control of their own bodies, to sisterhood, to women's self-organization, and to the struggle against patriarchy, as well as criticism of patriarchal religions.[120] *The Holy Book of Women's Mysteries* promises on its front cover 'Feminist witchcraft, Goddess Rituals, Spellcasting, and other womanly arts. . . .'[121]

It would be easy to dismiss the practice of feminist witchcraft now, as pseudo-science and mysticism. But it did a number of important things, including reaching back to the pagan religions before patriarchy and reintroducing some of their more female-positive traditions; affirming women's rights; building sisterhood and solidarity between women, which created social ties strong enough to carry political organizing through tough times; and it made feminism fun, by creating rituals and celebrations, and by giving social status to women (e.g. as priestesses) that may have been denied to them in the wider world.

Technological advances. Firestone's imagined solution was different, in that it was technological. She located the source of women's oppression in their reproduction, and the constraints that imposed for the duration of pregnancy, breastfeeding, and care of young children. She wanted reproduction outside of the woman's body, for example in the laboratory (this is now discussed under the term 'ectogenesis'). Freed from physical burden, a sex-based division of labour would no longer be necessary.[122] Some women worry about technological solutions to problems affecting women because technology is so often male-designed and male-controlled for male-profit. And there are a host of feasibility and ethical questions that this proposal raises. Is it really that the equality of the sexes is impossible so long as women still reproduce? Is ectogenesis technologically feasible, at scale? What moral responsibility does a person who contributes genetic material (sperm or eggs) have over the baby that results?[123] Will corporations be allowed to control this lab-based reproduction, or is this a matter for the state? Will sex selection be allowed? Can we expect this system to reproduce existing social injustices? Was Dworkin right to fear this technology, on the grounds that 'when women no longer function as biological breeders we will be expendable'?[124]

Changes to language. Yet another group of radical feminists were focused on what today we would probably call 'linguistic activism', a kind of activism focused on words, concepts, and meanings. Together with Jane Caputi, Mary Daly wrote *Webster's First New Intergalactic Wickedary of the English Language*. This was full of new words, and new meanings for old words. Insults were reclaimed: 'catty' became 'Self-reliant, independent, resilient; having the Wild, Witchy, and Wicked characteristics of a cat'.[125] New concepts helped women to come to terms with their history and see themselves as a caste, for example 'gynocide' was coined to mean 'planned, institutionalized spiritual and bodily destruction of women; the use of deliberate systematic measures (such as killing, bodily or mental injury, unliveable conditions, prevention of births), which are calculated to bring about the destruction of women as a political and cultural force, the eradication of Female/Bio-logical[126] religion and language'.[127] Thousands of years of male domination can be expected to have become entrenched in language; this was a direct attempt by women to rewrite some of the more obvious patriarchal words and concepts, and to make a feminist contribution to language.

The limits to this kind of solution are that language cannot generally be changed by decree, but depends upon uptake by the rest of the language community.[128] Furthermore, it's not clear how much changes in the material reality of women experiencing domination or discrimination as a result of language change. J. K. Rowling puts this perfectly through the character of detective Cormoran Strike in *Troubled Blood*, when he says to student activists 'Reclaim... language all you fucking like. You don't change... real-world attitudes by deciding slurs aren't... derogatory'.[129]

Consciousness-raising. Catherine MacKinnon argued that while some of women's oppression was material, some of it was also psychological. She wrote about 'the pain, isolation, and thingification of women who have been pampered and pacified into nonpersonhood—women "grown ugly and dangerous from being nobody for so long"'.[130] The remedy for psychological oppression is consciousness-raising, which means women coming together in small groups to talk about their experiences. MacKinnon says that in consciousness-raising 'the impact of male dominance is concretely uncovered and analyzed through the collective speaking of women's experience, from the perspective of that experience'.[131] In the editor's note to her paper, consciousness-raising is described as 'challeng[ing] traditional notions of authority and objectivity and open[ing] a dialectical questioning of existing power structures, of our own experience, and of theory itself'.[132] Consciousness-raising was a way to start unmaking feminine socialization, first by becoming aware of it, and then by beginning the work of throwing it off, with support from and in solidarity with other women. This solution was distinctive to the radicals; it functioned as a response to their diagnosis of women's socialization into femininity as running especially deep, as something that would hold her in place even when her material constraints were lifted.

As a solution, consciousness-raising was most crucial when feminism was new. In a context in which feminist ideas are widespread, and in which we have good explanations of the mechanisms by which women's oppression is sustained and women are made (or attempted to be made) feminine, it is likely to be less central. However, it may earn its place again in contemporary feminism, as part of a pushback against socially dominant feminist ideas.

The end of sex differentiation. Some radical feminists thought the solution to women's oppression was to end the social practice of classifying people by sex. Marilyn Frye takes as one of her projects an explanation of sexism, ending up at the idea that 'individual acts and practices are sexist which reinforce and support... cultural and economic structures which create and enforce the elaborate and rigid patterns of sex-marking and sex-announcing which divide the species, along lines of sex, into dominators and subordinates'.[133] Resistance to sexism undermines those structures, and engages in the project of 'reconstruction and revision of ourselves'.[134] Frye anticipates Judith Butler when she says that we 'perform' gender:

> It is quite a spectacle, really, once one sees it, these humans so devoted to dressing up and acting out and 'fixing' one another so everyone lives up to and lives out the theory that there are two sharply distinct sexes and never the twain shall overlap or be confused or conflated... It is wonderful that homosexuals and lesbians are mocked and judged for 'playing butch-femme roles' and for dressing in 'butch-femme drag', for nobody goes about in full public view as thoroughly decked out in butch and femme

> drag as respectable heterosexuals when they are dressed up to go out in the evening, or to go to church, or to go to the office.[135]

She spends much of the essay pointing to the ways in which sex is 'announced' through dress, comportment, speech, and behaviour; making clear that we make a big deal of marking our own sex and of knowing others'. Her point is that there could not be a dominance-subordination structure without caste boundaries, and these particular caste boundaries depend on the constant identification of sex.[136] And here's the kicker: the oppression of women '*could not exist were not the groups, the categories of persons, well defined*... the barriers and forces could not be suitably located and applied if there were often much doubt as to which individuals were to be contained and reduced, which were to dominate'.[137]

Frye is pointing towards the solution that many feminists seem to have taken up with enthusiasm today, namely the project of blurring or entirely getting rid of sex categories. Sex-announcing and sex-marking is deliberately confounded by some gender non-conforming people. Some have argued that we should stop announcing sex in language, by shifting to gender-neutral pronouns for everyone.[138] Some claim that sex is a social construct,[139] or sex is much more complicated than we have assumed,[140] or that sex is a spectrum.[141] Indeed, Frye herself makes a version of this claim when she says 'There are people who fit on a biological spectrum between two not-so-sharply defined poles'.[142] So does MacKinnon, when she says 'Sex, in nature, is not a bipolarity; it is a continuum. In society it is made into a bipolarity'.[143] If it is sex that the hierarchy is imposed upon, one solution is to 'disappear' sex (or 'abolish' sex, as Monique Wittig put it).[144]

There are some reasons to think this is not a good solution. First, sex is *not* socially constructed. In philosophy, when we talk about 'social construction', we're generally talking about thoroughly social entities: paradigmatically, money, universities, corporations.[145] For example, if people didn't together believe in the authority of the university to award degrees, universities would not have that authority. There would not be such things as degrees, conferring status upon people and making them more employable. There are rocks, mountains, and lakes out there in the world, and they would be there whether we did anything or not. But 'universities' and 'degrees', and the 'authority to award degrees', are all in the world because of us, because of our shared beliefs and attitudes. Sex is like rocks and trees; gender is like money and universities. Sex is out there in the world, whether we choose to care much about it or not. Gender depends on us (or depends in large part on us).[146] The content of feminine socialization has varied across time and place. We've created a world that limits women's opportunities, and then we've pointed to the lack of women's accomplishments to justify keeping those limits in place. We've constructed women as passive, as objects, as people whose existence is literally *for* men (while men are constructed as active, as agents, as people who exist for themselves).[147] When radical feminists say that *gender* is socially constructed, they mean to highlight the special sense in which some things come entirely from social attitudes. The 'glue' that holds gender together is our human attitudes, beliefs, and expectations. The same is not true for sex.

Pointing to the fact of social construction when the meaning of a thing is pernicious, or hurts people, is often a first step in finding a way to *deconstruct* it. This is exactly what the second-wavers were trying to do when they first made use of the sex/gender distinction. This strategy makes sense when it's deployed against things like money and universities (although once made, it is not necessarily easy to unmake). But it's absolutely hopeless against things like rocks and trees. Imagine saying that because people have been tripping over rocks and falling over, we're going to stop noticing rocks and referring to them. That's going to result in nothing but a bunch of people pretending not to see something that they very much do see in the short term, and it's unlikely to stop people tripping over. Given that we have noticed rocks, we'd be better to clear them out of the way. If it's really *sex* and not *gender* that's hurting people, which is doubtful, we'd do better to raise awareness about what does and doesn't follow from being of a particular sex (which is what the gender abolitionists do, on which more next), rather than arguing that sex doesn't exist.[148] Because sex is not 'socially constructed' in the first place, deconstructing it—including abolishing it—is not possible.

Second, as above, it's not clear whether changing our terms and concepts really precedes meaningful political change, which requires change to people's beliefs, attitudes, and actions. Perhaps people will stop referring to sex, because they learn that this attracts social sanctions. But this doesn't mean they'll stop perceiving sex, or responding to sex, or having sexist beliefs or expectations. Forcing linguistic or conceptual change does not necessarily correspond to securing real moral or political change.

Gender abolitionism. An alternative to 'disappearing' sex is to 'disappear' the mistaken expectations that we pile onto sex instead—all the assumptions about what follows from the reproductive and other bodily differences between the sexes. John Stuart Mill[149] (ahead of his time), Beauvoir,[150]

Frye,[151] and others have all argued for the following sceptical conclusion: we just can't know that there are differences in men's and women's behaviour or capacities or interests resulting from their biology, because we've never had a context in which that biology was free of structural constraints.[152]

Many of the second-wavers saw gender as channelling people into sex roles, creating a hierarchy that perpetuates male dominance.[153] This view places a heavy emphasis on the environment women are in, and how they are socialized. They argue that we *impose* gender onto male and female people, creating different broad social roles. Worse, these roles are not equal; women are considered inferior. Atkinson writes in the essay 'Radical Feminism and Love' that 'A woman can only change her political definition by organizing with other women to change the definition of the female role, eventually eliminating it, thereby freeing herself to be human'.[154] Similar comments are made by Firestone.[155] This is the project of dismantling feminine socialization and freeing women to be *whatever* they want to be. For those radical feminists who understood gender to be the socialization of the sexes into social roles (femininity and masculinity), the solution was obvious: gender abolitionism (sometimes also 'gender annihilation').

But the *way* some radical feminist women interpreted gender abolition or gender annihilation was as integrating both femininity and masculinity into a kind of harmony referred to as 'androgyny' or 'unisex'. For example, Carolyn Heilburn wrote a book called *Toward a Recognition of Androgyny* and talked about 'the realization of man in woman and woman in man'.[156] Betty Roszak wrote in an essay called 'The Human Continuum' that 'Perhaps with the overcoming of women's oppression, the woman in man will be allowed to emerge'.[157] In *A Room of One's Own*, Virginia Woolf talked about there being two powers in the brain, the male and the female, where one predominates. She wrote hopefully of a time where the two powers would be more in balance: 'the normal and comfortable state of being is when the two live in harmony together, spiritually co-operating'.[158]

Other radical feminists, among them Janice Raymond, Mary Daly, and Jeffner Allen, criticized this vision of gender abolition.[159] Rather than seeing current forms of masculinity and femininity as natural aspects of the human personality that are cultivated and magnified through socialization and so could exist in different proportion in each person, we should see current forms of masculinity and femininity as artefacts of patriarchy, which might be completely different—and indeed completely absent—without it. Instead of abolishing gender by incorporating both masculinity and femininity into each individual, we can search for new conceptualizations of how people can be *without gender*. Raymond compared androgyny as an aspiration for abolition to putting the concepts of master and slave together to define a free person.[160] Still, androgyny as a vision of what a gender abolitionist future might look like should not be confused with gender abolition itself, which is compatible with a number of different futures. We can agree with Raymond, Daly, and Allen that the harmony version of androgyny or unisex won't work, without throwing out the understanding of women's oppression and the proposed solution of gender abolitionism entirely.

We won't know how different masculinity and femininity will be, and indeed *whether* they will be much different, until we can 'run the experiment' in a human society without patriarchy. Frye agrees with this when she says

> we do not know whether human behaviour patterns would be dimorphic along lines of chromosomal sex if we were not threatened and bullied; nor do we know, if we assume that they would be dimorphous, *what* they would be, that is, *what* constellations of traits and tendencies would fall out along that genetic line.[161]

My own suspicion is that physiological differences will create some social differences between men and women, on average, in any possible future. The pain and inconvenience of menstruation; the different phenomenology of sexual intercourse; the fear of rape (even when its incidence is much lower); the possibility of pregnancy; the facts of pregnancy, breastfeeding, and the dependency of young children (even when the labour of childrearing is more equally shared); the impacts of pregnancy on the body (even when feminine beauty norms have been eroded); the incidence of menopause; these must all have an impact on what it is like to be female, which may in turn impact preferences and interests to at least some extent.

There will be many exceptions—just as there are to average differences between men and women even under our current non-utopian conditions[162]—but it remains plausible to expect some average differences. Still, once society is no longer marked by male dominance, these differences are unlikely to have much in common with the current content of 'femininity', which expects women to be, for example, beautiful, warm, supportive, nurturing, submissive, and self-effacing.[163]

It's worth noting that of all these solutions to patriarchy or ways of challenging patriarchy, two in particular are not likely to succeed unless they are 'women-only'. These are women's religion and consciousness-raising.

Arguably, women's religion is about creating spiritual bonds between women, bonds of sisterhood and solidarity. Women return to women some of the social status that they have not been given by men. In consciousness-raising, women discuss their *experiences* of domination under patriarchy, and try to find ways forward to free and recreate *themselves*. Having men involved in these practices is likely to undermine their aims. This is not obviously true for the other solutions—men can participate in challenging patriarchal language, and in working on technologies to free women from reproduction, for example. (This will be relevant in Chapter 3, when we come to the place of men in gender-critical feminism; and Chapter 5, when we talk about the tensions between gender-critical feminism and gender identity activism.)

3
Gender-Critical Feminism

> No amount of calling myself 'agender' will stop the world seeing me as a woman, and treating me accordingly. I can introduce myself as agender and insist upon my own set of neo-pronouns when I apply for a job, but it won't stop the interviewer seeing a potential baby-maker, and giving the position to the less qualified but less encumbered by reproduction male candidate.
>
> (Rebecca Reilly-Cooper, 'Gender is Not A Spectrum')[1]

3.1 Sex Matters

It should be clear from Chapter 2 that biological sex—being female—mattered to radical feminists. (As mentioned already, some people use both 'female' and 'woman' to refer to gender identity; but given that 'male' and 'female' are the standard scientific terms for the biological sexes, and especially given that there are no other terms to refer to the sexes, I am rejecting that usage here.) Sex was key to every explanation offered for the origins of women's oppression, whether it related to their reproductive capacities or to their comparative physical strength or to their sexuality. It was also a key feature in every explanation of the mechanisms by which women's oppression is sustained, however it got started. Babies are channelled into sex roles depending on what sex they are observed as being. Children are socialized according to socially constructed ideas about gender that are attached to people on the basis of sex. Sex is a necessary ingredient in gender, because it tells us what it is that the social meanings are attached *to*. There is no way to eliminate or displace sex—as some of those committed to gender as an identity want to do[2]—without a massive loss of explanatory power.

We can make this point about the importance of sex without any of the theoretical commitments of radical feminism, though. It's enough to simply notice that sex categories have political importance. They allow us to name a

Gender-Critical Feminism: Holly Lawford-Smith, Oxford University Press. © Holly Lawford-Smith 2022.
DOI: 10.1093/oso/9780198863885.003.0003

caste of people who have been oppressed and excluded from public life. It is *female people*, not people who perform femininity or people who identify as women, who were denied the vote, until 1893 in New Zealand (the first country to grant full suffrage to women), until 1920 in the United States, and until 2015 in Saudi Arabia. It is female people who have struggled since the end of the 16th century to secure rights to abortion, with abortions of all types (including as a result of rape or incest) still being illegal in twenty-six countries today.[3] It is female people who were excluded from work and from public life, for example in Australia women were not elected into the Commonwealth Parliament until 1943; didn't have the right to drink in a public bar until 1965; and were forced to resign from their jobs in the public service or in many private companies when they got married during the 1960s. Women are still paid 17.5 per cent less than men who do the same work.[4] Women are persistently sexually objectified throughout the media, and socialized to believe their primary value is in their appearance and in their capacity to reproduce. I could go on, and talk about sex-selective abortions; female genital mutilation; human trafficking, the great bulk of which is women into sexual slavery; prostitution and pornography; the distribution of domestic labour; career choice and remuneration; risk of male violence; underrepresentation in high-status employment fields; underrepresentation at the higher levels of almost all employment areas; underrepresentation in politics; underrepresentation in sports…but I am sure the point is clear enough.

Because women have historically been the victims of subordination and exclusion from public life, and because the effects of this subordination and exclusion have far-reaching implications which are still being felt today (even where the formal obstacles have been removed), it remains important to protect this caste of people. The international law Convention on the Elimination of all Forms of Discrimination Against Women (CEDAW) was adopted in 1979 in recognition of the fact that existing human rights law had not succeeded in protecting women. One way to protect women is by acknowledging relevant differences, e.g. the physical differences between male and female people that lead to the former's having a competitive advantage in sport.[5] Another is by implementing affirmative action policies in order to increase women's participation or representation in areas where they have been historically excluded and remain underrepresented.[6] Yet another is by providing (or maintaining) women-only spaces, services, and provisions, e.g. women's gyms, women's health services, women's consciousness-raising groups.[7] We cannot offer these protections if we cannot clearly identify the class of people to whom they apply. Radical feminists think sex is important, but you don't have to be a radical feminist to think this.

Reaffirming the political importance of sex also continues the radical feminist project of correcting for the disproportionate emphasis placed on the mind over the body, which was a legacy of classical liberalism. Alison Jaggar calls this 'normative dualism', the idea that not only is there a mind/body divide, but that the mind is the more important and more deserving of value. Jaggar criticized this view as male-biased, on the basis that men and women have very different physical experiences given the difference in their reproductive role.[8] A mind-focused approach to equal employment policy might overlook the distinctive bodily needs women have relating to menstruation, pregnancy, breastfeeding, and menopause. Bodily differences between men and women also matter particularly in the political debate over sports inclusion policy today. Because going through male puberty produces a set of physical differences that give men a competitive advantage in most sports, sports have tended to be sex-separated in order to allow fair competition. This sex-separation is being challenged today on the grounds of transgender inclusion, with some arguing that transwomen should be allowed to compete in women's sports.

Physical differences also matter for the politics of language. Some organizations are rewording sex-specific language to make it gender neutral, in order to accommodate 'gender minorities'. Women may get pregnant and breastfeed, women are at risk of cervical cancer, and women are most at risk of breast cancer. But if transmen are men, and non-binary females are not women, then to be maximally accurate and inclusive, we have to say things like 'people who get pregnant', or 'people with cervixes'.[9] This makes invisible the fact that it's only a very specific group of 'people' to whom these things happen, namely female people.

Female people have shared interests, as female. It is reasonable for people with shared interests to organize politically around those interests. This does not require that all women have the exact same experiences, which they obviously do not.[10] It is enough that there exist patterns that create a shared threat to them. There can be differential exposure to that threat while it still being the case that the threat is shared. Rape, for example, can happen to a woman regardless of whether she is advantaged in ways not relating to her sex.

Given everything I have said so far, hopefully the need and justification for a theory and movement that names the female sex caste and the oppression of its members is clear. That theory is radical feminism, and its latest incarnation, gender-critical feminism. It is an advantage of this type of feminism that there are few hard questions about group membership,[11] and so no pressure to throw our hands up and repudiate all attempts at a (non-circular) definition of 'woman'.[12]

It is important to note that while sex is the trait that gender is imposed on the basis of, sex itself does not have to be part of every specific way that women are marginalized. In this way, gender-critical feminism has a broader remit than (some versions of) radical feminism. Pressing women into the unpaid domestic service of men in many countries means they cannot engage in paid work, and those women have much less money than men, and are economically dependent upon men. Some of those women might have succeeded in disengaging from their male partner sexually, however, and may be childless. So it's not adequate to say that their oppression is based in their sexuality, childbearing, or childrearing. It's really not about their female *body* at all. Rather, it's about the way that people with those kinds of bodies have been subject to certain kinds of expectations and pushed into certain kinds of roles on the basis of them. We need to understand gender norms, the content of women's subjection to norms of femininity.

3.2 Gender Norms

In Chapter 2, I quoted Marilyn Frye on the point that it is social threats that protect against deviation from gender-conforming behaviour (by which I mean, men being masculine and women being feminine), and that the patterns of femininity and masculinity would not be there but for those threats.[13] And I mentioned that although she does not use the idea of norms, that is nonetheless a helpful conceptual framework for understanding what she was getting at.

Rebecca Reilly-Cooper, writing for *Aeon* in 2016, explains gender in this way. Gender is a set of norms that are applied to people on the basis of their sex, prescribing one set of behaviours to female people as desirable and proscribing another set as undesirable; and prescribing another set of behaviours to male people as desirable and proscribing another set as undesirable.[14] What is desirable for one is undesirable for the other. Reilly-Cooper explains:

> Not only are these norms external to the individual and coercively imposed, but they also represent a binary caste system or hierarchy, a value system with two positions: maleness above femaleness, manhood above womanhood, masculinity above femininity. Individuals are born with the potential to perform one of two reproductive roles, determined at birth, or even before, by the external genitals that the infant possesses. From then on, they will be inculcated into one of two classes in the hierarchy: the superior class if their genitals are convex, the inferior one if their genitals are concave.[15]

Most females are raised to be 'passive, submissive, weak and nurturing', while most males are raised to be 'active, dominant, strong and aggressive'.[16] This system constrains human potential and creates social hierarchy.

It is important to distinguish between two different types of norms: social norms and moral norms. Moral norms are personal. They can differ from person to person, and do not depend much upon what other people think. They are requirements we impose on ourselves, and failure to live up to them can be a cause of guilt or shame. Social norms are social. They are held in place by social beliefs, social conformity, and social policing. Social norms start with normative expectations, which means expectations that have value judgements attached. Cristina Bicchieri gives an account of social norms as rules of behaviour that people prefer to conform to because they believe that most other people conform to them, and most other people believe they ought to conform to them.[17] When Bicchieri talks about 'most people', she doesn't mean most people in the whole world. She means, in a 'reference network', which is something like, in the group of people you're embedded in. This might be your country, your state, or your community.

For an example of a social norm that fits this account, in Japan, there is a norm (although it is currently being challenged) of women wearing high heels to work, usually between 1.9 and 2.75 inches in height.[18] For any given woman who does this, she is likely to believe (because she observes it) that other women do in fact wear high heels to work, and likely to believe that people think that women *ought* to wear high heels to work. Perhaps she has seen other women get in trouble with their bosses when they don't wear high heels, or she has read opinion pieces in the media about the importance of women wearing high heels, or has heard other women express negative thoughts about women who don't wear high heels to work. (The #KuToo movement is an attempt by Japanese women to raise awareness about the discomfort of working long hours in high heels, and to change this norm in Japan).[19]

Gender norms are social norms, but they may also be internalized as moral norms for many people. Perhaps a woman works to stay in shape, and does that because she sees a lot of other women doing it, and because she knows that a lot of people believe women ought to be physically attractive. But she may also believe that regardless of what any other woman is doing, *she* ought to stay in shape, and if she goes through a stressful period where she cannot exercise as much and gains weight, she may feel ashamed for failing to live up to this standard that she has imposed upon herself.[20] Because gender norms are so pervasive, and because women are enculturated into the norms of femininity since birth, it is not uncommon for at least some gender norms to be internalized as moral norms, and not just social norms. When norms are social, they can be changed by challenging conformity (for example, getting a lot of women in Japan to stop wearing high heels to work), and by challenging the idea that conformity is *valuable* (for example, by pointing out how much discomfort it causes women to be in high heels through long days on their feet, and showing how unfair it is that women are expected to suffer this discomfort while men are not).[21] When they are moral, things are more complicated.[22]

This should not be taken to suggest that if women were to stop conforming to gender norms and everyone were to stop policing norms of femininity tomorrow, women's oppression would suddenly dissolve and women would be liberated. The historical imposition of these norms has created a legacy of 'structural injustice', which is injustice that has been embedded into the law, culture, and major social institutions. For example, norms about marriage and homemaking imposed historically upon women meant there were *no* women in medicine until a particular point in time, and then *few*, and now still a minority in some areas (like cardiothoracic surgery, vascular surgery, and orthopaedic surgery).[23] Women form roughly 30 per cent of medical leadership in Australia (medical school deans, chief medical officers, medical college boards, and committee members).[24] This has meant that medical research has been androcentric to a very large degree throughout history, and to a significant degree even today. The fact that there is a lack of research into specific women's health issues creates disadvantage for women that suffer those issues (against a counterfactual baseline of there being no historical injustice, and so no transformation of historical injustice into structural injustice).

Feminist philosopher Katharine Jenkins, writing in defence of gender as identity, acknowledges that gender is a system of norms in roughly the way Reilly-Cooper has in mind, but argues that gender identity is *taking these norms to apply to you*. Jenkins writes 'to say that someone has a female gender identity is to say that she experiences the norms that are associated with women in her social context as relevant to her'.[25] But she also notes that one may take certain norms to be relevant while also knowing that 'other people judge their behaviour by reference to norms of (say) masculinity'.[26] According to Riley-Cooper, there is a system of norms that tell female people to be feminine;[27] according to Jenkins, anyone can take the norms of femininity to apply to them, and that's an explanation of what it is to have a gender identity. But Jenkins is making a mistake about how norms work. As Reilly-Cooper said, norms are 'external to the individual and coercively imposed'. If they were just *ideas*, out there in the world and freely available for people to take to apply to themselves or not, they wouldn't be norms, and there would be nothing to explain women's oppression. It's the *coercive imposition*, what Frye referred to as 'penalties' and 'threats', that make gender a system of norms in the first place. So a person who is not female can take feminine norms to apply to them all they like, but as long as they're recognizably male, they won't actually be subject to those norms (they'll be subject to the norms of masculinity instead).

A judge in a recent case in the United States involving discrimination on the basis of transgender status seems to agree with this. Aimee Stevens was employed at a funeral home while still presenting as male. Stevens told her employer that she was planning to transition and wanted to start adhering to the female dress code rather than the male one, and then was fired.[28] Elizabeth Hungerford quotes Justice Kagan, whose interpretation of a prior case was 'there is another trait…conformity to traditional gender roles'. Kagan joined the opinion of the court, which found that the firing of Stephens was unlawful for multiple reasons, one of which came from a legal precedent against sex stereotyping. Hungerford agrees with Kagan when she writes:

> Under a gender non-conformity analysis, Aimee Stephens' firing was clearly unlawful. Again, this reasoning requires that we hold Stephens' biological sex as male in order to assess which gender roles he is expected to conform to and/or has deviated from. It also avoids creating an assumption that people with 'transgender status' are more harmed or

> more burdened by the enforcement of gender roles than other people are, specifically those people who share the trait of gender non-conformity.[29]

When we understand gender as a system of norms imposed on the basis of sex, we are able to make predictions about how people will be policed. It is because Stevens was male that she was fired for wanting to dress in male-atypical clothing. If we suppose that Stevens was female, then it's a mystery why she was fired, given that no other women in the workplace were fired for wearing male-atypical (i.e. female-typical) clothing. If we suppose that this was about transgender discrimination, then we miss the fact that a gender non-conforming woman (for example, a butch lesbian)[30] who wanted to adhere to the male dress code in the same workplace might similarly be fired. This is an important point: it is not just trans people who face discrimination on the grounds of gender non-conformity. And yet it is only trans people who there is a serious social effort to protect from this kind of discrimination.

Some will argue that it can't be *sex* that norms are imposed on the basis of. After all, some people are routinely mis-sexed. The feminist philosopher Lori Watson writes:

> more often than not, I am identified by others, who do not know me, as a man; I would conjecture that in everyday interactions with strangers, I am taken to be a man over 90 percent of the time. This identification started happening regularly about sixteen years ago when I cut my hair very short. (I had always dressed in 'men's clothing' since my teenage years. Add to this that I am nearly six feet tall and have broad shoulders and a 'healthy' frame. This is the body I was given.) In fact, others so routinely identify me as a man that I am often caught off guard and surprised if someone correctly identifies me as a woman . . . I am not a man. I do not identify as a man. I don't want to be a man, trans or otherwise. I am a woman . . .[31]

Does this show that it's not sex, but something else, that norms are applied on the basis of? Feminist philosopher Sally Haslanger, in a well-known paper on race and gender, seemed to think so. She seemed to roughly agree with the norms picture, describing being a woman as being marked as a target for subordinating treatment. But she claimed that women were not marked as targets because they were *female*, but because of 'observed or imagined bodily features presumed to be evidence of a female's biological role in reproduction'.[32] Haslanger is one of the philosophers who decoupled sex from gender, and used 'woman' as a gender term, so that 'one can be a woman without ever (in the ordinary sense) "acting like a woman", "feeling like a woman", or even having a female body'.[33] Because she takes gender to be a social position (a position in a social hierarchy), she's interested in how people are viewed and treated, and how their lives are structured. So long as someone is viewed and treated in the way that female people generally are, and has one's life structured as female people's lives generally are, one can be a 'woman' even when one is not 'female'.

This might initially seem appealing. After all, it will be true that the norms of masculinity are applied to some people who are female (like Watson, above), and the norms of femininity are applied to some people who are male. But what is the ultimate explanation of *why* they are applied? Is the norm that 'female-looking people ought to be feminine'? Do pretty boy babies get channelled into the female sex role? The answer is no, in either case. The reason why people apply norms of masculinity to male-looking people is that they assume they are male. When they find out they had made a mistake, they generally don't continue to apply the norm (as long as they believe what is being said). Suppose a female-looking male person is taking an Uber Pool with a few other male passengers when the driver's GPS messes up. One of the men jokes that he'll navigate, because 'she' probably isn't any good with maps. All the female-looking male person has to do is point out that he's in fact male for this sexist assumption to fall away.

To make the point in a slightly sillier way, suppose that there is a black market in zebras because people will pay excellent money for their striped hides, and an entrepreneur comes up with the idea of painting donkeys to look like zebras and then charging hunters for access to the land where these 'zebras' are.[34] If we wanted to describe the killing of zebras for human economic gain as morally repugnant, would we say, 'zebras are hunted because hunters can make serious money from selling their hides', or would we say 'animals are hunted on the basis of observed or imagined bodily features presumed to be evidence of being a zebra, because hunters can make serious money from selling their hides'? It seems quite obvious to me that we wouldn't say the latter, which raises the question of why Haslanger introduced this cumbersome locution in the first place. Perhaps it is because by 2000, the feminist desire to be 'inclusive' when it came to the category 'woman' and the constituency of feminism was already well on its way to being fully internalized.

Understanding gender as a system of norms imposed on the basis of sex helps to make clear that gender is a social problem. Radical feminism and gender-critical feminism are in agreement that we need social solutions to social problems, not individual solutions to social problems. Women are a social group (class/caste). That group has a history of oppression. Its members are likely to face many of the same issues and obstacles. This makes it important for women to organize politically in order to advance their interests as a group. And it makes it important for women to describe *patterns* of abuse, harassment, exploitation, discrimination, disadvantage, etc., to understand where these are feminist political issues, rather than issues merely arising for individuals within their specific contexts and relationships. One of Janice Raymond's complaints about the phenomenon of transsexualism (which she refers to as 'transgenderism') during the second wave was that it proposed individual, medical solutions to the social problem of constraining ideas about gender.[35] This was also Reilly-Cooper's complaint against so-called 'nonbinary' or 'agender' identifications. She describes individuals' claims that they are nonbinary or agender as 'try[ing] to slip through the bars of the cage while leaving the rest of the cage intact, and the rest of womankind trapped within it'.[36]

3.3 What Radical Feminist Ideas Does Gender-Critical Feminism Leave Behind?

I've said already that virtually none of the ideas put forward by the radical feminists of the second wave are *necessary* to radical feminism as a theory and movement. This is even more the case for the proposed solutions they offered. Many of these were 'experiments in living', and not all of those experiments had positive results.

Gender-critical feminism leaves behind the strong belief in women's difference as it relates to personalities and preferences. It does not believe that women are naturally better with intuition, feeling, or emotion. This does not leave us committed to the view that the human mind is a 'blank slate' just waiting to be imprinted by different sets of social arrangements; but the sex differences gender-critical feminism can accommodate are unlikely to provide a rationalization of many of the social differences between the sexes we have seen in the past, or still see today. For example, it is highly unlikely that any 'innate', 'hard-wired', or 'predisposed' traits in female people would be sufficient to justify women's underrepresentation in politics, or in leadership positions in the business world, or throughout science, technology, engineering, and maths (STEM) subjects.

Gender-critical feminism leaves behind women's religion, and all of the spiritual aspects of 'women's culture', including witchcraft, that some radical feminists were concerned to build.[37] (It is only incompatible with such practices, however, if/when they conflict with a scientific worldview and a receptiveness to empirical evidence.) Its concern with women's culture is limited to a concern to protect women-only spaces, services, and provisions (which includes events aimed at celebrating femaleness and aspects of womanhood that have been devalued by men), and is rationalized by women's right to establish and enforce boundaries—important when so many women have had their personal boundaries violated by acts of childhood sexual abuse, rape, domestic violence, sexual harassment, and so on—and by women's right to freedom of association and self-determination.

Gender-critical feminism is supportive of lesbianism, but it has no commitments that make it unacceptable (or a betrayal) for women to have sexual or romantic relationships with men. On this point, it is in agreement with the criticism of earlier radical lesbian feminism made by intersectional feminist bell hooks, who says that the suggestion that real feminists are lesbians alienates too many women from feminism.[38] Far from thinking that all feminists *ought* to be lesbians, gender-critical feminists have an internal disagreement over the moral status of political lesbianism, with some vehemently rejecting the idea that it is possible for a woman to choose to be a lesbian.[39] Gender-critical feminism is also not separatist more generally (sex/romance aside) when it comes to feminist theory or activism. Gender-critical feminists will generally work with men and appreciate the support of male allies. Again this puts gender-critical feminism in agreement with criticism made by hooks, in this case that separatism is most appealing to white women, who do not feel solidarity with white men in the way that black women do with black men, or as do other women who share an axis of oppression with men.[40] (Note that the fact that gender-critical feminism is not separatist in the strong sense, advocating for women's withdrawal either entirely or as much as possible from men, doesn't mean it never values separation. Gender-critical feminists value female sex-separated spaces, which means that separation from men *is* a commitment, just in a much more limited number of domains).

Finally, gender-critical feminism has a broader remit than at least some versions of radical feminism. While it cares a great deal about biological sex and the female bodily experience, it does not restrict its attention to women's sexuality, or women's childbearing or childrearing. The explanation for this is somewhat complicated, and relates to the feminist idea of 'intersectionality'. (I take up this issue in detail in Chapter 7.) Gender-critical feminism focuses on a single axis of oppression, namely sex. That means it neither considers multiple axes of oppression in one movement nor focuses on the intersections of multiple axes.[41] Examples of the former include ecofeminism (combining environmentalism and feminism), black feminism (combining black liberation and feminism), and socialist feminism (combining class liberation and feminism). An example of the latter is focusing on the way that being working class and being female can interact to create negative stereotypes of working-class women. One study from 1985, for example, found working-class women to be rated higher than middle-class women as being each of 'confused, dirty, hostile, illogical, impulsive, incoherent, inconsiderate, irresponsible, and superstitious'.[42]

This helps to illuminate one of the major disagreements gender-critical feminists have with other types of feminists, who tend to be intersectional. But it goes further than that too, because some women who consider themselves to be gender-critical feminists also consider themselves to be intersectional. In Section 7.6, I defend a limited way in which this is possible, but in general I will argue that gender-critical feminism is *not*, and need not be, intersectional.

If you think oppression depends upon the complex combination of features a person has, then you'll need to be sensitive to all the ways in which a person might be oppressed, both visible and invisible. Combine this with two further influential feminist ideas—one, that we should focus on the situation of the worst-off women; and two, that marginalized people have specialist knowledge and should be deferred to—and you get a situation in which *within* feminist groups, white women are supposed to defer to black women, able-bodied women are supposed to defer to women with disabilities, straight women are supposed to defer to lesbians, white straight able-bodied women are supposed to defer to black lesbians with disabilities…and so on. Someone who is oppressed across multiple axes may fill the position of 'the worst off' in a particular feminist group and thus have a claim to their issues receiving the bulk of the group's attentions and energies, and their testimony being deferred to. Contingencies about which women happen to be in the group will determine the feminist agenda of that group.

If we instead maintain that feminism is a single-axis movement for women's liberation, then the members of feminist groups are *equals* in that context, so long as they're all women. If we changed the context so that all the same women were at a Black Lives Matter meeting, the white women would need to learn to be quiet and find out how to be good allies to black people.

But in the context of a feminist meeting, where the focus is and should be on sex-based oppression, there is no further hierarchy between women *that is of relevance to the feminist movement.* No one needs to apologize and defer within such a group; women have done enough apologizing and deferring in human history to last a lifetime.

A feminism that refuses to combine multiple issues, and refuses to be intersectional, is actually less hubristic. It is hard enough to get a firm grip on the mechanisms by which women are oppressed as a caste, and the things that need to change in order for women's liberation—*as women*—to be secured. Feminism hardly needs the added challenge of figuring out class liberation at the same time. That is not to assume that 'we' feminists are not working class; it's to assume that there is one set of questions about what the origins, sustaining mechanisms, and solutions are when it comes to sex oppression, and another set of questions when it comes to class oppression. Answering these questions deserves the full attention of a social justice movement. When these movements each come up with good answers, they can form alliances with each other to boost political support and solidarity.

This is a vision for feminism which sees it as just one piece of the puzzle when it comes to social justice. Its contribution affects half of the human population, but it does not affect them in all aspects of their lives. Furthermore, this approach helps to avoid the politics of deference that can distort debate and undermine political progress. The fact that someone is a member of a marginalized group is a reason to think they know *something* about being a member of that group, from experience. But it is no reason at all to think that they are an expert in the issues facing that group, or that they are well-informed about the political disagreement between members of that group, or could fairly and accurately represent the group to others. When intersectional feminists inside an activist group defer to one woman *because she has a disability*, for example, rather than *because she can reasonably claim to represent a community of people with disabilities*, they risk making things worse, not better, from the point of view of social justice.[43] And when disability activists inside a feminist group, for example, add sex-neutral disability issues to the feminist agenda, they risk making things worse, not better, from the point of view of justice for women as women.

Still, gender-critical feminism is left with the challenge of articulating what it is for feminism to be about 'women's liberation' when so many women are also unfree in virtue of their race, class, or other social group features. I'll give a fuller answer to this question in Chapter 7, but very briefly, we can give a theory of what it means to be oppressed as a woman by having a clear definition of 'woman' and a clear understanding of the ways that women are socialized into femininity. ('Woman' is a contested term. It is less important that people sign up to our usage of it, than that they agree the group we refer to with it has interests worth protecting.) For gender-critical feminists, 'women' are adult human females.[44] This became a classic assertion of gender-critical feminists' during the UK consultation over the Gender Recognition Act, made prominent by grassroots feminist campaigner Posie Parker's billboard featuring the definition.[45] Adult human females are people most of whom[46] have faced lifelong and concerted attempts at socialization into femininity. So gender-critical feminists consider something to be a feminist issue (aimed at the liberation of women *as women* rather than as persons more generally) whenever it relates to that socialization.

3.4 The Constituency of Gender-Critical Feminism, and Its Relation to Men

> Men are the enemy in much the same way that some crazed boy in uniform was the enemy of another like him in most respects except the uniform. One possible tactic is to try to get the uniforms off.
>
> (Germaine Greer, *The Female Eunuch*)[47]

As we have seen, gender-critical feminism accepts the radical feminist focus on female people as a class/caste.[48] The constituency of feminism, for gender-critical feminists, is female people. We do not apologize for this, no matter how hard anti-feminists and non-radical feminists work to extract such an apology (on which more in Chapter 6). Its central goal is abolition of the norms of femininity (of gender in its entirety), one of the most pervasive of which has been self-effacement. Gender-critical feminism, like radical feminism before it, does not apologize for putting women first. It does not see itself as a small part of another, bigger movement. It sees women's liberation as an important movement in its own right.

Contrary to the representation of radical and gender-critical feminism coming from some quarters as 'SWERFs', or 'sex-worker-exclusionary radical feminists',[49] gender-critical feminists do include prostituted women/sex workers in their constituency. They are female, and they are some of the worst-off women in the world, so they are not only included but often prioritized (the work of women like Catharine MacKinnon and Andrea

Dworkin during the second wave, and the work of women like Kajsa Ekis Ekman, Julie Bindel, Meagan Tyler, and Caroline Norma today is an example of this).

But the accusation behind 'TERF', or 'trans-exclusionary radical feminist', is partly correct. Gender-critical feminists are not exclusionary of trans people per se, but they include in their constituency transmen rather than transwomen, and female nonbinary people rather than no/all nonbinary people. Gender-critical feminists do this because our constituency, as already explained, is female people. Far from excluding trans people per se from the constituency of feminism, gender-critical feminists are very concerned with the situation of transmen and female nonbinary people. We are very concerned with the massive increases of young girls reporting to gender clinics,[50] with the risk clinical 'affirmation' policies for trans people pose to young lesbians and to lesbian culture, and with the increasing numbers of detransitioned women speaking out about their experiences.[51]

What about men? (*What about men?!*) Deborah Cameron makes a distinction between different ways to think about what feminism is, which are helpful in thinking about the place of men.[52] Feminism might be a collective political project, an idea, or an intellectual framework (a 'mode of analysis'). If it is an idea, for example that women and men are moral equals, then clearly men *can* be feminists. If it is a collective political project, or an intellectual framework, then it depends on the details of these things. For some ways of understanding what the project or framework is, men can be feminist allies at best. (One role of an ally is to amplify women's voices, particularly to demographics that might be more responsive to men.)

Finn Mackay's book *Radical Feminism* contains interviews with British women who have been involved in the 'Reclaim the Night' protest, and does a nice job of tracking some of the disagreement over the place of men in feminism.[53] The point about men's place is well made in relation to that particular protest. The point of Reclaim the Night is for women to access public space that is ordinarily denied to them as a result of narratives about keeping themselves safe from assault. If an individual woman had a male chaperone, she wouldn't have any problem in accessing that space. So the symbolism is in women together reclaiming the streets and the night. If men join them, even with the best intentions, they undermine the very reclamation women are setting out to pursue.

What if the collective political project is women's self-determination? Women's oppression has literally determined their self-conception, which means that women's liberation centrally involves self-determination, recreating what it means to be a woman. Men who attempt to participate in that self-determination—again, even with the best intentions—undermine that very self-determination. They are a part of the 'other' who had been determining woman all along. So if feminism is a collective political project, and that project is self-determination, then men *can't* be feminists. The same is true if feminism is an intellectual framework, and that framework is consciousness-raising. The whole point is for women to reveal their experiences *as* women living in a male-dominated society. Including the experience of men will distort the mosaic that is pieced together from those experiences, and will affect women's collective self-understanding.

For these reasons, most gender-critical feminists think that men cannot be feminists, only allies. But I think it would be too strong to say that if you don't accept this, you are not a gender-critical feminist. A gender-critical feminist could formulate her position as an idea, e.g. that women are a sex caste, or as a collective political project, e.g. that feminism requires working for the protection of sex-based rights and the elimination of sex-based marginalization, and cheerfully accept men as gender-critical feminists. Nothing about these specific understandings of the gender-critical feminist idea or project precludes men's involvement.

This question of the place of men in feminism is a source of tension between gender-critical feminists and other types of feminists. Many of the former relegate *all* male people to the position of ally, at best. Most of the latter include transwomen (and sometimes nonbinary people) as part of the group concerned to self-determine, or raise consciousness. Yet those same feminists may simultaneously be happy to exclude all people who *identify* as men. For the gender-critical feminists committed to the exclusion of all men, this is aggravating. The explanation of why the collective political project, or intellectual framework, is needed has nothing to do with identity and everything to do with treatment as a sex caste.

Marilyn Frye wrote in *The Politics of Reality* that there is a distinction between being male, on the one hand, and being masculine or 'a man' on the other. Here she does as some feminists do, and uses 'male/female' as sex terms and 'man/woman' as gender terms, rather than both as sex terms. The distinction creates a way for a male person to work to avoid complicity in women's oppression. Frye says 'I have enjoined males of my acquaintance to set themselves against masculinity. I have asked them to think about how they can stop being men, and I was not recommending a sex-change operation'.[54] She draws a parallel between being a man and being white, accepting a similar responsibility in herself to avoid complicity in racial oppression, and commenting 'I do not suggest for a moment that I can disaffiliate by a private act of will, or by any personal strategy. Nor, certainly, is it accomplished by simply thinking it possible. To think it thinkable shortcuts no work and shields one from no responsibility'.[55]

Although she's reflecting in that paragraph on disaffiliating from whiteness, the same point can be made for masculinity. One cannot escape masculinity by fiat, or with a simple thought; with masculinity comes responsibility and to escape it takes work. This point applies to all those socialized into masculinity who would call themselves feminists or feminist allies, including transwomen and male nonbinary people. Gender identity cannot circumvent sex-based privilege and complicity in women's oppression. This is what Frye describes as 'a private act of will', a 'personal strategy', a thinking possible, an attempt at a shortcut, an avoiding of responsibility.

There are open questions that remain to be resolved in figuring out what it takes for a man to disaffiliate from masculinity.[56] Resolving these would allow gender-critical feminists to articulate their disagreement with other feminists and gender identity activists, about their disagreement with the claim that a transwoman is, in virtue of being a transwoman, already disaffiliated from masculinity in the way that feminists want all men to be. Disaffiliating is not as easy as merely disclaiming or repudiating; there is some work to be done in shrugging off the impacts of a lifetime of socialization into masculinity, and it remains to be seen exactly what that work consists in and how women can reliably identify those who have done it and those who have not. If gender-critical feminists do not ask and answer these questions, they risk taking the ham-fisted approach of rejecting the involvement in feminism (whether as feminists or as allies) of anyone who has been socialized into masculinity.

3.5 Procedural Commitments

Three quick final points, all relating to issues internal to feminist activism: equality, leadership, and criticism.

Radical feminism's commitment to real equality led to policies like having no leaders, or having no specialist roles. For example, The Redstockings in their 1969 manifesto say 'We are committed to achieving internal democracy. We will do whatever is necessary to ensure that every woman in our movement has an equal chance to participate, assume responsibility, and develop her political potential'.[57] Such a group might have a system of rotating roles, where someone who had not been in the role before would get it next, so that all women had a chance to increase their skills, and no woman gained power through being irreplaceable.

These groups often didn't last long. Some roles require specialist skills—like treasurer, for example—and so passing them to someone new every month will generally mean many more mistakes, some of which could be serious. There's inefficiency in 'flat hierarchy', which many women who have been involved in feminist activism will attest to. Even Firestone, who writes approvingly of radical feminism's commitment to internal democracy, comments that 'it goes to (often absurd) lengths to pursue this goal'.[58] Gender-critical feminism should learn from these experiments, and try to strike the right balance between principles and productivity rather than sacrificing productivity at the altar of principle.

In *Feminist Theory: From Margin to Centre*, bell hooks criticizes the feminist movement for its mistaken conception of power. She says feminists have confused leadership qualities in women with attempts at domination, which means they have worked to cut down or cut out women who could have made valuable contributions.[59] Jo Freeman's essay 'On Trashing' from 1976 makes a similar point, although it extends to other ways women cut each other down.[60] In her memoir, Phyllis Chester writes:

> Feminists spent years accusing each other of being 'male identified' and elitist. According to Ruth Rosen: 'One of the strangest consequences of such anti-elitism was that activists pressured one another to write without bylines. Writing anonymously has been required of modest ladies of the nineteenth century. Now, in the name of solidarity, some women's liberationists asked that no woman take credit for her work'. My friends...were, like me, subjected to these insane pressures. Charges of plagiarism, especially against Robin, were fierce. But at the time it was impossible for me to know what or whom to believe. That was what the radical feminists were doing—eating their leaders, destroying their own best minds.[61]

Gender-critical feminism should not make this mistake. So far, leaders have emerged naturally from grassroots activism, but there has not been a complete absence of trashing. Insofar as this is motivated by an incorrect perception that any leadership is domination, it should not be any part of gender-critical feminism. (Neither should trashing more generally, but that's another story.)

A final important procedural commitment is the welcoming of constructive criticism and disagreement. Christina Hoff Sommers' book *Who Stole Feminism*? is a ruthless fact-checking and debunking of data frequently cited by feminists, on the silencing of women in the classroom, domestic violence, and rape, among other hot-button feminist issues. If we are to retain credibility we must respond to critics not as villains, but as people interested in what the truth of the matter is, so that they or others can make informed decisions about where to put their energies. If Sommers is right, for instance, that campus rape-prevention activism is a privileged people's hobby, then perhaps we'll want to pour our feminist attention into other areas.[62] This kind of evidence-responsiveness will help prevent gender-critical feminism from becoming ideological in the pejorative sense; it cares about women's sex-based rights and interests because they are necessary for women's liberation. If it could be established that women weren't oppressed, or women were in fact already liberated, or women had no distinctive sex-based interests, then there would be no need for gender-critical feminism. These questions have to be settled by evidence, not assumed to be settled in advance as though tenets of faith.

All of this means that as gender-critical feminists, we should make a conscious decision to seek out, engage with, and respond to criticism, whether from anti-feminists, feminist-agnostics, or feminists of other types. We shouldn't dismiss anyone who disagrees with us as acting in bad faith; we should try to get comfortable with respecting and even admiring each other *despite* our disagreements, rather than only when there is agreement. As Jane Clare Jones puts it, gender-critical feminists can and do disagree with each other, because 'we're not a frickin cult'.[63] Back in 1859, John Stuart Mill celebrated dissent as creating value at the social level by making truth more likely to emerge. Some on the left have lost sight of this contribution today, and tend to treat critics of social justice movements as morally abhorrent people who need to be shut down as quickly as possible. Gender-critical feminists can set a (re)new(ed) precedent, celebrating its apostates and heretics rather than trying to cancel them.

3.6 Paradigm Issues

As we saw in Chapter 2, the radical feminists were concerned with an impressive breadth of issues. But perhaps paradigmatic among them was their concern with prostitution and pornography, which they saw as seriously harming the women directly involved, and as degrading to all women. (Before the third wave, there was more widespread agreement among feminists of all types about the harms of prostitution and pornography.) There's a widespread perception that gender-critical feminism is 'about' opposition to trans rights, which is inaccurate, but somewhat understandable given the amount of space the trans issue is taking up inside gender-critical feminism at the current moment. A way to gain more insight into each, then, is to consider in more detail these two paradigm issues. This will also help to make clearer the continuities between the two, and to establish the claim that gender-critical feminism is concerned about gender identity ideology *because* it is concerned with women as a sex class/caste, and the ongoing fight for women's liberation. It will also help to bring back into focus one of the huge issues waiting for gender-critical feminists' attention when the fight against gender identity ideology is exhausted. Rather than simply survey existing views on these topics, I will take these topics up afresh, from the perspective of a feminism committed to sex class/caste. In Chapter 4, I'll talk about the challenges to women's liberation posed by the sex industry (combining prostitution and pornography), and in Chapter 5, I'll talk about the challenges to women's liberation posed by contemporary gender identity ideology and its accompanying activism.

4
The Sex Industry

> It is his false consciousness that is the basis of all prostitution because he shuts his eyes to what he knows to be true: that she does not desire him or even like him.
>
> (Kajsa Ekis Ekman, *Being and Being Bought*)[1]

There is vitriolic disagreement between feminists of different types about the sex industry. Feminist activists on either side of this disagreement tend to pay selective attention to particular figures within it. Those in favour of the industry often rely on the figure of the empowered student who chooses sex work as a way to put herself through college. Those against the industry often rely on the figure of the 'exited woman', a woman who has left prostitution, and carries a litany of abuses. Despite these different narratives, it is clear that *both* types of women exist, and they experience the sex industry in very different ways. Contrast the following first-personal accounts, for example:

> I had a roommate at the time, um, that was a dancer, and she knew an agent his name was Jim South. He said hey, there's a producer that saw your picture and he'd like you to come do a movie, how would you like to do a movie? And I said, ah, well I've never done a movie before, but sure I could do it, no problem. I went down, and I had braids like Bo Derek at the time and, did my first scene. It was a three-way. I had never even been with a woman, I didn't know what to do with a woman. I had no idea what I was doing. But the minute those lights hit me, I swear that was where I was supposed to be. Everyone said do it, do it, do it. And the more you do the more money you can make dancing on the dance circuit, the more magazines you can do, the more you're exposed, you can, I mean gosh, 'have a sex toy line! Now we want to do an action figure of you!' All of it was just like, cool, yeah, sign me up. I was just having a blast.[2]

Gender-Critical Feminism. Holly Lawford-Smith, Oxford University Press. © Holly Lawford-Smith 2022.
DOI: 10.1093/oso/9780198863885.003.0004

And:

> Drug and alcohol abuse are endemic. We are all used to the stereotype of the heroin addict who enters street prostitution to feed her habit. This happens in prostitution, I've seen it; but what I've seen far more regularly is women developing addictions in prostitution that they never had in the first place, usually to alcohol, valium and other prescription sedatives, and to cocaine. These substances are used to numb the simple awfulness of having sexual intercourse with reams of sexually repulsive strangers, all of whom are abusive on some level, whether they know it or not, and many of whom are deliberately so. These substances offer an effective release and escape.[3]

The first comes from a porn actress known simply as 'Houston', who is best known for the 1999 pornographic film *The World's Biggest Gangbang 3: The Houston 620*, in which she broke the world record at the time for the greatest number of sexual partners in a single day (apparently 620 in under eight hours).[4] Interviewed in the Netflix documentary *After Porn Ends*, Houston's narrative is one of enthusiasm and ambition; glad of opportunities and active in expanding her own career. We can try to tell stories about how women like this are brainwashed by the patriarchy but such an explanation sits uneasily: there doesn't seem to have been an obvious 'patriarch' on the scene exercising undue influence at the time, and if it's *the patriarchy* more broadly, why is Houston enthusiastically pursuing the idea of having sex with 620 men in a single day, while other women aren't?

The second comes from Irish woman Rachel Moran, a survivor of prostitution who is now an anti-prostitution advocate, who tells her story in her 2013 book *Paid For*. Moran became homeless as a teenager after having problems at home, entered street prostitution and then later brothel and escort prostitution, working across all three areas (which, she says, is unusual). She describes how she felt about prostitution and how she and the other women felt about the men who paid for them. Contrary to popular narratives about indoor sex work being better, Moran comments that of all the men she met for paid sex, some of the most brutal and contemptuous men were at high-end hotels.

These two women's perspectives couldn't be more different, and the difference is not only whether or not there's a camera on the scene while the sex is happening. Women enter the sex industry for very different reasons; some become trapped in it and cannot leave while others actively choose to remain; some can exercise control over where and how they work, and which clients they take, and others can't (or cannot to any significant degree); some are protected from abuse and can make use of formal systems when they are subject to crime while others can't; some have many other options, while others have none. These are the real differences that make a difference to women's experiences in the sex industry. And they create the possibility of feminists talking past each other, because they're paying selective attention to women with very different experiences of the sex industry.

Phyllis Chesler describes the debate over pornography during the second wave of feminism as 'diverse and highly charged'.[5] She distinguishes five factions. The first were concerned about state censorship and eager to avoid a repeat of history where women's sexuality was under the control of men. The second were concerned about the battered wives and the women who were victims of child abuse being used in pornography. The third were focused on the positive possibilities of pornography, in leading to arousal or enjoyment that might not otherwise have been had. The fourth thought pornography could be educational, and might reduce rape.[6] And the fifth maintained that pornography caused men to see women as sex objects and led to the degradation of all women.[7] The first, second, and fifth concerns apply equally to prostitution.

There is something that these factions have in common with each other, though, namely that some (the first, third, and fourth) are concerned with the positive potential of pornography, while others (the second and fifth) are concerned with its negative actualities. In discussing this subject of disagreement among feminists, Jessica Joy Cameron argues that we should think not only about the content of a theory or position but about its *affect*. How do these theories make the women who hold them feel about themselves? She argues that quite aside from what Andrea Dworkin, for example, might have gotten right in her characterization of heterosexual sex, women don't want to see themselves as passive objects that become property through being fucked by men; don't want to think of themselves as participating in their own oppression when they enjoy heterosexual sex. Cameron says 'false consciousness arguments'—*you think you're enjoying this but really you've just internalized a patriarchal view of what women are for*—'are condescending and infantilizing'.[8]

The view of pornography (and prostitution) that focuses on its transformative and educative potential involves more positive affect: it lets women feel like 'active social agents capable of making informed, self-affirming decisions'.[9] Feminists with this view can work on making pornography better. This might mean featuring more diversity in who has sex and how they have it, or broadening out what 'sex' means from penetrative, penis-in-vagina intercourse to all forms of sexual pleasure-giving and -receiving, including self-administered.[10] It might mean featuring more content that is explicitly educative, teaching men how to give women pleasure—something that is sadly lacking in heterosexual sex, with a recent study in *Archives of Sexual Behaviour* reporting that while 95 per cent of heterosexual men said they orgasmed during sexual intimacy, only 65 per cent of heterosexual women could say the same.[11] It might mean creating porn in a way that is palatable to women who for religious, cultural, or other reasons have been sexually repressed and are under-informed about the capacities of their own bodies.

But a point Phyllis Chesler makes about the *hijab* (in the context of a Women's March in the United States) provides a helpful analogy here:

> As to the hijab: I know too much about girls and women who are beaten, even murdered by their families for refusing to cover their head, face, and body properly; thus, I view veiling as the sign and symbol of women's subordination. The sight of American women virtue-signalling by donning headscarves or hijab (a symbol of oppression) as if it were a gesture of solidarity with freedom fighters and opposition to alleged Islamophobia was both alarming and Orwellian. Confusing conformity with resistance is unwise.[12]

We can make the same point about a feminism that supports prostitution and pornography by maintaining that 'sex work is work!'.[13] We might say that we know too much about the girls and women who suffer childhood sexual abuse, domestic violence, drug and alcohol addiction, and severe poverty who end up being exploited in prostitution or pornography.[14] And we might say that we have come to view the sex industry as the sign and symbol of women's subordination. That is compatible with there being women who freely choose it, just as there are undoubtedly women who freely choose the *hijab*. Feminists holding placards proclaiming that 'sex work is work!' at marches and demonstrations, who have themselves never been involved in sex work and did not experience the conditions that make women and girls vulnerable to sexual exploitation, are doing the equivalent of what the American feminists wearing headscarves at the Women's March were doing. They're attempting to virtue-signal. But signalling support for a global industry that involves the trafficking and brutalization of women is not virtuous.

4.1 Self-Ownership as a Red Herring

In the context of discussing surrogacy,[15] Chesler makes the following comment: 'I knew that many feminists supported surrogacy for another reason too: They believed that women own their bodies and therefore have the right to an abortion, the right to sell sex, the right to rent out their wombs, and the right to sell the fruit of their womb's labour'.[16] This is the philosophical conception of self-ownership, which says *my body is my property and I can do with it what I like*. Many people have this view. But there is serious opposition to this view, too. Its opponents put forward difficult cases in order to argue that the principle of self-ownership has its limits. Can a person really sell herself into slavery? Can she offer herself up to a cannibal? Can she choose the time and manner of her own death? Or more to the focus of this chapter, can she sell herself into *sexual* slavery? Can she exchange sex, whether on-camera or off-camera, for money or for economic security (or for other material rewards)?

But focusing on what *she* can do with her own body, although it has dominated feminist discussion of prostitution and pornography, is actually a red herring here. When we think about the selling of organs, we don't waste time arguing that desperately poor people have the right, grounded in the principle of self-ownership, to sell off parts of their bodies so that they can pay the rent or buy food or support their families. It can be perfectly rational to make choices like these, and we need attribute no 'false consciousness' to the people who make them. When we focus on the choices of the exploited we deflect from the real issue, which is the actions of the exploiters. Let's keep our attention squarely where it should be: on the question of what people with money and power should be able to buy. We surely think it is morally unacceptable that wealthy people should be able to simply replace their non-working body parts with those of people less fortunate. Most countries make a trade in organs illegal for precisely this reason.

There are obviously differences between a trade in organs and a trade in sexual access to women's bodies, not least in that there is a much more limited possible supply of organs. But they have in common that the more important question is about what (privileged) people should be able to *buy*, rather than what (marginalized) people should be able to sell. One of the great tricks of the pro-prostitution activists is that they have managed to keep men almost entirely out of the question.[17] But men are crucial to the question. Exited woman Michelle Mara, in an interview with radical feminist journalist Meghan Murphy about decriminalization in New Zealand, says the following about the men who buy women:

> It's not like you see warning signs in one in a hundred men, you see it in every second dude. It's not like these are just, you know, nice guys on a day out. They are men who do not respect women. They are men who obviously don't respect their partners, because they're out there cheating. They are men who want to experience what it's like to do certain things they can't do with 'normal' women. They…the reason they're there is because they can't get access to whatever they want to have access to without paying for it.[18]

The moral question here is, what are the moral limits to what people may do with other people's bodies, even when the other person consents to it being done? Some people think there is no such limit, that consent is everything. Others think there are many such limits. Courts have found a number of actions impermissible in spite of consent, notably cannibalism.[19] One of the current preoccupations of feminists is whether men may choke women during sex, a question that has arisen given the increasing numbers of women dying during sex, with their male partners alleging 'sex games gone wrong'.[20] Radical and gender-critical feminists say that he should not be inflicting this kind of violence on her during sex, no matter what. Intimate partner strangulation is now a distinct offence in New Zealand, having been found to be one of the most lethal types of domestic violence.[21]

Is the sexual use of another person's body the kind of thing that is appropriately commodified for exchange in a market? Is it morally permissible for men to buy sexual access to a woman, as in prostitution; or to pay[22] to watch other men rape, brutalize, or use women's bodies, as in pornography? Money changes incentives, and so its involvement can lead to coercion or exploitation. One way to safeguard against this outcome is to rule money out of the picture.

Our answer to the moral question (and whether taking these industries off the market would be a good way to support that answer) does not necessarily settle the policy question. Public policy is a matter of the public good, which means we need to think carefully about the balance of benefits and harms. It might be that alcohol does so much harm that it should not be available on the market, but that people are so adamant about drinking that any attempt to take it off the market will fail and just bring about more harm (as attempts at prohibition demonstrated).[23] If we end up being anti pornography and prostitution because we're anti harm to women, then it would be rather absurd to endorse a policy that will ultimately bring about *more* harm to women. So once we've considered the moral question and its implication for whether sexual use is appropriately commodified, we need to consider the policy options and their likely harms independently. This is in line with the procedural commitment outlined in Section 3.5, that gender-critical feminism prioritizes empirical evidence over ideology.

4.2 What We Cannot Buy

In this section, I'll draw on three different discussions where there is controversy about what people should be able to buy. The first is persons and parts of persons. I'll talk about both slavery and the buying of other people's organs. The second is entertainment in the form of sports that involve a high risk of physical injury to their players. I'll focus on boxing and draw a parallel between boxing, on the one hand, and prostitution and pornography, on the other. The third is access to competitive goods where there is an issue of merit. I'll focus on admissions to prestigious universities. Together, these parallels establish a strong case against men being able to buy the sexual use of women's bodies. I'll cement this case in the following section, where I survey the harms to women in the sex industry.

Persons and person-parts. Slavery was wrong for many reasons, but a fundamental reason was that it involved the buying and selling of persons. Alastair Campbell argues that for something to be *appropriately* treated as a commodity, it must meet three conditions. This is an evaluative rather than a descriptive claim, which means we can acknowledge that something *is* in fact commodified while asserting that it *should not be*, that it is inappropriate to commodify it. The three conditions are 'alienability', 'fungibility', and 'commensurability'. An object is alienable when I have the right to 'alienate' (i.e. separate) myself from it, to 'sell, mortgage, lease, give away or destroy' it. It is fungible when it is interchangeable with other objects of the same type. And an object is commensurable when it can be valued on a common scale with other goods, where that common scale is usually money. (Things are incommensurable when there is no common scale, for example in trying to 'rank' a beautiful sunset against a delicious meal.) When an object meets all of these conditions then it is a commodity, which means it is appropriate to think of it as having market value.[24]

Campbell considers the case of a 'desperate father selling himself into slavery in order to raise enough money to feed his family', to test the idea of persons as commodities, and says 'a human person is not an alienable object, which is fungible...and commensurable with a monetary sum'.[25] (He seems to be imagining a one-time payment for being sold *into* slavery.) In its most violent and degrading form, slavery involved the kidnapping of people from their home countries, their transport to other countries, and their forced labour for the profit of a slave-owner. Adding a pay cheque to these violations—whether before they commence or as they unfold—does not miraculously transform their status. Even if the labour the slave is forced to undertake is labour that he might have been prepared to undertake for fair remuneration in another context, the fact that he did not have that choice means we cannot treat the one case as the other.

But this has all the same features as human trafficking into sexual exploitation.[26] The woman is kidnapped, transported across state or country borders, and forced to work in prostitution and/or pornography. Generally she is not paid. But even when she is, that doesn't transform her situation into 'work'. If it is not permissible for the desperate father to sell himself into slavery, because this turns a human person into a commodity, then it is not permissible for the desperate mother (and any other woman) to sell herself into prostitution, because in exactly the same way, this turns a human person into a commodity. *Persons* are not things that anyone should be able to buy.

Campbell then asks, what if we're not talking about whole persons, but only body *parts*? Some such parts are alienable: I can choose to separate myself (with a little help from a surgeon) from my kidney, liver, pancreas, heart, and lung.[27] He thinks this doesn't help, because the parts of the body make up the whole body, and the body is fundamental to personhood. Still, he explains, those who think of personhood primarily in terms of the mind—reason and rationality—might not be particularly moved by this. If the person *really is* just the thoughts, or the thoughts are *more important than* the body, then why should we be particularly bothered about what happens to the body? For people who are inclined towards this view (in Chapter 3 we saw that Alison Jaggar called it 'normative dualism'), Campbell offers a second argument, this time based in opposition to exploitation.

This argument runs by way of considering the likely impacts of a legalized market in organs. Sellers are likely to be socially and economically vulnerable people. In Iran, 'the market has resulted in widespread pleading by the poor to have their organs purchased'.[28] And this exploitation cannot even be given a consequentialist defence in terms of making more organs available and thus saving more lives: research has found that when there is a market in organs family members are less likely to donate and people are less willing to donate after death.[29] Instead of trying to solve the problem of demand for organs with legalized markets that commodify persons and exploit the poor, we might make public health interventions to reduce the *need* for organ transplants, or initiate campaigns to increase the rate of organ donations after death.

The exploitation argument is equally applicable to prostitution, which will become clearer in the next section, where we talk about who and what men are actually buying. It is not wealthy women with stable family backgrounds, generally, who are working as prostitutes. As Moran put it, women enter street prostitution because they are *destitute*, and escort or brothel prostitution because they are *desperate*.[30] So when men are enabled to buy access to women's bodies, it is the worst-off women who will end up being bought.

Human persons are not the kinds of things that should be bought and sold. Intimate access to one's body is not 'alienable', one's body cannot be parted with. There is no separation of body and self; the body and the self are one.[31] Intimate access to one's body is not 'fungible', either, because it *does* come with a loss to the 'owner'/person (these losses are catalogued in more detail in Section 4.3). And intimate access should not be commensurable, despite a long history of its being treated as such. Just as wealthy people who drink too much and ruin their livers shouldn't be empowered to simply purchase the livers of the world's poor, so too the sexually entitled men who treat women in a way that leaves few or any willing to have sex with them shouldn't be empowered to simply purchase the use of a woman's body to masturbate with.[32] (I think the same is true, in both cases, for people who are not responsible for the fact of their need/want).[33] The moral costs of commodification and exploitation are too high.

Entertainment with high risk of physical injury. Should sports fans be able to pay to attend live boxing matches, or for subscriptions to watch televised matches? We can argue that they shouldn't, *because of* the physical harm to, and exploitation of, the boxers themselves. Boxing involves blows to the head, and blows to the head cause chronic brain damage. Studies from the 1980s found that 64–87 per cent of then-current and former boxers had measurable brain damage. Boxing can also result in cuts, fractures, and eye damage. The American Medical Association proposed in 1984 that boxing be banned.[34]

Precisely because professional boxing involves taking these risks in order to acquire wealth, Nicholas Dixon focuses on the moral case against professional boxing (rather than including amateur, and therefore all, boxing). Many if not most boxers will be under-informed about the risks and long-term health impacts of the profession; their managers have an interest in not informing them. Boxers often come from disadvantaged backgrounds,[35] such that the sport may represent 'their only means of escaping from dangerous, poverty-stricken neighbourhoods'.[36] If boxers were mainly in it for the love of boxing, we'd expect to see more representative demographics, whereas in fact most boxers come from poor backgrounds. For many boxers, then, boxing is exploitative.[37]

But all of this is true for prostitution. It comes with high risk of physical harm (rape, sexual assault, physical assault) and long-term health impacts including disassociation and post-traumatic stress disorder (PTSD). Many prostituted women are likely to be under-informed about the risks or are too desperate to be able to afford to care about them. They are very often from disadvantaged backgrounds (having experienced e.g. homelessness, child abuse, or domestic abuse). Most prostituted women don't independently desire to have sex with either the punters (in the case of prostitution) or their on-screen partners (in the case of pornography). 'Sex work' is coercive. Even sex worker rights activists Juno Mac and Molly Smith[38] do not seem to disagree with this: they say repeatedly in their book *Revolting Prostitutes* that sex work is a survival strategy which allows women to secure resources.[39]

Paying to watch a boxing match is a better parallel to paying to watch pornography than it is to paying for the sexual use of a prostitute. In both boxing and pornography, the 'entertainment' involves another person being physically and/or psychologically harmed. In prostitution, it is more like a boxing fan paying to get in the ring and punch the other guy, while the other guy has to put up just enough of a resistance to make the consumer feel like he's genuinely won the match. The 'entertainment' is actually doing physical and/or psychological harm to another person. While many consumer industries involve risks of harm (e.g. workplace injuries) few involve injury as so central a part of what is being consumed.

Dixon ultimately defends a compromise solution: rather than a complete ban on professional boxing, 'a complete ban on blows to the head'.[40] This leaves the sport largely intact while taking out the worst of its physical harms. But if it's the constant sexual use by men that leads to drug addiction,[41] disassociation, and PTSD[42] in prostituted women, then there's no way to ban the worst of the physical harms of prostitution without also banning prostitution. Sexual use is not an aspect of prostitution that can be removed, leaving the rest of the practice intact. It *is* the practice. This is an argument for banning it.

Distortions of meritocracy. At first glance, it might seem that the question of buying admission to university (usually a parent buying a place for their child) has little to do with prostitution and pornography. After all, this isn't a question of generally desperate people selling something that is either a part of their body or at least the use of their body for a period. It's not bodily at all. When it comes to buying university admission, the controversy is usually around the use of wealth and power to secure something that is *unearned* or *undeserved.* Robert Goodin and Christian Barry, for example, discuss the moral issue of benefiting from others' wrongdoing using the running case of a person who discovers later in life that his father bribed a Harvard official in order to secure his (the son's) admission. They write 'it was…wrong that you were admitted to Harvard (your test scores just didn't merit admission)'.[43] They argue that because the first person's Harvard education benefited them, at a cost to a second person whose deserved place was lost, the first person is morally obliged to disgorge the benefits. This means something like, attempt to quantify the benefits in monetary terms and then pay this in compensation to the person whose place was taken.

This is actually a surprisingly helpful way to think about men buying sex from women. As Michelle Mara said of men who use prostitutes, 'they can't get access to whatever they want to have access to without paying for it'.[44] Sex, like admission to a university, should be the kind of good that a person gets access to for reasons that have nothing to do with money. Universities have entry requirements that must be met, and prestigious universities offer limited places to exceptionally well-qualified individuals. If you do not earn your place, you should not have a place.[45] Similarly, women have individual tastes and preferences and boundaries and desires, all of which determine who she will be interested to have sex with and what kind of sex she wants to have. It might be with a long-term partner who she is in a loving and committed relationship with, and it might be with an attractive stranger who she thinks is a good prospect for a mutually enjoyable one-night stand. While women do in fact tolerate large quantities of bad sex with men,[46] few if any would actively seek it out.

If a man is to have sex with a woman, it should be because a woman desires him; not because he wants access to a woman's desire, cannot get it, and so bribes her for it. Sex should be mutually desired and mutually beneficial. But the idea that a woman's pleasure has any role to play in prostitution or mainstream pornography is unrealistic. The reporter on the *World's Biggest Gangbang III* filming talks about one of the 'few men'—in this case man number 407 out of 620—who goes down on Houston during the gangbang.[47] He comments, 'Houston does not come once during the day'.[48] It seems the event has nothing to do with her pleasure and the men involved all found that unremarkable. In fact, it was the man who thought it *did* have something to do with her pleasure that attracted attention.

When wealthy parents in the United States—including celebrities and CEOs—were discovered to have been buying university admissions for their children, they were charged and many will spend time in prison.[49] This sends a strong signal that those with wealth and power are not beyond the law; the same rules that apply to everyone else apply to them. If they want their children to go to university, they had better teach those children to work hard enough to earn a place. What they cannot earn on their own merits, they should not have. So too for sex. Socialization into masculinity inculcates the belief that women owe men service, sexual and otherwise.[50] But women are not *for men*. Women are not *for* anything. What he cannot earn on his own merits, he should not have. If he is not funny, or charming, or likeable, or intelligent, or interesting, or fit, or handsome, then he will have to limit his sexual pleasure to what he can provide himself. The sooner that men reconceptualize sexual pleasure and sexual access in this way,[51] the better for women.[52]

Noxious markets. In her book *Why Some Things Should Not Be For Sale*, Debra Satz provides a way to unify some of the considerations above, by offering a set of parameters for when a market is 'noxious' and therefore a candidate for being banned or constrained. The parameters are *harmful outcomes for individuals, harmful outcomes for* society—particularly where the market 'undermine[s] the social framework needed for people to interact *as equals*', *weak/asymmetric knowledge/agency*, and *extreme vulnerability*. Selling person-parts involves all four parameters—it is one of the clearest cases of a noxious market.[53] Boxing involves harmful outcomes for individuals (the boxers), and to the extent that boxers are drawn from a marginalized social group, for society. It also involves asymmetric knowledge. Buying university admissions involves harmful outcomes for society.

In her chapter 'Markets in Women's Sexual Labour', Satz addresses prostitution specifically, saying that it counts as a noxious market in virtue of the social harm it causes. Against a backdrop of sex inequality, prostitution sustains the social subordination of women and in doing so harms women as a class. It has effects on how men perceive all women, and how women perceive themselves. She says 'prostitution is a theatre of inequality'.[54] This is an interesting argument because it takes social structures seriously (on which, more in Chapter 9), but does not require any claim about the buying/selling of sex being *intrinsically* wrong. There could be some possible, sex-equal future, where buying/selling sex did not harm women as a class, and did not meet any of the other parameters, so did not count as a noxious market.

4.3 Who and What Are Men Buying?

Many people think it's morally impermissible to buy factory farmed meat, because of the suffering the animals experience. Many people think it's morally impermissible to leave greenhouse gas emissions unchecked, because of the suffering people in low-lying countries and poor countries experience, and future people will experience. Many people worry about sweatshops and blood diamonds and conflict minerals and unfair trade, for all the same reasons. In this section, I want to show that consuming the products of the sex industry is unethical consumption par excellence, and belongs in the same category as these other, more familiar, cases. At the start of the chapter, I said it's clear that the types of women held up by different groups of feminists, in the first case to defend the sex industry and in the second case to argue against it, both exist. In this section, I will show that nonetheless, the type of women the radical and gender-critical feminists are worried about are the large majority of all women used in the industry.

Let's start with prostitution alone (prostitution without filming). In the European Parliament's 2014 report 'Sexual Exploitation and Prostitution and Its Impact on Gender Equality', authors Erika Schulze, Sandra Isabel Novo Canto, Peter Mason, and Maria Skalin lament the lack of reliable data on prostitution and sexual exploitation. They say 'There is no clear picture of the number of prostitutes and their clients, and their revenue and profits (including for the pimps)'.[55] This means policy-makers are forced to rely on estimations. They note that qualitative social research on the selling of sex is often biased, towards either the regulatory or the abolitionist approach (on which more soon). They quote one of the researchers they take to be an exception to this bias, saying 'the knowledge base for evidence-based policies on prostitution is weak'.[56] They comment that the abolitionist data unhelpfully blurs the distinctions between 'women selling sex and women [who are] sexually exploited'.[57] They seem to have in mind the difference between a woman selling sex consensually who is subject to violence at the hands of clients, and a woman who is trafficked or pimped[58]—although they do include earlier in the report that there are issues with whether any consent to prostitution can be authentic.[59] Finally, they recognize that the evidence on men buying women is also scarce, and relies on estimations, which range from 'few' to 'one third' of all men.[60]

Prostitution is estimated to involve forty to forty-two million people globally, 75 per cent of whom are between 13 and 25 years old, and 90 per cent of whom depend on third parties (pimps and madams).[61] On the most conservative estimate, roughly 14 per cent of prostitutes being sold in Europe are trafficked; on the estimates of some European Community countries between 60 and 90 per cent of the prostitutes being sold in their countries are trafficked. Most trafficking is for sexual exploitation.[62] The United Nations' 'Global Report on Trafficking in Persons' gathered data from 155 countries, finding that 79 per cent of human trafficking was for the purpose of sexual exploitation, and that the predominant victims of sexual exploitation were women and girls. Based on aggregated data from 2006, 66 per cent of trafficking victims were women and 13 per cent were girls. Other purposes of trafficking included exploitation as domestic servants and wives.[63]

A Dutch study published in 2000 reported 79 per cent of the women in their study being in prostitution by force.[64] An interview-based study of 854 people (mostly women) in prostitution across nine countries found that 65–95 per cent were sexually assaulted as children; that 70–95 per cent were physically assaulted in prostitution; that 60–75 per cent were raped in prostitution; that 75 per cent of those in prostitution had been homeless at some point; that 89 per cent of 785 people interviewed wanted to escape prostitution; that 68 per cent of 827 people interviewed had severe symptoms of PTSD; and that 88 per cent experienced verbal abuse.[65]

Things will be different in each country, and in some cases in each state of each country. But we can learn something about the commonalities by considering some specific cases.

Eaves Housing for Women, a London-based charity focused on violence against women which closed in 2015, attempted the ambitious project of mapping the sex industry across London in the second half of 2003. Their key findings were that between 2,972 and 5,861 women were selling sex from 'flats, parlours and saunas' in London, and between 1,755 and 2,221 women were selling sex as escorts in London; that only 19 per cent of the former women were from the United Kingdom (they found 25 per cent were Eastern European; 13 per cent South East Asian; 12 per cent Western European; and smaller numbers of people from other regions),[66] and only 20 per cent of the latter women were from the United Kingdom (33 per cent were Eastern European, 13 per cent South East Asian, 12 per cent Western European, and there were smaller numbers of people from other regions).[67]

A detailed study of street-based sex workers conducted through a series of interviews in the British city of Stoke-on-Trent in 2007–8 found that drug dependency was the primary reason why women in that cohort entered street-based sex work, and that other reasons included being coerced by pimps, and needing money to pay off debts, or to pay for rent or food. Homelessness was a pathway into prostitution, with most women homeless at the time that they started selling sex (this was Moran's pathway: running away from an abusive home as a teenager, becoming homeless, and eventually turning to prostitution).[68] Debt, whether drug debts, missed rent payments, or police fines, kept women in prostitution even after they managed to kick their drug habits. Violence and rape at the hands of punters was routine.[69] The researchers in this study also found that the key triggers of homelessness were leaving home as a result of sexual abuse, physical abuse, neglect, and other problems/conflicts; domestic abuse by a partner; leaving state care and not maintaining contact with social services; and the impacts of traumatic experiences.[70] Fifty-seven per cent of their cohort were homeless by age 16, and some left home when they were as young as 10 years old.[71] These women were 'a very vulnerable population with significant and extensive welfare and support needs', almost all of whom had a criminal record and most of whom had been in prison, most of whom had drug dependencies, and most of whom had experienced domestic violence.[72]

In Australia, the Prostitutes Collective of Victoria in 1990 received up to fifteen reports a week of rape and violence against prostitutes.[73] Research undertaken in Victoria with twenty-three women in 1996 found that *all* had been raped, bashed, or robbed by a punter and *all* had been forced to have sex without a condom.[74] A study run by the group Child Wise in 2002 found there to be 1,205 children under 18 working as child prostitutes in Victoria.[75] Research from 1994 found that of the street-based prostitutes in St. Kilda in 1994, 80 per cent were drug addicted, 70 per cent were homeless, 25 per cent had a psychiatric disability, 20 per cent were addicted to alcohol, and 10 per cent had an intellectual disability.[76]

So, who or what are men buying? There are no definitive statistics on the ratio of women who are trafficked compared to women who entered prostitution in another way, or the ratio of women whose reasons for entering and staying in prostitution severely compromise the validity of their 'consent' to sell their bodies compared to the women who can genuinely be said to consent. But we have enough information to know that the odds of any given man encountering a non-exploited and genuinely consenting woman when he goes to buy sex are very poor. In fact, the website punternet.com includes reviews of prostitutes' services written by punters, and 'frequently refers to men buying sex with women who are clearly unhappy, unwilling, frightened and/or in pain.'[77] The chances are that what the man is buying is sexual access to someone who has been trafficked, and/or who is from an abusive background (whether at the hands of her family or her intimate partner), and/or who is or has been homeless and desperate, and/or who is addicted to drugs or alcohol. These are women who are in a precarious social and economic position and who generally have no other way of meeting their basic needs.

This is not to say that there are *no* women working as prostitutes who have a range of decent options and nonetheless choose prostitution. There surely are a few. But we can hardly justify the existence of a huge global industry absolutely full of female suffering by holding up a few happy 'workers' and pretending that the *literally millions* of other women don't exist. There might be someone in the world who would be enthusiastic about selling a kidney for a decent price rather than working the hours it would take to earn the equivalent sum. He has two; he'll probably get by just fine with one; and he quite likes the idea that one of his organs might be used to save a life. (Not quite enough to donate it, though.) We don't hold this man up as our sole argument for establishing a legal trade in organs. We think that the actual and likely harms to the global poor outweigh whatever weak reasons this man's mere preference might have given us.

Is it the same story for pornography? There are more possible defences here: some pornography *is* focused on the woman's pleasure, and so is reciprocal and mutually pleasurable in a way that makes it more like sex should be (although the *vast*, vast majority is not like this). But again, we should not let these rare exceptions obscure what the great majority of women inside the industry are actually experiencing.

A 2015 documentary *Hot Girls Wanted* follows 18–25-year-old women in America, working in the porn industry. The film explains the huge demand for 'amateur' pornography with young girls. It tells the story from the girls' perspective, their hopes for making big money, having fun, and becoming famous. One of the most disturbing parts of the documentary is its study of 'forced blowjobs', which involve men grabbing women roughly by the heads, and fucking them in the throat until they vomit. This is male violence against women and girls. Some porn apologists will try to say that some women like to be dominated, and this is something that the women being filmed might find a turn-on. But this claim is quickly dispelled when the two women involved in such scenes talk about them. One says 'the physical part it's just…' (someone off-camera suggests 'temporary') '…yeah. I'm here to put on a show, I'm not here to be comfortable. I come and put on a show and make myself uncomfortable, so you can get off so I can get paid and be comfortable on my own time'[78]. Another woman talks about being flown in to film a blowjob scene, and only being told after arriving that it would be forced. These are not women who are *enjoying* what they're doing, they're women who are *willing* to do it for other reasons, not least to get paid.

It's also important to note that porn is addictive.[79] In order to keep receiving the 'hit' of arousal, novelty is required, which means new girls, and new things being done to them. This demand for 'innovation' in porn has driven producers to ever more violent and degrading extremes (the forced blowjobs mentioned already are one example—in a scene featuring the woman quoted above, after she has thrown up, a man off camera can be heard directing her to 'lick it up'; another example mentioned in the Netflix series *Hot Girls Wanted: Turned On* is pushing a girl's head into a toilet bowl and flushing it while fucking her from behind (episode 1). This stuff is brutal. Women and girls are being treated in ever more creative degrading and demeaning ways, in order to satisfy *men's* constantly ratcheting-up sexual demands.

In summary, the men who buy the use of women's bodies (or who watch other men having access to women's bodies that others have paid for the use of), are using (watching the use of) women who are much more likely than not to have been trafficked, abused, homeless, destitute, and/or drug-addicted, and to be suffering from severe PTSD. Even those who entered prostitution or pornography as the result of an apparently free choice are likely to have been coerced into doing things that they are not comfortable with. There is so much harm in the sex industry and so little good that considering the industry in isolation seems to give us sufficient reason to shut it down.

Still; the argument is not won simply by cataloguing the harms of the sex industry, either globally or within a particular country. A further question has to be asked: what is the expected harm reduction—and what are the independent harms likely to be caused by—the policy models we might use to address these identified harms of the sex industry? There's no point ending one lot of harms by replacing them with another, or attempting to end one lot of harms with a proposal that in fact just ends up making them worse. So we have to think carefully about what's being proposed and whether it works. That is the focus of the next (and final) section.

4.4 Policy Models

It is common for feminists to distinguish three policy models: legalization, decriminalization, and the Nordic Model. Many feminists today tend to support decriminalization[80] while radical and gender-critical feminists tend to support the Nordic Model.[81]

In *Revolting Prostitutes*, Mac & Smith argue that this typology misses important distinctions.[82] They survey five policy alternatives instead, all implemented in different parts of the world: partial criminalization, full criminalization, asymmetrical criminalization (also known as the Nordic Model), legalization, and decriminalization. These are basically what they sound like.

- *Partial criminalization*: criminalizes some aspects of prostitution and not others, as in England, Scotland, and Wales where it is legal to buy and sell sex, but illegal to solicit clients, facilitate the buying/selling of sex, or work indoors with others selling sex.
- *Full criminalization*: criminalizes all aspects of prostitution, including all parties involved in it (e.g. sex workers, managers, landlords, advertisers), as in the United States, South Africa, Russia, and China.
- *Asymmetrical criminalization*: (the Nordic Model) criminalizes the buyers of sex, but not the sellers, aiming to eliminate demand. This is the model in Sweden, Norway, Iceland, France, and Canada.
- *Legalization*: makes all aspects of the sex industry legal, but usually comes hand in hand with regulations like mandatory health checks or registration as a sex worker (perhaps for this reason, Mac & Smith refer to it as 'Regulationism' instead). This model is in place in Germany and the Netherlands.
- *Decriminalization*: shifts sex work entirely out of the criminal law and makes regulation a matter of labour law. It has in common with legalization that involvement in the sex trade is no longer criminal, but it tends to avoid the bureaucracy that comes along with legalization in

> the countries that have implemented it. This is the policy model in New Zealand.[83]

Mac & Smith—both themselves sex workers, and to all appearances both extremely well-informed about, and well-networked into, sex worker collectives and communities around the world—defend a clear ordering of these policy models from worst to best. Criminalization (full, partial, or asymmetric) is the worst, driving sex workers into increasingly unsafe and risky practices, empowering police and officials to do further harm to already extremely marginalized communities (e.g. confiscation of earnings as the 'proceeds of crime', eviction, deportation), and making it even harder for desperate people to meet their basic needs. Legalization is better, but still bad for all the women who can't or won't meet the bureaucratic requirements, who are then still criminalized. Decriminalization is by far the best, because it gives sex workers labour rights, it makes them safer, it removes the power of police to interfere, and it increases workers' bargaining power with managers and negotiating power with clients. (Although the authors are keen to stress that there are still improvements that can be made upon the way decriminalization has been implemented in New Zealand.)

This might be taken to imply that Mac & Smith are *pro* sex work, but that's not entirely obvious. Although they are sex worker rights activists, and critics of the anti-prostitution positions of many radical and gender-critical feminists, they still imagine a future that is largely without sex work:

> To make sex work *unnecessary*, there is much work to do…If everybody had the resources they needed, nobody would need to sell sex…If we are then able to end poverty and borders (and the litany of other ills discussed here), sex work might indeed whither *[sic]* away and effectively be abolished for all but the small number who genuinely love it.[84]

This shows that abolitionism is not synonymous with the Nordic Model; feminists of very different types can hold abolition as an end goal, while disagreeing about the policy pathway we should use to get there.

Mac & Smith make a persuasive case for decriminalization, based on a concern to alleviate the material harms currently experienced by sex workers, but see this as *a way* (together with other policy measures like poverty reduction and reduced border control) to work towards a future in which there is virtually no sex work. There may be some talking past each other between feminists of different types depending on whether they're talking about the ideal end state, or the policy measure we should use to get to it. But the main disagreements between those who side with Mac & Smith and those who side with their radical and gender-critical counterparts seem to be in two areas. First, Mac & Smith focus on mitigating harm to sex workers, rather than on the balance of harms to *all* women.[85] Second, they are more or less fatalistic about women entering prostitution, given socio-economic precariousness (they mention the deterrence effects of alternative policies only a few times in their book, and never with any concrete data). Kajsa Ekis Ekman comments on the 'myth of the sex worker' (prostituted woman as *worker*) that 'There is resignation, cynicism, and an absence of hope for a better world. The best thing that could happen, according to this story, would be if prostitutes were murdered a little less frequently and had somewhat nicer places to work in'.[86] While Mac & Smith do have hope for a better world, they are not unreasonably characterized by Ekman's description of the best thing that could happen anytime soon.

We make a value judgement about *the best* policy pathway by thinking about who is harmed and who is helped, and by weighing up harms, whether the same types of harms (more straightforward) or different types of harms (more difficult). Are we thinking about the *most marginalized* women, and therefore focused on the sex workers themselves, or are we thinking about *all women*, and therefore interested in the impacts of prostitution on women more generally? Are there some lines we will not cross (e.g. no woman can be 'sacrificed' to deportation or a high risk of rape or murder in order to secure fewer women working in prostitution), or is everything thrown into the utility calculation? What do we hold fixed, in terms of thinking about *what human societies are like*? Assumptions of the following kinds are frequent throughout Mac & Smith's book, and largely unacknowledged: that police will always abuse their power; that criminalization will not stop women selling sex but only make it more dangerous for them; that mandatory health testing will not stop infected people working but only drive them away from health facilities; that drug users will not stop using no matter how high the financial and physical price of securing drugs; that migrants will not avoid prostitution just because it is illegal, but rather will just do it under more dangerous conditions; and so on.

Mac & Smith argue that radical feminists have been too concerned with the 'symbolic' aspects of prostitution, to the exclusion of how sex workers are materially impacted by particular policies in the here and now.[87] And indeed, in a review of their book on the Nordic Model Now! webpage, Anna Fisher writes that:

> prostitution works to subordinate women *en masse*... [because it] implicitly positions women and girls as objects for male sexual consumption, rather than as subjects in their own right. This implies that men are human and women are lesser, sub-human, or second class, and it affects how all men see women and how women see themselves. This is strengthened and legitimised whenever prostitution is normalised, for example, by considering it a form of regular work.[88]

We can accept that subordination is harmful while agreeing that it is a harm of a different quality to material impacts. In 1993, feminist philosopher Rae Langton defended the idea that pornography is a 'speech act', combining a judicial decision that pornography is *speech* with Catharine MacKinnon's argument that pornography is an *act*.[89] Since then, it has been common to consider pornography as a speech act, focusing either on its 'locutionary' effects (what that speech *means*), its 'illocutionary' effects (what that speech *does*), or its 'perlocutionary' effects (what that speech or speech act *causes*, downstream). For example, when a woman is depicted as an object to be moved around at will and fucked for the man's pleasure, the scene may *mean* that women are objects for men's sexual gratification. The same scene may *degrade* or *defame* or *oppress* female people. Rosemary Tong, writing in 1982, argued that hardcore pornography was 'harmful to all women to the degree that [it is] meant to degrade and defame females'.[90] And the same scene may *cause* the men watching it to later treat women in real life in sexually demeaning, disrespectful, or harmful ways. The links between the first two categories and the last are difficult to establish. A person who wishes to make a decision about policy based on *material* harms will not be able to do much with the meaning and the doing of pornography. It might be true that pornography does symbolic harm in sustaining the idea that women are sex objects, and true that pornography degrades women, defames women, oppresses women, and yet *not* be true that either of these things cause women material harm. Unless Fisher connects the subordination of women to material outcomes, she is vulnerable to Mac & Smith's objection.

Fisher responds to Mac & Smith by saying that the existence of prostitution does do material—not just symbolic—harm to women, citing research on the correlation between rape, sexual harassment, and violence perpetrated by men against women, and their buying of sex. She points to a study by the United Nations of violent men across six countries which found that men who buy sex were almost eight times more likely to rape than other men, and that buying sex was the second most significant factor that men found guilty of rape had in common.[91] This shows that in order to defend an alternative policy model against Mac & Smith, we don't need to defend merely symbolic harms as outweighing harms like the deportation of migrant women for sharing a flat while selling sex (which in the UK is classed as brothel-keeping).[92] We can compare the whole slew of harms to both women involved in the sex industry and women impacted by the sex industry's existence, to the likely harm-alleviation of decriminalization.

So the question becomes, do prostitution and/or pornography lead to material harms against women? A similar question arose over video games in the mid-2000s: does playing violent video games make players more violent? Controversy arose when it was revealed that Grand Theft Auto let its players

> pick up a hooker, take her out in the woods, have sex with her many times, then let her out of the car. Then you can shoot her, pull over, beat her with a bat, then you can get into the car and run her over. Oh, and don't forget to pick up the money you paid her for sex.[93]

These games clearly have locutionary and illocutionary effects, the question is whether they have perlocutionary—i.e. causal—effects too. Meta-analysis of empirical studies reported on in 2003 found that violent video games were 'significantly associated with' increased aggressive behaviour, and decreased prosocial behaviour (which means, behaviour that involves helping others). Frequent exposure to violent video games has been linked to fighting at school and violent criminal behaviour like assault and robbery.[94]

Is the same true for prostitution and pornography? Are the (heterosexual and bisexual) men who watch porn more likely to subject women to bad sex? Are the men who watch violent porn more likely to be sexually violent with women? Are the men who use prostitutes more likely to violate women's boundaries in sex, to care less about real consent, to be sexually violent? We know that younger and younger people are accessing porn, and that porn has become, for many people, sex education. This surely has negative effects on the sex that is being had. But is there evidence?

Paul Wright and Robert Tokunaga gathered data from college men attracted to women, aiming to test the thesis that 'the more men are exposed to objectifying depictions, the more they will think of women as entities that exist for men's sexual gratification...this dehumanized perspective on women may then be used to inform attitudes regarding sexual violence against women.'[95] They were interested in objectifying media more broadly, including pornography but also reality television and men's magazines. The most important attitudes for our purposes were those 'supportive of violence against women'. They found that, indeed, 'men who viewed women as sex objects had attitudes more supportive of violence against women.'[96] This meant agreeing with statements like 'Being roughed up is sexually stimulating to many women', 'Many times a woman will pretend she doesn't want to have intercourse because she doesn't want to seem loose, but she's really hoping the man will force her', 'Sometimes the only way a man can get a cold woman turned on is to use force', 'When women go around braless or wearing short skirts and tight tops, they are just asking for trouble', and 'A woman who is stuck-up and thinks she is too good to talk to guys on the street deserves to be taught a lesson.'[97]

This does not yet show *actual* violence against women; it is conceivable that men with high exposure to women-objectifying media are more likely to condone other men's violence against women but do not perpetrate it themselves. Given that sexual assault is a crime, it will be a lot harder to get reliable data on the causal connection that matters the most. A meta-analysis of nine studies involving 2,309 participants got a little closer, in that three of the 'attitudes' it covered were about *likelihood* of performing certain acts: likelihood of rape, likelihood of sexual force, and likelihood of sexual harassment. As the researchers explain, these are scales 'used to measure the hypothetical potential of a man to rape or commit similar sexually aggressive acts given the assurance that he would face no punishment.'[98] They found a significant correlation between the consumption of pornography and attitudes supporting violence against women, and further that violent pornography was more likely than non-violent pornography to have this association.[99]

A 2018 study in South Korea looked at the connection between men using prostitutes and men committing sex crimes in order to challenge the common argument that prostitution reduces the incidence of sexual violence against women. Seo-Young Cho looked at a sample of 480 men imprisoned for sex offences, and found that 'buying sex significantly increases the probability that one commits various further forms of sex crimes—sexual assaults in general and forced sex with a stranger or partner',[100] and that 'furthermore, the experience of paying for sex with an underage prostitute exacerbates the severity of sex crimes committed by sex offenders.'[101] (A limitation of the study was that there *could be* a common cause of a person's use of prostitutes and committing of sex crimes.)

Finally, Paul Wright and his colleagues conducted a meta-analysis of twenty-two studies from seven countries to try to answer the hardest question, namely 'Is pornography consumption correlated with committing actual acts of sexual aggression?' They understood physical sexual aggression as the use of threat or physical force, and verbal sexual aggression as verbally coercive but not physically threatening (for example, threatening to break up with your partner unless sexual intercourse is had). The researchers found significant associations between pornography consumption and physical sexual aggression (more so in the case of violent compared to non-violent pornography),[102] but concluded very cautiously, saying only that 'violent content *may* be an exacerbating factor'.[103]

Given all of this, and given what prostituted women say about their experiences even when they are 'high-end',[104] it seems to me highly unlikely that decriminalization is going to emerge as the preferable policy. The industry permits men to buy what no one should be able to buy, the sexual use of women who are highly likely to be extremely vulnerable. It involves serious harm to the women working in it, and that harm is integral to the nature of the work, making reform impossible. And its existence may be contributing to male violence towards women who are not part of the industry, too. Decriminalization focuses too much on harm reduction in the short-term and for a narrow group of women, rather than in the short- *and* long-term and for *all* women.

It is useful at this point to make a distinction between the 'perfect' and the 'good'. The perfect is the thing that is morally desirable in principle. For radical and gender-critical feminists concerned with the trafficking, coercion, exploitation, domination, and abuse of women across the sex industry, and the impacts this industry has on all women (materially and symbolically), what is *perfect* is sex industry abolitionism. Women's liberation is ultimately incompatible with the existence of prostitution, or with pornography in anything like its current form. The buyer is the problem, for his sexual entitlement is what creates demand. The Nordic Model is a policy pathway that responds to this without further harming the women caught up in the sex industry. So the ideological commitment of gender-critical feminism should be to abolitionism via the Nordic Model. But what is *good* depends on what will do the most to reduce male violence against women and girls, and advance the cause of women's liberation. If sufficient evidence can be provided to show that decriminalization beats the Nordic Model on these measures (unlikely, but possible), then gender-critical feminists ought to choose to support it. Not letting the perfect become the enemy of the good means that we shouldn't let ideological commitments get in the way of reducing harm and advancing women's practical interests. We should always remain responsive to the evidence about what will bring more good to women.

5
Trans/Gender

> The oppressed is keenly aware of the humanity of the privileged. For the privileged, on the other hand, the oppressed is an enigma living in a magical, half-human world.
>
> (Kajsa Ekis Ekman, *Being and Being Bought*)[1]

At the heart of the disagreement gender-critical feminists have with other types of feminists over trans issues is 'the woman question', which is, what does it take to be a woman? A lot depends on the answer to this question, for it tells us who feminism is for and what it is about. Our answer to this question has implications for what we think about the permissibility of excluding certain people, and certain issues. As we have seen, gender-critical feminists think that to be a 'woman' is to be an adult human female; a member of a sex class that has a history of oppression and whose members are still oppressed in some countries, or are dealing with the lasting structural effects of historical oppression in others. For gender-critical feminists, feminism is about female people. We use the terms 'female' and 'woman' interchangeably to refer to these people. Gender-critical feminists do distinguish sex from gender, viewing sex as a biological fact and gender as a system of norms imposed on the basis of sex. But these distinctions pick out the same class of people, not different ones. So even if gender-critical feminists were to use 'female' for sex and 'woman' for people subject to certain norms and expectations on the basis of that sex, they'd still ultimately be talking about female people in both cases. (Most gender-critical feminists instead use 'femininity' to talk about the gender norms imposed on females.)

Importantly, this is not a mere disagreement about words. Gender-critical feminists think there are good reasons for female people to hang on to the word 'woman', not least because it is used synonymously with 'female' throughout domestic and international law designed to protect sex-based rights. But even if they were to cede the word 'woman', they would *still think* that female people were a subordinated class[2] in need of its own theory and

Gender-Critical Feminism. Holly Lawford-Smith, Oxford University Press. © Holly Lawford-Smith 2022.
DOI: 10.1093/oso/9780198863885.003.0005

movement. For them, the fact that some activists today are trying to change the meaning of the word 'woman' doesn't change any of the underlying facts about the importance of sex and the history of sex-based oppression. At best, it would simply create a new social group, and new questions about whether this group was itself subject to any historical or contemporary injustice.

Some feminists, though, think 'the woman question' is different from 'the female question', because they use 'woman' as a gender term *and* reject the understanding of gender as a system of norms imposed on the basis of sex. Some think that gender, rather than being something that is done to us, is something that we do, something that we 'perform, produce, and sustain' through our voluntary actions.[3] Others think that gender is an identity, a way that we feel about ourselves and that we alone have authority over.[4] When pushed, many of the feminists who subscribe to either of these views will admit to a sex/gender distinction. But at the same time, many support legal and political reforms that effectively eliminate sex and replace it with one of these views of gender. For example, there was considerable support among British feminists for changes to the UK's Gender Recognition Act (GRA) that would make self-declared gender identity the relevant attribute for almost all social and legal purposes where sex had formerly been relevant (with a narrow range of exceptions where sex was still considered relevant).[5] Or to give an example from my own state, many Victorian feminists supported the Births, Deaths and Marriages Registration Amendment Bill 2019, which made it the case that legal sex could be changed on the basis of a statutory declaration of belief. For example, any male person could declare that he believed himself to be female, and thereby secure the legal status 'female'. This gives that person access to all and any spaces, services, and protections available to female people, with the sole exception of competition in elite sports. So even if the feminists who support these changes admit to sex as a biological category, they repudiate its significance or importance as a political or social category.

For feminists who think gender is a performance or an identity, anyone who performs femininity or identifies as female/woman *is a woman.* For them, feminism is for all of these people. So feminism is for some males (although many would refuse to call them that, given the close association between 'male' and 'man' in ordinary language). From the perspective of these feminists, the gender-critical feminists' attempt to restrict the constituency of feminism to female people is exclusionary, keeping some women out of a political project that is meant to be for all women. Very often, both sides lose sight of the fact that they disagree about what it means to be a woman, and fall into accusing each other of various transgressions against the sisterhood. Gender-critical feminists are accused of failing to learn from feminist history, and treating men with gender identities in just the way that the 'white feminists' (read: white, middle-class, etc., feminists) treated more marginalized women in the past.[6] Other types of feminists are accused of being such victims of feminine socialization that they have become handmaidens for the patriarchy, so self-effacing that they're willing to put men first even inside feminism.[7] The debate is ugly, and it has been ugly for a long time.[8]

The feminists who think gender is a performance or an identity appear to believe that there is no loss to women in shifting to an alternative understanding of gender, and therefore a new constituency for feminism (and in many places, redrawn boundaries of the group eligible for protection as female/woman under the law and in social policy). The aim of this chapter is to show that they are wrong. Gender-critical feminists, following radical feminists, are concerned with women as a sex class. We care deeply about harms to this group. 'Gender identity' is an imprecise term given to a cluster of very different people with very different underlying issues. There are no diagnostic criteria for gender identity; we are simply asked to take a person's word for it that they have one, and what it is. In the law in my state, 'gender identity' is an attribute protected from discrimination, but its definition is 'a person's gender-related identity', and 'gender' is not defined.[9] The ideology of gender as identity, and the activism that doggedly pursues its introduction into law and policy, is harmful to women, and creates a conflict of interest between women as a class and trans people as a social group.

Although considerable energy has been expended by opponents of gender-critical feminism characterizing it as 'anti-trans',[10] this conflict of interest does not put gender-critical feminism and support for trans rights in tension. While gender-critical feminists reject legal conflation between sex and gender identity, and advocate for continued protection of sex under the law, there is no tension with *also* supporting the protection of gender identity, transgender status, or gender expression.[11] The limit to our support for these things is that we do so *without* believing that they change a person's sex. Gender-critical feminism is not anti-trans. In fact, characterizing it as 'anti-trans' is a kind of anti-feminist propaganda, distortion of a movement and theory for women and women's sex-based rights by labelling it according to what it is not about (more in Chapter 6). It would be like the 'pro-life' side of the abortion debate insistently referring to the 'pro-choice' side as 'anti-foetus'. Just as a woman does not terminate a pregnancy because she hates foetuses, and it would be patently absurd to claim that she does, a gender-critical feminist does not deny 'transwomen are women', or reject sex self-identification in law, because she hates transwomen. There is no hatred or other 'anti' sentiment anywhere in the view.[12]

In the first part of this chapter, I'll focus on the harms of gender identity ideology to gender non-conforming women and girls, in the second part of the chapter on harms to women and girls more generally.

5.1 Gender Non-conforming Women and Girls

Danish comedian Sofie Hagen, one of the founding members of The Guilty Feminist podcast, announced in 2019 that she was 'non-binary', giving as reasons that people in comedy paid a lot of attention to her sex, which felt wrong, and that wearing trousers 'felt so right'.[13] In societies that value males more, and that give opportunities to males that are not given to females, is it any surprise that women and girls would come to dis-identify with femaleness, and identify more with maleness? In a 1946 poll, a *quarter* of the women respondents said they wished they'd been born the opposite sex.[14] Are we to believe that a full quarter of women were transgender then? Radical feminist Shulamith Firestone made this point in 1970 (in the section this passage comes from she's giving a feminist reinterpretation of Freud):

> As for the 'penis envy', again it is safer to view this as a metaphor. Even when an actual preoccupation with genitals does occur it is clear that anything that physically distinguishes the envied male will be envied. For the girl can't really understand how it is that when she does exactly the same thing as her brother, his behaviour is approved and hers isn't. She may or may not make a confused connection between his behaviour and the organ that differentiates him.[15]

Firestone's point is that what Freud called 'penis envy' wasn't literally envy of the penis, but rather envy of males' superior social status. Simone de Beauvoir made the same point in 1949 when she said: 'if the little girl feels penis envy it is only as the symbol of privileges enjoyed by boys. The place the father holds in the family, the universal predominance of males, her own education—everything confirms her in her belief in masculine superiority'.[16] Clara Thompson and Karen Horney made the point as early as 1939 (summarized a little later by Thompson): 'that cultural factors can explain the tendency of women to feel inferior about their sex and their consequent tendency to envy men; that this state of affairs may well lead women to blame all their difficulties on the fact of their sex'.[17] Feminists have been making this point for a long time, but back then they were making it against insufferable male theorists like Freud and Sartre, not—as they must do today—against clinicians, mental health professionals, counsellors, teachers, and all the other professionals who support the affirmation of any young girl's claim that she is really a boy. Radical feminist Janice Raymond criticized the medicalization of what was at her time of writing transsexualism rather than transgenderism (the difference being whether mere self-identification, as opposed to having undergone sex reassignment surgery, was taken to be sufficient for trans status) as being an individual solution to a social problem.[18]

Gender-critical feminists do not find it surprising that girls wouldn't identify with their gender. On the contrary, that is exactly what our understanding of gender predicts and explains. If all women were naturally inclined towards femininity, there wouldn't need to be so much effort expended in policing conformity, in offering social and economic rewards for conformity and punishments for non-conformity. Some women might get lucky, and happen to genuinely prefer what they would be pushed into even if they didn't prefer it. But we can expect many women not to be in this position. Those women are not all transgender. Gender non-conforming women, that is, women who are not feminine in every or even any respect, are not a minority variation on the statistically normal feminine woman.[19] Gender non-conforming women are normal.[20]

We seem to have utterly lost sight of this basic feminist point today. Clinicians, school counsellors, mental health providers, and other professionals are being increasingly encouraged to 'affirm' the beliefs of children who claim to be the opposite gender.[21] As I was finishing the writing of this book, law was introduced in Victoria, Australia, condemning failure to 'support or affirm' a person's gender identity.[22] An affirmation-only approach makes it more difficult, when a female child claims to be a boy, to question them about other aspects of their life, in order to try to rule out other possible explanations than that they are transgender for why they might be thinking of themselves this way. There are high rates of mental health issues,[23] family dysfunction,[24] childhood sexual abuse,[25] autism,[26] and same-sex attraction[27] within cohorts who identify as trans, any of which might be a better explanation of their wish to transition than that the individual is, in fact, trans.[28]

One clinician, interviewed anonymously by Michele Moore, an Honorary Professor in Health and Social Care at the University of Essex, and Heather Brunskell-Evans, who was a Senior Research Fellow at King's College London, said:

> You don't just see one child and understand gender identity is not innate, but once you've seen a hundred you've seen 'the Reddit kid', you've seen 'the teenager with autism', 'the one who might be gay', you've seen 'the girl who was sexually abused and hates her body', or whose mother has been sexually abused and hates her body and doesn't want the same for her child. We know that by not examining what is behind the onset of dysphoria, and going straight for 'self-affirmation' that the patient is transgender, we are subjugating children's needs to an ideological position.[29]

'The Reddit kid' here refers to the likelihood of a social contagion around identifying as transgender. In a (2018) paper, Lisa Littman introduced what she called 'rapid onset gender dysphoria', identification as trans that appears suddenly during or after puberty (rather than from a very young age), and generally after exposure to transgender-identifying peers or transgender social media content.[30] In the friend groups reported in Littman's study, the average number of friends in the same group who began to identify as transgender was 3.5, and 60.7 per cent of those adolescents and young adults who announced that they were transgender experienced increased popularity among their peers.[31]

In the UK, there has been a 4,400 per cent increase in girls being referred for transitioning treatment in ten years, with drugs (specifically puberty blockers) being offered to children as young as 10.[32] In the five years between 2015 and 2020, there was a 400 per cent rise in referrals to the Tavistock centre in the UK, which is the only public health clinic treating children with gender identity issues.[33] The majority are girls who identify as boys, generally without having shown signs of dysphoria in childhood.[34] In Sweden, there has been a 1,500 per cent rise between 2008 and 2018 in the diagnosis of girls aged 13–17 years old as having gender dysphoria.[35] This suggests we're going to be seeing more and more 'trans kids', mostly identifying as boys. It is unlikely that these kids would have met older diagnostic criteria.[36]

In February 2020, the well-known gay Australian writer Benjamin Law tweeted (from his account with 106K followers) 'And even if there were more trans people in 2020, what would be the problem exactly? Let's face it: so much of this conversation stems from an aversion to—and hatred of—the existence of transgender people'.[37] This makes use of a familiar idea from the gay rights movement, namely that when people worried about 'social contagion', or gay adults influencing children to be gay, there was no real explanation of why it should be objectionable that there are more gay people *unless* there's something wrong with being gay.

As we have just seen, there are a lot of different explanations for why people might wish to transition. Now imagine there's a similar range of explanations available for why people claim to have feelings of attraction to the same sex, many of which suggest that they are not actually gay. Perhaps of all the people claiming to be gay, some of these were only bisexual, some were straight but just experimenting, some were rebelling against their parents, some were avoiding partners of the opposite sex because of past sexual abuse by people of that category, and so on. Imagine there were peer group incentives to claim to be gay, and this was especially appealing to people who had no other marginalized identities and were sick of being accused of being 'privileged'. Suppose there was a kind of social contagion where groups of kids were coming out as gay at the same time, in groups of friends, after exposure to online information about gay communities.

What's the worst that can happen during a period of a person thinking they're gay when they're not? They experiment with some people of the same sex, who they will later end up ruling out as sexual or romantic partners. Is this a bad thing? It doesn't seem so. Experimentation, sexual and otherwise, is commonplace. There's no harm at all to affirming as gay people who are not gay. On the other hand, there is risk of serious harm in refusing to affirm such people. At worst there is 'conversion therapy', where gay people are subject to attempts to make them straight. This has been linked to depression, suicidal ideation, suicide attempts, low self-esteem, sexual dysfunction, harm to interpersonal relationships in particular with partners and parents, alienation, loneliness, and social isolation.[38] Short of conversion therapy, refusal to affirm may cause a gay person to experience shame and self-loathing, to remain 'in the closet' for a long period, to feel unconfident about trusting others—which can negatively impact the quality of their interpersonal relationships, and to miss out on caring romantic and sexual relationships. Ultimately, there is no reason at all to refuse to affirm claims about sexual orientation on the basis of wanting there to be *fewer gays*.

More gays, fewer gays, it doesn't matter. No one is harmed by being gay (except, of course, by people who don't like gays and are willing to act on that).

But the idea doesn't apply to trans people as straightforwardly as Law seems to assume. The potential harms of affirmation are very different when it comes to gender non-conforming kids who consider themselves trans. First of all, they may fail to receive support for possible underlying issues of the kinds mentioned already, including autism, histories of childhood sexual abuse, mental health problems, family dysfunction, and same-sex attraction.[39] Second of all, they may start taking harmful drugs. Kids who consider themselves trans may be prescribed puberty blockers[40] (these do what they say, and block the onset of puberty) and later, cross-sex hormones. In the UK, cross-sex hormones have been prescribed to kids as young as 12.[41] Much of this medical treatment is experimental. Despite the World Professional Association for Transgender Health recommending the use of puberty blockers, there is disagreement among paediatric endocrinologists, psychologists, psychiatrists, and ethicists about whether they should be used.[42] The UK National Health Service (NHS) website used to describe the effects of Gonadotropin-Releasing Hormone agonist (GnRHa) treatment as 'fully reversible', but this was changed in late May 2020 to say 'little is known about the long-term side effects of hormone or puberty blockers in children with gender dysphoria', 'it is not known what the psychological effects may be', and 'it's also not known whether hormone blockers affect the development of the teenage brain or children's bones'.[43]

One key study looking at puberty blockers suggested that they might contribute to gender dysphoria persisting.[44] This study looked at seventy young people between 12 and 16 years old, who had started on puberty blockers. *All* of these children went on to the next stage of transitioning.[45] In the UK, evidence assessed by the High Court showed that 'practically all children / young people who start P[uberty] B[locker]s progress on to C[ross] S[ex] H[ormones]'.[46] This suggests pathway dependence: that once children take the first step (puberty blockers) they are highly likely to take the next (cross-sex hormones). (Although the Court of Appeal has recently provided evidence suggesting the connection is less strong.)[47] There are eleven papers showing that children with strong feelings of childhood gender dysphoria tend to 'desist' when left unmedicalized.[48] Canadian psychologist James Cantor says that the studies all come to a very similar conclusion, namely that 'very few trans-kids still want to transition by the time they are adults'.[49] If most of the children who are put on puberty blockers and/or cross-sex hormones persist as trans, and most of the children who are not put on puberty blockers and/or cross-sex hormones end up desisting, then *whether* we put a kid on puberty blockers and/or cross-sex hormones or not determines to a large extent whether or not they will be trans as an adult. This medicalization doesn't *treat* trans people, it *creates* trans people.[50]

The High Court in the UK in a case at the end of 2020 stated that in order to demonstrate the competence to consent to puberty blockers, a child would have to 'understand, retain and weigh up' the following relevant information:

- The immediate physical and psychological consequences of the treatment.
- The fact that most children who take puberty blockers then go on to cross-sex hormones (so, understand that puberty blockers are a pathway to greater medical intervention).
- The relationship between cross-sex hormones and later surgeries, and the implications of those surgeries.
- The potential loss of fertility caused by cross-sex hormones.
- The impact of cross-sex hormones on sexual function.
- The impact of puberty blockers as the first step along this pathway on current and future relationships.
- The unknown effects of puberty blockers; and the fact that the evidence base for puberty blockers is 'as yet highly uncertain'.

They found it to be unlikely that people under the age of 16 would be able to understand all of these things, and so unlikely that they have the competence to consent to puberty blockers.[51] The Court of Appeal later found that the High Court should not have made this declaration, which effectively directed children and young people wanting puberty blockers and cross-sex hormones to the courts, instead of leaving the matter with children and young people, their parents, and their clinicians. But they did not disagree with the reasoning in terms of what consent would involve,[52] and urged that clinicians 'take great care before recommending treatment to a child and be astute to ensure that the consent obtained from both child and parents is properly informed by the advantages and disadvantages of the proposed course of treatment and in light of the evolving research and understanding of the implications and long-term consequences of such treatment'.[53]

There is also ongoing debate over the effects of puberty blockers on bone density,[54] and interest in the question of whether hormonal treatment impacts brain development.[55] A study on a nonbinary teenager taking puberty blockers reported that 'their bone mineral density has regularly fallen and is now in the lowest 2.5 percentile'. The authors go on to explore the risks of impaired fertility and low bone density, as they trade off against the benefits of treating the teenager's 'gender dysphoria and anxiety'.[56]

Gender non-conforming kids who consider themselves trans may also end up getting invasive surgeries and other cosmetic interventions. Most common among transmen are chest surgery reduction or 'reconstruction' (a euphemism for double mastectomies) and hysterectomy,[57] and most common among transwomen are electrolysis and vaginoplasty.[58] It's noteworthy how much more common invasive interventions on girls and women are compared to boys and men: 36 per cent of transmen in the United States have had chest reduction or reconstruction surgery while only 12 per cent of transwomen have had vaginoplasty or labiaplasty. That's three times as many transmen as transwomen undergoing invasive surgeries. (Although one explanation for this may be that breasts are physically obvious and make it harder for transmen to pass as male).

What about the harms of refusing to affirm as trans people who are in fact trans? There is little data on this. Although legislation is being introduced in multiple countries to prevent 'conversion therapy' on the basis of sexual orientation and gender identity, the legislation seems to be justified with reference to research that is disproportionately about sexual orientation.[59] Furthermore, refusal to affirm a gender identity is not equivalent to rejection or outright disbelief. The clinical alternative to the 'gender-affirmative' model is the 'watchful waiting' model, which explores with the child in therapy their other issues, and makes sure to affirm a trans identification only if and when other explanations are ruled out. As Diane Ehrensaft—Associate Professor of Pediatrics at the University of California San Francisco (UCSF), and Director of Mental Health at the UCSF Benioff Children's Hospital Child and Adolescent Gender Centre—explains, 'Since a large majority of gender nonconforming young children seeking services at gender clinics desist in their gender dysphoria by adolescence, best practices would be to wait and see if the child persists into adolescence before making any significant changes in the child's gender identity'.[60] The harms of affirming kids who are not trans as trans are likely to far outweigh the harms of failing to affirm as trans kids who are trans, especially if the alternative is watchful waiting.

If being trans were just like being gay in that it didn't impact a child's health, then affirming everyone who considers themselves trans *as* trans might not be a problem. More trans people, fewer trans people, who cares. But it's not like being gay, because it tends to involve medical interventions, invasive and painful surgeries, and uncertain long-term health impacts. Kids who consider themselves trans are at risk of being put on a conveyor belt to a lifetime of medical dependency. And these negative outcomes are now disproportionately impacting girls. A 2017 UK government survey on 108,100 lesbian, gay, bisexual, and transgender (LGBT) or intersex individuals in the UK found 57 per cent of trans respondents under the age of 35 to be non-binary,[61] 26 per cent to be transmen, and 17 per cent to be transwomen. Other studies have found between two and five times more females than males identifying as nonbinary.[62] The authors note that the percentages are in line with referrals to gender identity services, 'where the majority of referrals in 2016–17 were for people assigned female at birth (1,400 of the 2,016 referrals—69%)'.[63] This reveals a generational shift in trans identification, with more girls than boys now considering themselves trans.[64]

We also find disproportionate impacts when we look at sexual assault in trans communities. As we might have expected given what we know about the differential rates of sexual assault outside of trans communities, female people face disproportionate impacts. An Australian survey from 2018 showed that trans people experienced sexual violence at higher rates than the general public, but it was transmen and female nonbinary people who experienced the highest rates, with 61.8 per cent of those respondents answering 'yes' to the question 'Have you ever been forced or frightened into doing something sexually that you did not want to do?'.[65] Of the transwomen and male nonbinary participants, 39.3 per cent answered 'yes' to this question. Female nonbinary people were the most at risk (66.1 per cent), followed by transmen (54.2 per cent), then male nonbinary people (44.5 per cent), and finally transwomen (36.1 per cent).[66] Feminists who consider transmen to be men cannot consider this to be a specifically feminist issue, even though it is a rate of sexual coercion *three times higher* than that experienced by female people neither trans nor nonbinary.

The UK government survey mentioned above found something similar, asking trans people about their experience of 'incidents' including verbal harassment, coercive or controlling behaviour, physical harassment or violence, and sexual harassment or violence. They found that 'trans men were notably more likely to have experienced an incident (58%) than trans women (40%) and non-binary respondents (47%)', and that '6% of trans men said they had experienced physical harassment or violence, compared to 4% trans women and 4% of non-binary respondents'.[67]

Accepting the redrawn boundaries of 'woman' and therefore the new constituency of feminism proposed by those feminists who think that gender is an identity or a performance would therefore lead to the dismissal of significant harms at the intersection of being female and being trans-identified, as not being feminist issues. Gender-critical feminism accommodates the interests of the most vulnerable people in the trans community. Trans *is* a feminist issue, just not in the way that most feminists today think it is.

5.2 Identifying into Women-Only Spaces

In Iran in 2015, the national women's soccer team had eight transwomen players.[68] In the UK in 2017, a transwoman was elected to Women's Officer for the Labour Party for the constituency of Rochester and Strood,[69] and in 2018 the same transwoman was elected National Women's Officer for Labour Students.[70] A transwoman was appointed as the keynote speaker for the British Film Institute's 2018 'Woman with a Movie Camera Summit'.[71] One of the 'lesbians' acting as an advisor to Stonewall, the UK's most prominent LGBTQI+ (lesbian, gay, bisexual, transgender, queer, and intersex plus) charity, is a transwoman.[72] There was a transwoman on the 'Top-100 Female Champions' list, produced for the annual ranking 'HERoes: champions of women in business' (which has a separate male list).[73] There are transwomen in women-only prisons—including in Australia one who struck two people in the head with an axe, in Sweden one who went to jail for murdering and mutilating their girlfriend, and in Canada one who raped and murdered a 13-year-old girl.[74] Transwomen have been admitted to women's shelters, for example at a shelter for women recovering from substance abuse in Canada.[75]

The explanation of why there are so many transwomen in women-only spaces today is the influence of gender identity ideology, the idea that what it is to be a woman/female (man/male) is to identify as a woman/female (man/male), and that this subjective identification supersedes facts about sex class membership. Identification as a transwoman is allowing male people to be included in spaces and services originally designed for and dedicated to women, understood as members of the female sex.

In *Sister Outsider*, radical feminist Audre Lorde wrote 'I grew up in largely female environments, and I know how crucial that has been to my own development. I feel the want and need often for the society of women, exclusively. I recognize that our own spaces are essential for developing and recharging'.[76] She went on to make a similar point about black-only spaces:

> As a Black woman, I find it necessary to withdraw into all-Black groups at times for exactly the same reasons—differences in stages of development and differences in levels of interaction. Frequently, when speaking with men and white women, I am reminded of how difficult and time-consuming it is to have to reinvent the pencil every time you want to send a message.[77]

Many women value sex-separated spaces. If a 'woman' is anyone who identifies as a woman, then women-only spaces are no longer female-only spaces. If the space only serves its purpose when it is single-sex, then this undermines it.

In a piece for the *Verso* blog in 2018, feminist philosophers Lorna Finlayson, Katharine Jenkins, and Rosie Worsdale summarized (in order to oppose) what they took to be the feminist case against transwomen's inclusion as women in the context of reform to the UK GRA:

> The argument runs as follows. Men as a group systematically oppress and inflict violence on women. And trans women—or at least some of them—share, albeit to varying extents, in the features which make men more likely to inflict violence against, and otherwise to oppress, women. First, they may have certain bodily features, such as a penis, testes, and higher levels of testosterone. Second, they have been treated for at least part of their lives as boys or men. The first factor is often referred to by saying that trans women (or some trans women, at least) are 'biologically male' (or simply 'male'). The second is expressed in the statement that trans women have a 'history of male socialisation', and in the associated claim that they are bearers of 'male privilege'. Note that this part of the argument doesn't rely on claiming that trans women are *more* likely than cis men to be violent or oppressive to women. The claim is that trans women (or at least, those who are substantially similar to cis men in the respects just outlined) are *just as* prone to commit violence against women as cis men are.[78]

This is a fair summary of the opposition to the reform, although gender-critical feminists wouldn't beat around the bush describing 'shared features' as though it's a surprising coincidence that transwomen and men both have these.

Feminist women opposing the GRA reform weren't worried about transwomen in particular; they were worried about male people in general, and didn't make an exception for those who identified as women. If there's a reason to keep sex-separated spaces, then there's a reason to worry about people identifying into them. Finlayson et al. do make an exception: for transwomen. They argue that while it's true that 'men commit violence against women at much higher rates than women commit violence against either women or men', we don't know that the *basis* of this difference lies in male biology or male socialization. They say that taking it to be biological risks naturalizing it (assuming it to be innate or hardwired, and thus excusing it), and that taking it to be socialized assumes that transwomen are socialized to the same effect. But the fact that transwomen identify as women, and other men don't, shows—those feminists think—that they can't have been socialized to the same effect. These authors say 'it is, to say the very least, not obvious that gender identity makes no difference to the way in which either biological and social factors manifest themselves'.[79] They are supposing that having a gender identity could make a relevant difference, one that would justify treating transwomen as exceptions to generalizations made about males.

It's hardly surprising that some feminists have been reluctant to take it on trust that transwomen don't share the propensities of males, given that what differentiates them—their 'gender identity'—is an imprecise and unverifiable idea that covers a range of very different people.

Maybe a review of the empirical evidence can help us to work out whether there are differences that should justify treating transwomen differently when it comes to exclusion from, or inclusion in, women-only spaces. From a gender-critical perspective, there is no automatic right to inclusion, because these spaces are part of a package of political provisions designed to improve women's participation in public life, or increase women's representation in areas where they have been historically underrepresented, or correct for structural, institutional, and interpersonal discrimination against women. But there might nonetheless be reasons to *choose* to include transwomen, if it can be shown that they are 'like women' or 'unlike men' in the respects that rationalize the spaces.

To try to resolve this question, I'm going to draw on work done by sexologists in the 1980s and 1990s. This is likely to raise the question, why not draw on work that is more up-to-date, given that we surely have a more sophisticated understanding of trans issues today? The problem lies in the conceptualization of 'trans' status over time, which has changed so much that there is very little overlap with the original cohort. There has been a shift away from the understanding of trans as 'transsexual', and towards an understanding of trans as 'transgender'.[80] A review of 2,405 articles on trans health published between 1950 and 2016 notes that 'there has been a massive shift in ideology and treatment', and further concluded that there was 'an overall lack of high-quality research'.[81] Trans identification has become politicized. As the transgender population expanded to include more people, differences were flattened out into a single notion of 'gender identity',[82] and attempts to complicate that picture vehemently resisted (as evidenced by, for example, the dogpiling of Lisa Littman when she published her study suggesting that social contagion might be playing a role in transgender identification today).[83]

In the 1980s and 1990s sexologists worked with trans*sexual* populations, and we have evidence from that time. We have no real way of knowing how many transwomen today would have been transsexual in the past, but the fact that 88 per cent today have not had sex-reassignment surgery suggests most would not.[84] It could be that people with the same underlying trait are now choosing not to have surgery; but it could also be that the underlying trait has changed as the group expanded, and/or there is no longer any underlying trait.[85] 'Gender identity' cannot play the role of an underlying trait, because it is a philosophical concept, not a scientific one. It is not useful to ask empirical questions about what makes someone trans, or whether trans cohorts share certain attributes, if the cohort itself is not unified by any underlying trait. (Compare this to asking empirical questions about what makes someone gay, or whether gay cohorts share certain attributes, while working with a concept of 'gay' that includes a mixture of gay and straight people).[86] Considering the evidence from a time where there was, arguably, an underlying trait (or two distinct underlying traits—as we shall soon see) is at least a start.

Prior to 1989, Ray Blanchard had been working with gender dysphoric males, and noticed that there seemed to be two distinct types. There were 'homosexual transsexuals', males attracted to males who tended to have feminine boyhoods and transition earlier in life; and there were 'non-homosexual transsexuals', males attracted to females, or to both males and females, or to neither, who tended to have masculine boyhoods and transition later in life. Blanchard's innovation was to suppose these two types of transsexualism to have different explanations and to correlate with different sets of behaviours and experiences. The most prominent of these differences was 'erotic arousal in association with cross-dressing'.[87] Blanchard divided a clinical population of transsexuals into groups according to their sexual orientations, and found that most non-homosexual transsexuals had a history of erotic arousal associated with cross-dressing, while most homosexual transsexuals did not.

Blanchard suggested that cross-dressing was a result of 'autogynephilia', a term he coined to mean 'love of oneself as a woman', rather than a result of feminine identification, and confirmed that non-homosexual transsexuals showed less feminine identification than homosexual transsexuals[88] (a finding already made in 1974 about asexual transsexuals). He proposed that in the diagnosis of transsexuals for clinical research, identifying 'fetishistic arousal' directly would be difficult, but that distinguishing according to sexual orientation would be a reliable proxy.[89]

Anne Lawrence, who self-describes as an autogynephilic transsexual, summarizes the two very different explanations as follows: 'Androphilic MtF [male-to-female] transsexuals were extremely feminine androphilic men whose cross-gender identities derived from their female-typical attitudes, behaviours, and sexual preferences. Nonandrophilic MtF transsexuals, in contrast, were conventionally masculine, fundamentally gynephilic men who resembled transvestites in that they experienced paraphilic arousal from the fantasy of being women (autogynephilia); their cross-dressing identities derived from their autogynephilic sexual orientations'.[90] She also notes that Blanchard found bisexual transsexuals to have the highest scores on the 'Core Autogynephilia Scale', and that he had hypothesized that they were *pseudobisexual*, meaning that they were actually heterosexual but had developed an attraction to men primarily motivated by seeking validation of their femininity.[91]

Michael Bailey advanced Blanchard's typology in his popular science book *The Man Who Would Be Queen* which focused on feminine boys, as did Anne Lawrence later in her book *Men Trapped in Men's Bodies*.[92] After publication of his book, Bailey was the subject of vicious personal attacks by several high profile transwomen.[93] Together with Kiiri Triea, Bailey argues that Blanchard's typology has greater explanatory value than two proposed alternatives, the 'feminine essence' narrative, and the 'brain-sex' narrative. The feminine essence narrative is basically gender identity, but ramped up to be considered innate. According to the brain-sex narrative, male transsexual brains are more similar to female brains than non-transsexual male brains. But it's pretty hard to make the latter work, given that there's a huge debate over whether it even makes sense to talk about male and female brains.[94] Bailey and Triea say that Blanchard's theory 'is based on far more data, with respect to the number of both studies and subjects; no published scientific data in the peer-reviewed literature contradict it; and other investigators in other countries have obtained similar findings'.[95]

There is some disagreement between Julia Serano (who is transgender) and Blanchard over whether his typology accounts for *all* transsexual people or only some. Serano thinks it's some and Blanchard thinks it's all; Lawrence provides some persuasive reasons for how it can be all even when the data don't show that (one being that in some clinics, access to treatment has depended on fitting a particular description).[96] But their disagreement is only about the comprehensiveness of Blanchard's typology. As Serano says, 'nobody seriously doubts the existence of cross-gender arousal',[97] and as Blanchard says, 'the existence of autogynephilia as a distinguishable form of sexual behaviour is scarcely in doubt'.[98]

Why is it so important to pay attention to this distinction, rather than collapsing it under the heading of 'gender identity' as is standard practice today? Because being aroused by the thought of being a woman doesn't make you a woman.[99] In a 1987 study, out of 125 males presenting to a gender identity clinic over a four and a half year period, fifty-two were homosexual and seventy-three were heterosexual.[100] *Less than half* of the transwomen at the time were homosexual transsexuals. Homosexual transsexuals have a claim to being 'like women' and 'unlike men', at least in some respects. (As noted above, Blanchard found that they showed more feminine identification).[101] Autogynephiles do not, or at least, do not in virtue of their autogynephilia. Perhaps there is some other trait that makes them 'like a woman', but it remains unclear what that trait could be. This ratio of homosexual to autogynephilic transsexuals is likely to be even lower today than it was then, as advances in gay rights and gay acceptance have removed some of the incentives for feminine same-sex attracted males to transition to live as women. Men who experienced feminine boyhoods may have experienced some socialization and some discrimination that is similar to what girls experience, so provisions set up to mitigate this experience may be fairly extended to them. But that doesn't get *transwomen* in general a foot in the door, it gets *a small number of* transwomen a foot in the door. Autogynephiles, who had masculine boyhoods and transitioned later in life, are not in this small group.

This point is further reinforced when we add in what we learned in Section 5.1 about changes to the transgender community since roughly

1990. It is clear that there's more going on today than just homosexuality and autogynephilia.[102] Other factors mentioned already include social contagion, autism, family dysfunction, and childhood sexual abuse. And there's *politics.* Sandy Stone and Leslie Feinberg popularized the idea that transgender is a political identity, and this continues to be influential today.[103] But no male who has merely adopted a gender identity for political reasons is going to have any legitimate claim to women-only spaces. I cannot see why we should expect any of those outside Blanchard's typology and captured by the 'more going on today' idea to be 'like women'.

It is unclear whether Finlayson, Jenkins, and Worsdale would accept that cross-gender arousal, social contagion, or political identity, for example, are enough to make a male into a woman. I suspect they would not. If that is right, then we should *only* be talking about the inclusion in women-only spaces of those transwomen who might have a better claim. But if they would accept that all of these things are sufficient to make a male into a woman, then we can return to treating transwomen as an undifferentiated community and simply ask for evidence of differences between this community and men in general that would justify including this community among women for all political, legal, and social purposes. There is little such evidence currently available. A Swedish study that compared rates of violent crime ('homicide and attempted homicide, aggravated assault and assault, robbery, threatening behaviour, harassment, arson, or any sexual offence')[104] in cohorts of trans*sexual* women to male controls found that transsexual women 'retained a male pattern regarding criminality'.[105] Even more striking were the study's findings comparing cohorts of transsexual women to female controls: adjusting for their higher psychiatric comorbidities, transsexual women were 18.1 times more likely than female controls to have been convicted for violent crime; and without that adjustment, transsexual women were twenty times more likely than female controls to have been convicted for violent crime.[106]

I noted earlier that most transwomen today are not transsexual, so it is not clear whether and to what extent we should expect the Swedish study's findings to generalize.[107] From the armchair, it seems we'd have substantially *less* reason to expect transwomen to be 'like women' and 'unlike men'. Consider those transwomen who only begin to identify as women in adulthood, having shown no signs of childhood gender dysphoria. We'd have to suppose that any influence of male biology, male puberty, and male socialization from birth to whatever age identifying as trans happened, were all rendered void by the mere fact of the sudden claiming of a gender identity. This is highly implausible.

There is no basis for a presumption of inclusion. The burden of proof lies with those who support including transwomen in women-only spaces.[108] Perhaps this will be the impetus the trans rights movement and its existing feminist allies need to stop opposing relevant research and the publication of research findings,[109] and to start producing research that actually supports the claim that 'gender identity', at whatever point it sets in, actually blocks the effects of male biology, male socialization, and/or the interaction of the two.

The point I am going to make now is speculative, but I think it's worth considering. We've talked a lot about the impact of gender norms on women, so far, but on the topic of transwomen including themselves in women-only spaces, or indeed identifying themselves *as* women, it's worth talking about the impact of gender norms on men. Suppose that the full spectrum of human expression left unchecked runs from what we today describe as 'masculine' all the way to what we today describe as 'feminine', and there are no reliable correlations between a boy child's sex and his interests, in how he wants to dress, what toys he wants to play with, how he wants to play, how extroverted or confident he is, what kinds of imaginative games he plays, what he says he wants to be when he grows up, and so on. All of the ways that people can be, which we today so doggedly categorize as either 'masculine' or 'feminine' and police departures from, would just be ways that humans can be.[110] If that is the unchecked expression of children, then there would need to be a lot of cajoling, sanctioning, suppressing, encouraging, and shaping going on to get them to fit into one or the other category. And indeed, there is evidence of this kind of pressure everywhere you look.

But people chafe under this kind of unfreedom. Eventually there will be people who feel strongly enough about what they want to do and how they want to be that they will do and be it anyway. It's an interesting separate question what makes some people willing to live as they want to regardless of social sanctions and other people not willing. Cristina Bicchieri calls the former 'trendsetters', and gives them a crucial role in bringing about social norm change in the context of global development.[111] Her general picture seems to be that there are just some people who are, for whatever reason, willing to do what they think is right for the world, or best for themselves, regardless of the social sanctions others will impose on them. Perhaps they do not feel those sanctions as much as others, being less sensitive to peer dis-esteem; perhaps they do but avoiding dissonance between their beliefs and their choices is more important to them.[112] Think, for example, about the first feminists, or the people who were openly gay when it was still illegal, or the people fighting for abolition when slavery was still legal, or even just the people willing to defy their parents' expectations to follow their own dreams.

If we ignore that this is a *general* character trait, we may be led to observe that gay people tend to feel so strongly about their sexual orientation that they will risk everything to express it, or that trans people tend to feel so strongly about their gender identification that they will risk everything to be recognized in that gender.[113] And this may lead us to think of being gay or being trans as innate identities that resist suppression and that matter enormously to the people who have them. But what if there are just as many—or more!—people who experience same-sex attraction, or who desire a different gender expression, but who don't have these 'trendsetter' character traits, and so who make different choices? If that's right, then it would predict that as the social sanctions reduce to nothing, more people emerge as having these statuses. We have certainly seen that in the case of sexual orientation; since the social sanctions reduced and the social protections increased (including legal recourse against discrimination) more people came out as gay.

Gender identity activists will say that it's just the same for trans—as the stigma reduces, more people will come out as trans. But if trans just is strongly felt gender non-conformity, then the categorization of these people as trans in the first place depends on keeping strong norms of gender in place. (If it has more to do with bodies, as it did on the older diagnostics, then it does not.) If we retain highly rigid ideas about masculinity, then more and more men will not identify with the norms of masculinity, and as the social sanctions against non-conformity reduce, more and more men will come out as non-masculine. Depending on the direction we've taken, perhaps they will come out as non-men or non-males too—the rising numbers of nonbinary people show that this is already starting to happen. And at this point it depends on the numbers. If most men are non-masculine, and most women are non-feminine, what's the point of having 'trans' or 'nonbinary' as categories? This is not to rule out that there can be oppressed majorities; the question will be whether there are still social rewards attached to being a feminine woman and a masculine man, despite the change in demographics and social attitudes. More colloquially, gender non-conformity is ordinary and should be expected. If everyone is trans then no one is trans.

5.3 Policy Implications

There are two policy implications that follow from this discussion. The first is an answer to the question of what forms the legal protection of trans people should take.[114] The second is how to approach the issue of harms to gender non-conforming women and girls.

Legal protection. Is discrimination against transwomen related to women's sex-based oppression? Patriarchy began as the sexual enslavement of women, and developed through the control of women's reproductive labour, into a broader system of exploitation and control of women by men. The victims of patriarchy, and relatedly, sexism/misogyny, are women. Through an understanding of the origins and the sustaining mechanisms of patriarchy, we have a coherent explanation of why, on what basis, and how women came to be and remain (to a greater or lesser extent depending on the country) oppressed. We should not lose sight of this explanation.

Still, we can retain coherence while admitting that there has been collateral damage to other social groups along the way. Focusing on the primary victims of patriarchy means keeping the bulk of our attention on how feminine gender norms have been constructed to constrain and control women. But this shouldn't stop us noticing that in the policing of women, people may sometimes make mistakes about who in fact 'deserves' policing treatment (if a woman looks like a man she may evade that treatment, and if a man looks like a woman he may receive it). In devaluing femininity, men may come to devalue feminine aspects of persons whether or not they appear in female people. In asserting the superiority of male people and of masculinity (and in seeing the two as synonymous), men may come to feel anger or even rage towards males who they perceive as 'betraying' men by violating or repudiating masculinity.

Discrimination against 'passing' transwomen (transwomen who strangers perceive and treat as female) is related to women's oppression because those transwomen are assumed to be members of the class that is singled out for a particular type of treatment. Discrimination against 'non-passing' transwomen (transwomen who strangers perceive and treat as male) is something different, namely the sanctioning of males for violating the norms of masculinity. Those sets of norms are connected as two parts of a broader social system that keeps both male and female people 'in their places'. The difference is that these norms benefit men in general even as they harm some individual males. Is this connection enough to justify protecting transwomen as women?

If the argument for protection is based merely on being collateral damage in women's oppression, then it's not just transwomen who should be protected as women, it's also gay men, effeminate men, and gender non-conforming men as well. For they are all just as much 'connected' to women's oppression. This is a problem for the feminism that accepts gender as identity. It does not propose that *all* those negatively impacted by patriarchy be protected as women. What it wants is to class all female people together with all people who identify as women. But it cannot offer a coherent explanation of the oppression of that particular combination of people. There is no origin story for the oppression of *women and also people with feminine gender identities.*

As we have just seen, there may be a common system behind the mechanisms that sustain the oppression of *women and also people with feminine gender identities*, in particular, social norms that support the idea of males being masculine and females being feminine and so sanction deviations in both cases. But the people with feminine gender identities who are visibly male will be subject to different mechanisms than women, namely the mechanisms that socialize males as masculine and push men into a superior social position on the axis of sex/gender. This common system may give women and gender non-conforming men a reason to be allies in fighting for both groups' rights and interests, but it is not sufficient to show that gender non-conforming men need legal protection as the opposite sex.

Any story that gender-as-identity feminists can give is dependent on the one told by radical and gender-critical feminists, for example that the devaluation of women in combination with the constructing of women as feminine led to the devaluing of femininity wherever it was found. (This explains the mistreatment of effeminate gay men and transwomen.) But from this common devaluation, again, it does not follow that we should collapse the distinctions between the groups.[115] It is a good reason for those who have been collateral damage in the oppression of women to be allies to women in women's fight for liberation. After all, women's liberation will be good for them too. Unfortunately, though, this is not how things have gone. Gender-as-identity feminists have been so busy being allies to transwomen, that they've forgotten to ask transwomen to be allies to women.

Most trans people today are aptly described as gender non-conforming. That means they *do not conform* to the norms and expectations that are imposed on them on the basis of their sex. But there are, and have long been, plenty of gender non-conforming people. This is nothing new or different. Gay and lesbian people are gender non-conforming insofar as they defy one of the central norms of masculinity—namely to be attracted to women—and of femininity—namely to be attracted to men—respectively. Bisexual people are gender non-conforming insofar as they defy the norm of being exclusively attracted to the opposite sex. Butch lesbians and masculine-presenting women (including drag kings and transmen) are gender non-conforming insofar as they defy norms of appearance for female people. Effeminate gay men and feminine-presenting men (including drag queens, cross-dressers, and transwomen) are gender non-conforming insofar as they defy norms of appearance for male people.

Having had a double mastectomy and grown your body hair out while female (as many transmen and nonbinary females do) makes you gender non-conforming, but it doesn't make you a man, or not a woman: many lesbians and feminists have grown their body hair out and many breast cancer survivors have had double mastectomies. Having grown breasts and lasered your body hair off while male makes you gender non-conforming, but it doesn't make you a woman: many overweight men have breasts, and cyclists, some gay men, and some male models, have had their body hair lasered.

This means there's a large group which have something in common, namely non-conformity with the current norms of masculinity and femininity. This group might need political protection, for as long as it remains stigmatized. We can protect it by adding gender expression (or presentation) to the list of protected attributes in our countries' Equality Acts. This makes a lot more sense than saying that anyone who identifies as a woman should be legally protected as female, and able to access the full range of legal protections put in place to mitigate women's historical oppression and ongoing underrepresentation and disadvantage.

Regulation of medical and surgical transition. If we return to Satz's parameters for noxious markets from Chapter 4, we can see that the transitioning of girls is likely to count. There is weak and asymmetric knowledge and agency: they're not adults, their ability to make a fully informed decision is compromised by the long-term nature of the decisions (especially given pathway dependence), and they cannot have full information about the risks because some of the medical interventions are experimental. There is harm to transitioners, whenever the risks detailed in Section 5.1 materialize, and to detransitioners. There is vulnerability, in the fact of being children and adolescents. And there is social harm, in that girls are deciding, against a backdrop of sex inequality that subordinates females and elevates males, that they are *not girls*, and being 'affirmed' in this belief.

For these reasons, access to medical and surgical transition should be heavily regulated. This is the *opposite* of what many countries are doing with a clinical policy of 'affirmation', especially one backed up by the threat of criminal sanctions for 'conversion' of children's gender identities.[116] There should be *no* medical or surgical transition for people under the age of 18, at least not while there is a culture of fear and silence inside gender-based medicine which is likely to prevent clinicians from really making sure that a child who identifies as trans *is actually trans*.[117] Over the age of 18, we should think of surgical interventions similarly to how we think of cosmetic surgeries. Many feminists have argued that these are a harmful social practice.[118] Trans surgeries, which appear to be an increasing part of a social and political movement which confers social status and esteem,[119] may need to be considered in the same way.

If we want to reduce harms to gender non-conforming girls short of such policy measures (which may not be easily won), there are two things we can do. First, we can keep working against sex inequality, which creates the understandable response in girls that they 'are not female' or 'are not girls', because they dis-identify with negative stereotypes and expectations of femininity. Second—and this may be difficult for gender-critical feminists to swallow—we can *support* the trans rights movement's efforts to decouple sex and gender identity.[120] The more that gender non-conforming girls feel that they can be 'boys' or 'men' *without medical or surgical transformations*, the fewer harms of the kind outlined in Section 5.1 there will be. The fine line to get reduced harm to girls *and* protection of women's sex-based rights is to support the decoupling while insisting that both categories matter—rather than that gender identity displaces sex.

5.4 Is Gender-Critical Feminism 'Trans-Exclusionary'?

We saw in Section 3.4 and at the start of this chapter that gender-critical feminism is regularly accused by other feminists of being 'trans-exclusionary' and 'anti-trans'. Is it? My answer is 'no'. Gender-critical feminism is feminism for females, not feminism for feminine 'gender identities' or feminism for feminine 'gender performances'. Because of this, it includes transmen, and excludes transwomen. It does not exclude trans people in general: on the contrary, it is very concerned to include transmen and female nonbinary people, because it is concerned with the harms done on the basis of female sex and as a result of the (attempted) imposition of norms of femininity. Because some women don't fit those norms or find conformity to those norms comfortable, they end up thinking that they are *not women*, or being convinced by others that they are not women. When they then identify as transgender, whether as nonbinary or as transmen, this can come along with negative health impacts for the individual and have adverse consequences for society, impacting lesbian culture, diversity, and feminism.

Lesbian culture is impacted when lesbians repudiate this status and claim to be straight men instead. It is impacted when the lesbian partners of transmen feel under pressure to change their publicly claimed orientations because they no longer fit with those partners' gender identities. Diversity is impacted when women look around and see only a narrow version of femininity represented under the label 'woman', because non-feminine females now identify as nonbinary or as transmen. And finally, feminism, understood as a political project aimed at women's liberation, is impacted when its goal is downgraded so substantially, from gender abolitionism to a mild form of gender revisionism.[121] Gender abolitionism is the only sensible response to a harmful system of norms that constrains people's life choices and impacts on their well-being. Accommodating gender identity means leaving in place a system that harms women in general because that system is desirable from the perspective of a small group of trans people. No feminism worth its salt should be willing to make that trade.

6
Why Is Gender-Critical Feminism So Vilified?

There is an extraordinary amount of antagonism towards radical and gender-critical feminists. It stands in need of explaining. In 2020, J. K. Rowling was viciously attacked across social media, oftentimes with the worst misogynistic slurs, for stating that sex is real and matters.[1] She is the most high-profile target of abuse, but her targeting is illustrative of the targeting of gender-critical feminists in general. After giving some more detailed examples of how gender-critical feminists are treated, I will offer three explanations for this antagonism.[2] The first is that the gender-critical position on trans issues has been associated with 'exclusion' in a way that links it to previous failures of feminism for which there is justifiable moral indignation and resentment. The second is that such antagonism is in at least some cases the natural expression of fundamental moral disagreement, because moral commitments generally come with strong feelings, and yet when they are 'basic' they cannot be argued for, which causes frustration that tends to spill over as hostilities. The third explanation is more cynical: the vilification of gender-critical feminism is politically propagandistic, a manoeuvre by lobbyists for the sex industry and activists for gender identity to demonize their opponents as a way of putting off potential supporters and so making political gains.

6.1 Antagonism towards Radical and Gender-Critical Feminists

Antagonism and hostility towards radical and gender-critical feminism and feminists is widespread, and not only from the places you might expect. It would be natural enough to expect it from anti-feminists, and from those conservatives who see the threat to traditional gender roles as either dangerous or wrong-headed. But in fact the main sources are not these

Gender-Critical Feminism: Holly Lawford-Smith, Oxford University Press. © Holly Lawford-Smith 2022.
DOI: 10.1093/oso/9780198863885.003.0006

groups, but rather other feminists, and others from the allegedly progressive left. This hostility shows up in academia, in activism, on social media, and even sometimes manifests as violence against radical and gender-critical feminist women. Dehumanizing language has long been linked to violence; at the time of writing there was increasingly widespread dehumanizing rhetoric against so-called 'TERFs' (trans-exclusionary radical feminists) and 'SWERFs' (sex-worker-exclusionary radical feminists), but few cases of violence. Many women fear that a rise in violence is likely to follow. Consider the following examples of hostility.

Vaishnavi Sundar is an Indian filmmaker who spent three years creating a documentary about workplace sexual harassment, interviewing women from across all strata of Indian society. In a podcast interview with Meghan Murphy for *Feminist Current*, she says that the roadblocks she encountered in getting help from other feminists in India were immense. They refused to help connect her with women to interview, they refused to help her crowdfund, and later, when the documentary was finished, they refused to help her find places to screen it.[3] A screening of the film in New York was cancelled a week before the event. Why? Sundar is a women's rights activist. She says 'I spend my time advocating for equal opportunities, contraceptive rights, education and the empowerment of women and girls. I centre women in all my work.' Her film, *But What Was She Wearing?*, was the first feature-length documentary on workplace sexual harassment in India.[4] Surely she is exactly the kind of person who other feminists should be throwing their support behind.

The answer is that Sundar is a threat to the dominant form of feminism, being not just a heretic, but an apostate. She *did* subscribe to its perspective, but she saw problems and she talked about them, and eventually she repudiated that type of feminism entirely and became a radical feminist. Sundar doesn't pull any punches about that fact, recently describing culturally dominant feminism (she says 'liberal feminism', but we mean the same thing) in an article for *Spiked* as 'a cult that extols men, who are often not really "queer" but who want to take advantage of "self-identifying" as a woman in order to gain oppression points and external validation.'[5] She was openly critical on Twitter about the politics of gender identity, including raising questions about whether transwomen should be allowed to compete in women's sport, be housed in women's prisons, or use women's changing rooms.[6] The New York organizers of her film screening cited her 'transphobic views' as the reason for cancelling the event.[7] Sundar says 'I was simply not the right flavour of woke for the postmodern, queer-theory espousing desis[8] of Manhattan.'[9]

At a Vancouver event on gender identity and media bias, protesters expressed opposition to the panel, which featured Meghan Murphy (*Feminist Current*),[10] Anna Slatz (*The Post Millennial*), and Jonathan Kay (*Quillette*). One woman held up a cardboard guillotine—arguably a symbol of violence against women[11]—saying 'Step right up!' and down each side, 'TERFS' and 'SWERFS'.[12] Journalist Meghan Murphy was the woman being specifically targeted with the cardboard guillotine; first 'cancelled' in Canada for her views on prostitution and pornography, and later again for her views on transgenderism. While working for the Canadian online magazine *Rabble*, a petition was circulated to have her permanently deplatformed ('cease offering a platform for hate'), which included accusations of racism, bigotry, transmisogyny, whorephobia, and dehumanization of and disrespect for women.[13] *Rabble* later did an audit of her work and published a statement saying 'In our opinion, her writing is not transphobic or racist'.[14] Murphy holds views that would generally be described as radical feminist, although she does not use any particular label for herself.[15]

In *Being and Being Bought*, Kajsa Ekis Ekman writes about the cultural debate over prostitution '[t]here is hardly a text written about "sex workers" that doesn't vilify radical feminists; it doesn't even seem possible to tell the story of sex work without an introductory tirade about radical feminists who think that all prostitutes are victims and who prevent anyone else from speaking'.[16] She notes further that 'these tirades never include a definition of what radical feminism is, though; it is always portrayed by way of sweeping generalizations as an extreme approach: dogmatic, man-hating and sex-hostile'.[17]

This is something I noticed about the media debate over changes to the understanding of sex in the law, which were billed as positive for transgender people and inconsequential for women. Radical feminists were generally vilified, but no one writing the articles ever seemed to be able to say what radical feminism actually was, and actually answer the concerns that radical feminists have about the proposed reforms. Caricature and misrepresentation were rife. For example, in a piece for *The New York Times* in 2019, Sophie Lewis introduced her topic by talking disapprovingly about two British gender-critical feminist activists, Kellie-Jay Keen-Minshull (better known as Posie Parker) and Julia Long, then claiming 'The term coined to identify women like Ms. Parker and Dr. Long is TERF, which stands for Trans-Exclusionary Radical Feminist. In Britain, TERFs are a powerful force'.[18] At no point in the article are we told what this radical feminism—alleged to be trans-exclusionary—*is*. One could be forgiven for assuming that it's *about* excluding trans people, which, I've already argued, it isn't.

Lewis finishes her article by mentioning that Keen-Minshull spent time at the Heritage Foundation while in the United States.[19] Why bother trying to characterize the political, moral, and intellectual disagreement, when you can just namedrop a conservative boogie-monster and let that do the work of letting everyone know which side they should be on? Or in another *The New York Times* piece in 2019, Carol Hay does not bother to say what radical feminism is, but uses the slur 'TERF' throughout, and says she considers radical feminist Janice Raymond's 1979 book on transsexualism to be 'hate speech'.[20] Again, anyone reading this piece might think that radical feminism is all about excluding trans people. Again, it isn't.

Katelyn Burns, writing for *Vox*, does at least attempt to explain radical feminism, but she throws in a heavy dollop of misrepresentation when she writes of radical feminists who do not 'support trans women' that 'They now prefer to call themselves "gender critical", a euphemism akin to white supremacists calling themselves "race realists"'.[21] *What?* White people are *the* dominant social group when it comes to race, *and* 'races' have been shown not to be the precise biological categories they were at one time believed to be. White supremacists calling themselves 'race realists' in order to justify discrimination against people of colour is ignorant and propagandistic. For the parallel to gender-critical feminism to hold up, gender-critical feminists would have to be a dominant social group when it comes to sex/gender, the concept of sex would have to be based on outdated science, and calling ourselves 'gender-critical' (a name we chose for ourselves) rather than 'trans-exclusionary radical feminists' (a name made up by our opponents) would have to be a euphemism for *what we really are*.

Given that we're into the sixth chapter of a book about gender-critical feminism, it probably barely needs explaining that gender-critical feminists are not a dominant social group when it comes to sex/gender, we're part of a subordinated social group: women. The concept of sex is not based on outdated science, despite what a few academics desperate to be on 'the right side of history' may write in the opinion sections of prominent science journals.[22] And finally, we don't call ourselves 'trans-exclusionary radical feminists' because, as I have already said, gender-critical feminism is not *about* trans people. It has implications for trans people, in that it includes transmen and not transwomen. But those implications fall out of its larger feminist analysis, and are only important because they come into conflict with gender identity activism, which is currently enjoying widespread institutional power.[23] Our calling ourselves 'gender-critical' is not a euphemism for anything. Rather, the new generation of radical feminists tend to self-describe as gender-critical rather than radical in part to carve themselves some space to do things differently without being accused of getting radical feminism wrong. It's not surprising that when high-profile venues like *The New York Times* and *Vox* publish claims like these, an under-informed public end up siding with transwomen-including feminists and gender identity activists, and trans people themselves begin believing that they are under siege from parts of the feminist community.

It is unlikely that Yale philosopher Robin Dembroff labours under false beliefs about what gender-critical feminism is. Their (Dembroff identifies as nonbinary) representation of gender-critical feminism is strongly political in character. For example, in their recent reply to Alex Byrne's journal article 'Are Women Adult Human Females?',[24] Dembroff says '"woman are adult human females" is a political slogan championed by anti-trans activists, appearing on billboards, pamphlets, and anti-trans online forums'. Later they say 'Conservative groups insist that "there are only two genders", and that "a woman is an adult human female"; liberal groups claim that "trans women are women" and that "gender is not binary"'.[25] In the second sentence, Dembroff packages two sets of claims together which need not go together, and characterizes the first set as 'conservative' and the second set as 'liberal'.

In fact the slogan—which is actually 'woman: adult human female'[26]—originated with left-wing or 'politically homeless' women. ('Politically homeless' is a self-description used by women who are alienated by the left's uptake of identity politics and failure to advocate for women's issues, and who feel that there is no party that adequately represents them.)[27] The slogan has been used as part of a thriving resistance movement in the UK made up of mostly left-wing and trade unionist women. In Australia, *all* of the radical and gender-critical feminists I am networked with (a little under 600 women), self-describe as left-wing or politically homeless, and most endorse the slogan.

Dembroff is making an *affective* move here, which works first by packaging the claim about the gender binary together with the 'adult human female' claim, making it impossible to disagree with the one without the other so a reader feels compelled to reject both; and second by associating the two claims with 'conservatives' in readers who are likely to identify with left-wing politics, so that they think of the issue in polarized terms. '*We* reject the gender binary and a biological understanding of womanhood', the reader is supposed to think. '*They* do not'. But the two claims are not a package. Gender-critical feminists don't think gender is identity, but if they did they'd probably agree that there are more than two such identities (personalities). That would put them on the 'liberal' side in Dembroff's pairings: 'gender is not binary'. Gender-critical feminists think gender is a set of norms, and that there are two sets of norms. That would seem to put them back on the 'conservative' side in Dembroff's pairings: 'there are only two genders'. But if 'there are only two genders' refers to sets of norms, then it is false that conservatives believe this. For conservatives (or 'gender traditionalists'), gender is a set of innate traits determined by sex. So *conservatives* are not 'conservative' on this pairing.

There are at least three senses of 'gender' operating in Dembroff's sentence: a set of innate traits determined by sex (conservative), a set of social norms attached to sex (gender-critical), and gender as identity (trans activist). The meaning of a term should be held fixed across its use in a sentence or paragraph, but if 'gender' is held fixed in Dembroff's claim, using any one of those three senses, then what that claim says is false. The ambiguity creates plausible deniability. Pairing the claims means a negative reaction against one (*we disagree with conservatives!*) can be exploited to elicit a negative reaction against the other (*I guess we must disagree that women are adult human females, too*). This is the same type of strategy Kajsa Ekis Ekman describes being used by pro-prostitution feminists, who use particular words in describing prostitution that associate it in the reader's mind with luxury and status, thus obscuring the realities of what prostitution really is.[28]

Twitter has exacerbated this situation by introducing a 'Hateful conduct' policy intended to protect the participation of marginalized groups, but which has the actual effect of constraining open debate between feminists (and between feminists and other left-wing activists) and silencing one part of it. While the letter of the policy specifically includes prohibition of 'deadnaming' (using a transgender person's pre-transition name) and 'misgendering' (using sex-based pronouns to refer to a transgender person),[29] the policy appears to have been interpreted more widely, resulting in suspensions and bans from Twitter for people making claims about biological sex in dialogue with or about transgender people. The upshot is that feminists cannot use one of the world's most prominent open platforms for debate in order to advance or explore claims about the reality of biological sex as distinct from gender identity; the meaning of the words 'woman' and 'female' and 'lesbian' and 'mother', etc., if those don't include transwomen; or the meaning of the terms 'woman' and 'female' if those attach to sex rather than gender identity. I don't think progressive people should endorse these restrictions on debate, particularly as they conflict with and threaten to set back the women's rights movement. But before almost any of that discussion could be had, Twitter's policies have made particular feminist views practically unsayable on their platform.[30] This has the further effect that media outlets can report in shocked tones of people like Meghan Murphy (and me, for that matter) that we've been 'banned from Twitter for violating its hateful conduct policy',[31] without explaining what the hateful conduct policy is, whose interests it serves, and how many women are routinely silenced on its basis.

At an event I attended in Edinburgh in June 2019 on the future of women's sex-based rights, radical feminist speaker Julie Bindel was subjected to an attempted assault by a transwoman who uses the name 'Cathy Brennan',[32] who had been part of a protest against the event. Bindel says 'he was shouting and ranting and raving, "you're a fucking cunt, you're a fucking bitch, a fucking Terf" and the rest of it. We were trying to walk to the cab to take us to the airport, and then he just lunged at me and almost punched me in the face, but a security guard pulled him away'.[33] Bindel makes the point that this is not an isolated incident in which sole responsibility for the attempted assault lies with the perpetrator. Rather, she says, it was made more likely by the climate at the University of Edinburgh in the lead-up to the event. The day of the event, all twelve members of the university's staff pride network committee resigned after the university intervened on their vocal public criticism of the event, asking them to 'support the university... or be quiet'.[34] Bindel says 'I think the lecturers and other staff who stoked the flames of this by calling women bigots and fascists and Nazis because we were holding an event to discuss women's rights, should take responsibility for this'.[35]

The perpetrator had some time earlier incited violence against radical and gender-critical feminist women (those most frequently targeted by the term 'TERF') by tweeting 'any trans allies at #PrideLondon right now need to step the f**kup and take out the terf trash. Get in their faces. Make them afraid. Debate never works so f**k them up'.[36] And on another occasion, in reply to criticism, 'I am a member of the trans community and we are already in danger. Rather than blame me for endangering the trans community we should be seeking to deplatform the GC [gender-critical] movement which has fostered this hostile environment. *By any means necessary*'.[37] In the aftermath of the attempted assault, some criticized Bindel for 'misgendering' her would-be assailant,[38] this fact apparently being more significant that the fact that there had been an attempted assault on a feminist by a male, after a talk on violence against women, in the name of trans rights activism. Brennan was cautioned and charged with threatening and abusive behaviour by Police Scotland.[39]

In 2017 there was also an incident of violence after a meeting titled 'We Need to Talk about Gender' in Hyde Park in the UK.[40] Gender-critical feminist Maria MacLachlan, a 60-year-old woman, was kicked and punched to the ground by trans rights activists, in addition to having her camera smashed and its memory card stolen.[41] One of her assailants, transwoman Tara Wolf, was convicted of assault for the crime, and fined £430 in fines and court costs. Wolf was found guilty of 'assault by beating'.[42] Jen Izaakson writing for *Feminist Current* describes the bizarre atmosphere of the court case, in which Wolf was accompanied by twenty-four people, mostly anarchist men dressed in all black, three with fighting dogs, and the group carrying a sound system playing loud death metal.[43] One of the four witnesses who testified in Wolf's defence admitted to working to get the feminist meeting's original venue cancelled, and said 'TERFs hate trans people', 'TERFs are fascists', and 'TERFs are a danger to queers'.[44] This is interesting because it reveals that the media and popular misrepresentation of what it means to be a radical or gender-critical feminist (slurred with the term 'TERF') is actually feeding into a climate of fear and hostility in which male violence against women is perversely rationalized as self-defence. *They hate us, so we are justified in hurting them*, goes the thought.

This is far from an exhaustive catalogue of the ways that radical feminists have been treated by other feminists and by people who see themselves as progressives (anarchists, environmentalists, anti-racists, trans rights activists). Antagonism against radical feminism is real, and has very real consequences, from a chilling effect on feminist speech, through impacts on women's careers and livelihoods, to psychological health impacts in managing the stress of protest and vilification, to physical violence. *Why*, though, is there so much antagonism? On the face of it, these are groups that surely agree about a lot more than they disagree about. Moreover, the antagonism is asymmetric. It's not just that within social movements there are warring sub-groups and in some cases they can behave in absolutely vile ways towards each other. That would be less surprising. Attempts at silencing, cancelling, shunning, inciting violence, damaging careers and livelihoods, slurring, etc., are directed by some feminists, and by trans rights activists, sex worker rights activists, and other supposed 'progressives', at radical and gender-critical feminists; but *not* generally by radical feminists at other types of feminists and those in the groups just mentioned. In general, radical and gender-critical feminists are fighting for the right to speak at all. What explains this rather strange situation?

6.2 'Exclusionary' Feminism

In *Who Stole Feminism?* Christina Hoff Sommers talks about attending the National Women's Studies Association (NWSA) conference in Austin, Texas, in 1992:

> Being aggrieved was a conference motif. The keynote speaker, Annette Kolodny, a feminist literary scholar and former Dean of the Humanities Faculty at the University of Arizona, opened the proceedings with a brief history of the 'narratives of pain' within the NWSA. She reported that ten years ago the organization almost came apart over outcries by our lesbian sisters, that we had failed adequately to listen to their many voices. Five years ago, sisters in the Jewish caucus had wept at their own sense of invisibility. Three years later the disability caucus threatened to quit, and the following year, the women of colour walked out. A pernicious bigotry, Kolodny confessed, persisted in the NWSA. Our litanies of outrage overcame our fragile consensus of shared commitment, and the centre would no longer hold.[45]

Kolodny was attesting to a history of fragmentation in the NWSA: the lesbian caucus, Jewish caucus, disability caucus, and women of colour caucus had all aired grievances with the organization over the years. Note that the content of these grievances might have had to do with recognition and respect *within* the NWSA (which is to do with the relations between women within a particular women's group), and might have had to do with uptake of specific caucuses' interests within the aims, goals, and projects of the NWSA (e.g. in curriculum design or design of conference themes). This is an important distinction. Feminism can be accused of being 'exclusionary' either because the theorists who create it, or activists who practice it, have exclusionary attitudes or practices or because their focus excludes particular goals or projects.

Set aside the actual content of the caucuses' grievances for a minute, and imagine a way that things could have gone. Suppose, for the sake of argument, the lesbian and Jewish caucuses were making claims relating to being gay women and being Jewish women, while the disability and women of colour caucuses were making claims relating to being disabled and being black (or people of colour).

First, consider two complaints related to the women's studies curriculum. Suppose the lesbians thought that teaching on workplace sexual harassment was overly focused on women who conform to feminine gender stereotypes, and left as invisible the harassment of butch and masculine women. And suppose the Jewish women thought that teaching on marriage overlooked issues impacting Jewish women, particularly the Jewish religious law requiring a *get* (a document which must be presented by a husband to his wife in order to initiate divorce). This religious law permits men to keep women 'chained' in bad marriages (she cannot remarry, and the laws of adultery still apply to her). Imagine that in both cases, the accusations are presented in an antagonistic way: the lesbian and Jewish women are hurt and frustrated that their issues are never front and centre; and the straight and atheist (and other religious) women are defensive and embarrassed. But eventually it is agreed that these grievances are entirely justified, and the women of the NWSA vow to do better when it comes to gay women's and Jewish women's issues.

But now imagine that soon afterwards—with the women of the NWSA still reeling a little from the realization that no matter how progressive and inclusive of 'all women' they feel, they still make big, embarrassing mistakes—came complaints from two other caucuses, this time to do with conference themes. Suppose the disability caucus wanted a session on urban design and architecture, focused on the way that design and construction choices can lead to the exclusions of people with disabilities. And suppose that the women of colour wanted a session on institutionalized racism in education. I will argue in more detail in Chapter 7, Section 7.3 that if there are no sex differences when it comes to social group issues, then those issues are not within the scope of radical or gender-critical feminist theory or activism (its goals, aims, or projects). Supposing for the sake of argument here that I am right about that, then the disability and women of colour caucuses would *not* be justified in these grievances, because these are not feminist issues. (They are issues that affect some women, in virtue of their having disabilities or being people of colour, but that is not the same thing as their being feminist issues, or so I will argue later.)

The point I want to make here is that if these grievances are presented antagonistically, in much the same way as with the earlier groups, then we can imagine their being accepted more easily. After all, the women of the NWSA have now learned their lesson, and have a little more humility when it comes to their capacity to make mistakes. They are a little more deferential to women who are differently situated, and willing to hear their criticism. So instead of critically examining the content of the claims that the disability and women of colour caucuses are making, we can imagine that they simply wave them through. Indeed, taking time to critically examine them, rather than accepting the criticism and apologising immediately, may be seen as adding further insult to the injury of the original exclusion.

For all I know, the actual history of the NWSA was very different to this—perhaps all the caucuses' grievances were justified, perhaps none were. What actually happened inside the NWSA is not my main focus. The general point of the story I have imagined is that women accustomed to being accused of 'exclusion', particularly when they *actually were being exclusionary* and have learned from those mistakes, may be less critical about future accusations that share a similar pattern.

Here's Natalie Stoljar, explaining the exclusionary nature of feminism at one time: 'white middle-class feminism has developed a norm that is inapplicable to other *women*. Implicitly conceiving of all women as white and middle class, and developing a feminist politics on this basis, has excluded and ostracized other women to the extent that many now resist identifying with the feminist movement'.[46] Although 'white middle-class feminism' or 'white feminism' have become a frequent characterization of the second wave, it is worth noting the extent to which they may be overstated rather than simply accepting outright this narrative that feminism has been marked by exclusion.[47] There are many exceptions to this general characterization of feminism as white/exclusionary who are almost never acknowledged, such as Marilyn Frye in her essay 'On Being White: Toward a Feminist Understanding of Race and Race Supremacy',[48] or Gloria Steinem, who was known to insist on speaking alongside African American women, most often Flo Kennedy.[49] Even bell hooks, who has been one of the most outspoken critics of feminism's failure to fully integrate issues of race, seems to swing between blaming the low numbers of African American women in the American second wave on the racism and exclusion of white feminists,[50] and the more concessive acknowledgement that the opposition feminists created between themselves and men was difficult for black women, who were used to standing together with black men in confronting racism.[51]

So far, we have a partial explanation of how the agenda of feminism was broadened out, namely as a result of an increased sensitivity to accusations of exclusion. Feminists learned the important lesson that feminism must be for *all* women, not just some women. A succession of accusations of 'exclusion'—many of which were justified—established a general pattern in which feminists were open to criticism and committed to learning from their historical mistakes. But this created a situation in which they were not as vigilant as they might have been about *unjustified* accusations of exclusion. Women who have been marginalized within feminism may nonetheless present issues which are not strictly speaking feminist issues (on which more in Chapter 7), and people who are justifiably excluded from feminism, because they are not women, may present issues which feminists nonetheless take seriously because they appear to be structurally similar to other issues that they do take seriously. Prostituted women are marginalized, so when the collectives representing them say they want better workplace rights rather than campaigns to abolish prostitution, feminists may then be insufficiently critical about assessing how the demand of the group trades off against core feminist commitments. When transwomen showed up claiming that the feminist agenda was involved in 'trans(women's) exclusion', feminists acclimatized to charges of exclusion will have been primed to apologize and accommodate, rather than critically assess and potentially reject, their claims.

It is easy enough, given all this, to identify a source of antagonism towards gender-critical feminists. Women who are sensitive to the feminist capacity to exclude, or who belong to groups that feel themselves to be inadequately represented within feminism, will empathize with others claiming to be excluded. Claiming to represent the interests of prostituted women while working for policy solutions many of them actively repudiate will not look like appropriate deference. And on trans issues, because there is already disagreement over *whether* transwomen are women, due to the more basic disagreement about what it means to be a woman, some will view radical and gender-critical exclusion of transwomen as amounting to the exclusion of some women. In particular, feminists who think that gender is identity, who accept that we should generally prioritize the interests of the most marginalized women, and who believe the oft-repeated claim that trans people are the most marginalized social group (they are not),[52] will see transwomen as both a clear part of the constituency of feminism and a clear candidate for being prioritized within feminism. For those feminists, the gender-critical position is not just objectionable, it is repugnant. But it is important to remember that there is only 'exclusion' if those other matters are already settled, namely that transwomen are women; that we should prioritize the interests of the most marginalized women (rather than e.g. issues affecting the greatest number of women, or issues affecting some women in the worst ways); and that trans people are the most marginalized social group. None of those matters are in fact settled.

6.3 Fundamental Moral Disagreement

Sometimes moral disagreement is fundamental. It can happen that two people just can't get beyond the fact that ultimately they disagree. Is disagreement about what gender is, and so what it means to be a woman, like this?

In *On Certainty*, the philosopher Ludwig Wittgenstein put forward the idea of a 'hinge proposition'.[53] These are particular sorts of claims, specifically those where it is not possible to give further reasons in support of them. Ordinarily, the reasons we give to demonstrate the truth of our claims are stronger than the claim itself. For example, suppose I say 'this person is male', and then I am asked 'how do you know?' and I provide my reasons: 'his physique, his facial features, the pitch of his voice'. These reasons—referring to typical sex differences that are apparent in appearance and social interaction—are stronger than my initial assertion that the person is male.

But sometimes, the strongest reasons that we have are in the claim itself. In trying to defeat the sceptics who doubted everything including the existence of the external world, G. E. Moore asserted that he knew that he had hands. But although he can try to come up with things to say if he is asked how he knows *that*, Moore won't be able to come up with anything that's stronger. Or to put this another way, the plausibility of the reasons he can give, e.g. that he can see his hands, or feel them, will depend on the plausibility of his original claim to have hands, not the other way round.[54] But the job of reasons is to resolve doubts, and in order to do that, the reasons will need to be stronger than the original claim. Hinge propositions are the claims that cannot be supported by reasons (because no reasons are as strong as the claim itself) *and* yet that cannot be rationally doubted to be true. That Moore had hands is like this. But so is that the world has existed for a long time, and that 12 x 12 is 144.[55]

This idea is a bit stronger than what we need for the point I want to make in this section. It doesn't need to be that a person cannot rationally doubt a claim (which means, that if they were to doubt it they would be doing something irrational). But it does need to be that a claim is the 'end of the chain' when it comes to giving reasons. In the moral context, this is basically what moral philosophers like G.A Cohen refer to as fundamental moral values (principles, commitments), the things about which there can be fundamental moral disagreement, and that are at the end of the line once we exhaust a chain of 'why?' questions that might involve both empirical facts and moral principles, values, or commitments that are not fundamental.[56] Richard Rowland defines fundamental moral disagreements as disagreements that would persist even in ideal conditions, and says: 'I'll understand ideal conditions as conditions in which agents are fully informed of all the empirical and non-moral facts, are fully rational, are unaffected by cognitive biases, don't hold any conflicting beliefs, and have engaged in the very best reasoning processes about normative ethics'.[57]

Again, this is a bit stronger than we need. When moral philosophers talk about conditions like this they are usually trying to resolve the question of whether in an ideal world people would agree on moral issues, and it's just things like having biases, and being differently informed about the facts, that cause us all to disagree so much. But we don't need to resolve that question here. For our purposes, it's enough to note that when gender-critical feminists and our opponents disagree, there will be *some* cases of disagreement that are not explained merely by other things of the type Rowland lists. Rather, the end of the chain—the 'hinge proposition' in Wittgenstein's terms, the 'fundamental value' in Cohen's, and the 'fundamental moral disagreement' in Rowland's (with two of these ideas weakened appropriately)—is a moral disagreement about which it isn't possible to provide any further reasons or justifications. For simplicity, I'll refer to these as fundamental values.

A good example of a fundamental value is equality. A great many people are committed to this value and think for example that all humans are morally equal, and that this means we must work for equality between the sexes, and the races, and anywhere else where there is inequality without a good justifying explanation. Different people can be committed to the same fundamental value while having an ongoing discussion about what exactly it means, which is what we see in the discussion between moral philosophers over whether it should mean equality of outcomes, equality of opportunity, equality of recognition, or something else.[58] But if someone were to disagree, and say that they didn't care about equality and thought that instead *the best people* should have all the stuff (however they wanted to fill in the details of what makes you the best), there wouldn't be all that much we could say to them.[59]

While these fundamental commitments can't be argued for, they can be—and generally are—*felt*. Disagree with someone who is passionate about equality and expect for them to be angry with you, or even disgusted. Some, perhaps even many, people who discover that you do not share their basic value commitments will not be interested in having much more to do with you. This is part of the explanation of group polarization, where people tend to talk more with others who share their beliefs, which then reinforces those beliefs because there's no outside criticism coming in.[60]

Now all we need to explain the depth of feeling against gender-critical feminists is to notice that they *disagree with* particular fundamental values held by other types of feminists, gender identity activists, and other leftists. One such value is something like 'it is crucially important to respect people's self-identifications about sex/gender'.[61] Another is 'it is crucially important to respect women's choices about their bodies'. Yet another is 'priority should be given to the least-well off women' (where 'women' is transwomen-inclusive).[62] There is no arguing about these values, from some leftists' points of view. Many simply refuse debate.[63] If this is right, then what is being expressed by all the hostile and antagonistic rhetoric in this debate is no more or less than *we don't share the same values*.

Radical and gender-critical feminists can't stop asking questions at this point. It is not the 'end of the chain' *for us*. We value collective political self-determination, and so see blind acceptance of identity claims (at least supposing that they determine political inclusion) as a threat, not a value. We want to know why the importance of a woman's choices about her own body imply that we should care about *men's* choices to exploit women. We want to know why it would be out of the question to orient feminism around projects that are good for all or most women, rather than the worst-off women. We want to know why it is important to respect self-identification about sex/gender but not about any other axis of oppression (or why self-identification in every other case comes along with some material facts that make the identification justified, except in the case of gender). We want to know why 'inclusion' is given so much weight when there are other values that matter morally.

But asking these questions is generally met with moral outrage. In 2019, three leftist academics were so affronted by finding out they were featured on the same webpage as three gender-critical feminists (two academics and one journalist) that they *deplatformed themselves* by retracting their contributions. In a subsequent statement they wrote

> We considered our inclusion in the... 'debate' to have been a non-consensual co-platforming, for which we sought redress through the retraction of our contributions... We object... to any 'debate' that questions transgender people's fundamental legitimacy as people who are entitled to the same respect as any other person.[64]

For the record, none of the gender-critical contributions, which are still available, questioned the entitlement of transgender people to equal respect.[65]

This is roughly the kind of response we might expect from someone hearing that we do not care much for equality. But the fundamental values of these feminists are nowhere near as widely accepted. Encountering the pushback against radical and gender-critical feminists for the first time, you're likely to go one of two ways. If you happen to already share the values of those pushing back, then you're likely to perceive things in moralized terms and be morally appalled by gender-critical feminists. And if you don't share those values, you're likely to be left completely confused about the intensity of feeling coming from many feminists and other leftists over what seem like commitments that are somewhat plausible but certainly leave a lot to be discussed. Acting as though their values already enjoy the wide consensus of a fundamental value like equality is a way for those who disagree with radical and gender-critical feminists to strongarm the public discourse and subvert the usual mechanisms of open deliberation and consensus-building. New values need to be argued for, not stipulated.

6.4 Political Propaganda

In *How Propaganda Works*, Jason Stanley puts forward the view that there are two main kinds of political propaganda, 'supporting' propaganda and 'undermining' propaganda.[66] These are roughly what they sound like. Both are kinds of speech that sidestep rationality and use emotional or other non-rational mechanisms, the first to support or bolster particular ideals, the second to undermine or erode particular ideals. This speech might appeal to nostalgia, sentiment, fear, or other categories of affect (emotions or feelings).[67] An example of supporting propaganda is 'the use of a country's flag... to strengthen patriotism'.[68] Stanley thinks undermining propaganda is much more complicated than supporting propaganda, because it exploits existing 'flawed ideological beliefs'.[69] An example of a flawed ideological belief is 'the ideology of the corporate-funded anti-climate science movement', which can be exploited in undermining propaganda like the 'expertise' of someone working as a member of a climate change team yet 'declaring environmental concerns to be "junk science"'.[70] There is also a third type of propaganda, which Stanley refers to as 'technicist', which masks flawed ideology with scientific or technological language.[71] In a way, this can be understood as the inverse of 'supporting propaganda', in that instead of sidestepping rationality with emotion, it sidesteps emotion—where it would have been appropriate—with rationality.

It's easy enough to spot speech that sidesteps rationality. One recent example comes from Mark Lance, writing for *Insider Higher Ed*. Lance opens his essay by describing a 1702 'theological/philosophical reflection on the nature of the American continent and its inhabitants', which 'asserted that the heathen savages that Europeans had met here were probably put here by the devil, likely lacked souls, were more akin to beasts than humans and absolutely must be at least converted, and if not, removed (i.e. killed)'. His point is that in the context these remarks were made, namely 'the dawn of the 18th century, as a mass influx of Europeans are launching one of the largest campaigns of ethnic cleansing and genocide in human history', 'these remarks are violence. They are an endorsement of genocide and played a very real role in facilitating it'.[72] Lance then smoothly segues into the claim that 'Recently, a small but highly visible group of scholars has taken to arguing against the growing acceptance of the gender self-identifications of trans people'.[73] He's drawing a parallel between not affirming transgender people's identity claims, and *genocide*. Don't worry though!—he doesn't mean to suggest that what gender-critical philosophers are up to is '*as grim* as the genocide of Native Americans'. He says there are 'differences of quantity, and some of content' between that particular genocide and the gender debates.[74] Here emotional reactions to the thought of genocide are harnessed to build antipathy towards feminists.[75]

When this kind of tactic is used in support of the right ideals, then it is merely an example of 'supporting propaganda'. For it to be undermining propaganda, we'd need to establish a flawed ideology. But how do we decide what's a 'flawed ideology' and what isn't? For Stanley, a flawed ideology is a rationalization of undeserved privilege, likely to emerge in societies marked by injustice, particularly in the form of large material inequalities.[76] We know that there is exactly this kind of injustice between the sexes, so we can expect flawed ideology to emerge to protect threats to male interests. Assuming for the sake of argument that Stanley's accounts of both flawed ideology and propaganda are correct, do they help us to identify propaganda in the debates over the sex industry and trans/gender, and thus help to explain the apparent animosity against the gender-critical position on both?

Kajsa Ekis Ekman's book *Being and Being Bought* contains an extremely helpful set of explanations of how so many people have ended up supporting the sex industry, a particularly surprising change when it comes to feminists, who were generally united in fierce opposition to pornography during the second wave of feminism.[77] The first move was to distort the meaning of 'victim'. To be a victim is to have something unjust done to you by another. It is perfectly compatible with your exercising agency. For example, suppose you are confronted by a mugger, who points a blade at you and demands your wallet and jewellery. You can exercise agency by making the judgement that being stabbed is worse than being robbed, and so decide to hand over the goods. In being mugged, you have been made a victim, but you also exercised agency throughout the mugging. Ekman explains that pro-prostitution lobbyists have deliberately conflated the concept of 'victim' with ideas like being weak, passive, powerless, helpless. This makes it easy to argue that prostituted women are *not* victims, by demonstrating that they exercise choice and agency at various junctures. Prostituted women choose to sell sex, in order to make money. So they can't be victims.[78] This gets us on the path to the contemporary 'empowered woman' archetype of the prostituted woman.

Next, we get a commodification-inspired dualism where what is sold is turned into a product, which in turn allows those thinking about prostitution to abstract away from what is actually being bought and sold. First it was 'sex' that was being sold, a *product*; then it was 'sexual services', a *service*. This allows us to have a discourse about prostitution and pornography without talking about how 'sex' and 'sexual services' differ as products from most other things in the marketplace. Ekman reports on a conversation she had in Barcelona with a woman called Maria who worked in escort prostitution, who used the following example. When you are a chef, the product is *food*, and you can create it and have the waiters deliver it to the client. You don't need to like what you're cooking, you never need consume it yourself, and you need not ever interact with the people who *are* eating it. 'The chef can be a vegetarian and still prepare meat; s/he does it because it is their job'.[79] With prostitution, on the other hand, it 'is as if the chef were forced to sit down and eat with all the patrons and say that it was delicious, that it was the best meat s/he had ever eaten, even if they were a vegetarian'.[80] This obfuscation of what is actually being sold, namely the intimate use of one's own body, one's own self, serves the interests of those who wish to continue to use or profit from the sex industry.

But it is even more complicated than that. For it is not only that this is a convenient way for the discourse around prostitution and pornography to be reshaped from the perspective of consumers and other beneficiaries, but that sex workers themselves will tend to talk this way to preserve their own dignity, and this will mean that feminists committed to *listening to sex workers*, at least those feminists who don't have an understanding of what this kind of talk actually means, may end up buying into it. As interview-based research shows, prostituted women tend to distance themselves from what they are doing, they refuse to kiss, they mark parts of the body as off-limits to the client, they refuse to perform particular acts, they adopt fake names, they retreat 'into the head' while their bodies are being used.[81] This is an attempt to distinguish the 'body', the thing being prostituted, from the 'self', the thing the women are trying to protect through these various manoeuvres. Many prostituted women have 'somatic dissociative syndrome', which means they can no longer feel certain parts of their bodies.[82] On the basis of interviews with 854 prostituted women[83] across nine countries, researchers found that 68 per cent of 827 met the criteria for post-traumatic stress disorder,[84] and that prostituted women's symptoms were in the same severity range as combat veterans, battered women, rape survivors, and refugees from state-organized torture.[85]

When a feminist is committed to *listening to sex workers*, and she hears them say 'it's not me, it's just my body', she may need to go a little further than just hearing that and thinking *I guess prostitution is fine! Sex work is work!*—and consider what it could mean to separate 'me' and 'my body'. When she finds out it means that the 'work' is so repugnant and damaging to the 'worker's' dignity that she must take steps to distance herself from it, and that this may end up causing psychological damage, e.g. disassociation, in the long-term, she may need to revisit her commitment to 'supporting sex workers' by advocating for the prostitution industry.

Still, if we're going to blame anyone, we should start with the men who buy sex and buy the watching of sex that is bought for other men, the third parties who traffick and pimp women for other men to buy or watch being bought, and anyone else who profits from this industry which involves massive amounts of female suffering.

Are these three moves—conflating victimhood with passivity, presenting a man's use of a woman's body as a 'product' or 'service', and advancing the idea that we should defer to someone who has a self-protective reason to deflect—propagandistic? They certainly pretend to uphold ideals, like respect for a woman's agency, respect for market transactions, and respect for testimony or 'lived experience'. Do they undermine those ideals while pretending to uphold them? Do they exploit a flawed ideology? It's not hard to locate the flawed ideology, given the thousands of years of women's sexual subordination to men, which secures for men women's sexual service. Flawed ideology is likely to emerge to rationalize the sexual privilege men have, in the form of claims about what women want or what's good for women. And indeed it looks like it has; by waxing lyrical about 'agency', 'choice', and 'deference', these speech acts in fact undermine respect for women's choice, agency, and lived experience, and perpetuate sexual inequality.[86] The clinical descriptions of selling sex as a 'product' or 'service' are good examples of technicist propaganda.

Is the same true in the case of feminist uptake of gender identity ideology? One transgender philosopher seems to have seen the potential for a similar explanation, and attempted to get ahead of it by accusing gender-critical feminists of propaganda before they could accuse gender identity activists (and the feminists who support them) of it. Transgender philosopher Rachel McKinnon (who currently goes by 'Veronica Ivy'), a well-known advocate for transwomen being permitted to compete in professional women's sports, had a brief symposium piece[87] published in the journal *Philosophy and Phenomenological Research* in 2018 which claimed that in the corpus of 'TERF propaganda' are claims like:

> trans women are not, and never could be, women. At best, they're deluded men, playing at womanhood—or perhaps they're 'constructed' females, but not authentically female. Moreover, trans men are really women, deluded by the patriarchy into abandoning masculine (often butch dyke) *female* identities. This is the heart of the TERF (flawed) ideology.[88]

Radical and gender-critical feminists assert that the word 'TERF', which McKinnon uses freely, is a slur.[89] McKinnon says that *the claim that 'TERF' is a slur* is itself propaganda. If McKinnon has things right, then we're to believe that the claim that gender norms constrain male and female people in different ways, and the claim that we should keep our focus on these norms in order to free people—women in particular—from domination, are 'flawed ideology' because they do not immediately cede ground to the claim that gender is identity. This allegation is made in face of ample empirical evidence for the existence of gendered social treatment.[90]

The tactics that are used within gender identity activist and gender identity activist-supporting feminist rhetoric are much better candidates for being propaganda than are the radical and gender-critical feminist attempts to grapple with them. The most significant of these is pronouns. As a result of extravagant social media dogpiling, petitions, open letters, and the like, it has become a common perception that 'misgendering' is a morally egregious thing to do to a trans person. 'Misgendering' (more accurately, 'mis-pronouning') involves referring to a trans person by sex-corresponding pronouns rather than pronouns that refer to their gender identity, for example calling a transwoman 'he' rather than 'she'. Is misgendering morally egregious?

It might have been, *circa* the roughly thirty years 1960–1990 when there were small numbers of transsexual women many of whom had generally experienced severe and distressing gender dysphoria during feminine boyhoods, and most of whom transitioned surgically—which signals a very serious commitment, and for whom it would be psychologically painful to be denied recognition, or for it to be made evident that other people do not see them as they see themselves. But as discussed in Chapter 5, the community of people who count as 'trans' today is much broader, and contains people with none of this history. It even contains people who say explicitly that they are nonbinary *for political purposes*, as a way of 'dismantling . . . [the] gender system'.[91] It is just not plausible that people who are trans for political purposes, or who have been swept up in the social contagion of gender identity ideology, are seriously harmed by misgendering. It *is* plausible for the people who would have counted as trans on the older diagnostic criteria (i.e. who are transsexual). According to the figures in Chapter 5, that might be as few as 12 per cent of the current cohort. The question then becomes whether the hurt experienced by this much smaller group is a sufficient reason not to 'misgender'. If there were no countervailing reasons, then I think it would be. But there are.

These claims by activists have led to a widespread perception that misgendering is morally egregious, and that makes it very hard to do it. But 'misgendering' is accurately referring to sex, and the ability to accurately refer to sex can matter a lot. For example, female athletes in Connecticut recently initiated a court case to challenge transwomen's participation in their sporting category (which was permitted on the basis of identifying as female). The plaintiffs and their counsel referred to the transwomen athletes as 'male athletes' or 'males', and the court reprimanded this language and said that it was 'needlessly provocative', and that 'transgender females' should be used instead because that was 'consistent with science, common practice and perhaps human decency'.[92] A judge in the UK in late 2019 decided that referring to a trans person by their sex might be 'incompatible with human dignity', especially in cases where that person has a Gender Recognition Certificate.[93] But as soon as you're forced to talk about 'trans female athletes', it sounds a lot like one set of women showing prejudice towards another.[94] When we're trying to oppose the sending into a female prison of a male person who murdered and mutilated their girlfriend and we're forced to do this referring to them as 'she' or 'her',[95] or when we're trying to talk about male overrepresentation in politics and trying to defend female-only shortlists but forced to refer to a transwoman candidate as a 'woman' or as 'female', or we're trying to explain how women in rape shelters need to be away from men but we're made to refer to 'transwomen', the points become much, *much* harder to make. And that may be why activists for transwomen's inclusion in women's spaces are so insistent about that language.

If we're talking about a group of *women*, then picking up on the fact that some are trans to justify not letting them compete in women's sport, or not be housed in the women's prison estate, or not be elected to a women's officer position, or not be admitted to a rape shelter, looks like 'punching down'.[96] It may look like we're finding a further disadvantaging feature that some women have and then discriminating (by attempting to exclude) on the basis of it. But feminism is not supposed to be for *some* women, it's supposed to be for *all* women. As Jennifer Saul writes, in opposition to gender-critical feminism, 'I hesitate to attach the label feminist to any view that is committed to worsening the situation of some of the most marginalized women'.[97] It is this kind of reasoning that allows the parallel to past acts of exclusion or failure of consideration by more privileged women towards more marginalized women (as explained in Section 6.2). Middle-class white feminists haven't been sufficiently inclusive of lesbian women, black women, women with disabilities, or Jewish women in the past; isn't this just another example of (some of) them failing to be sufficiently inclusive of transwomen?

Except that it isn't, because we don't all agree that we're talking about a group of women. We're disagreeing about what it takes to be a woman, with some of us saying that it takes being a female person and therefore being a member of the class of persons to whom feminine gender norms have been systematically applied, and others of us having accepted the criterion of self-identification as a woman. Then on the basis of that disagreement, some of us are classing transwomen as male/men, and others of us are classing transwomen as female/women. *Only* if it's true that transwomen are female/women, which means *only* if it's true that gender is identity and nothing else, is it reasonable to consider attempts to exclude transwomen from women-only spaces, services, and provisions as discriminatory. But the enforcement of 'progressive' language choices, that transwomen must be referred to as 'women' not men, and must be referred to as 'she' and 'her' rather than 'he' and 'him', attempts to settle that argument in advance, because it implements the language of one side.[98] Twitter is perhaps the most prominent enforcer of this language, but it has been adopted across many (if not most) media outlets. (You may wonder why I have used this kind of language myself at some points in this book. I was asked to by my publisher.)

All of this is propagandistic. The social injustice consists in the norms of femininity that are imposed upon female people to channel them into the service of men; the idea that women are for *others*, particularly men and children, not for themselves; that refusing to centre men or service men is a violation of a right that men have. This can be expected to produce a flawed ideology in which men rationalize their own domination, for example seeing non-conforming women (in this case, radical and gender-critical feminist women) as selfish, exclusionary, hateful. Because those women are *bad* and *wrong*, it's justifiable that they be ignored, and even censured. It becomes possible to claim that *they're* the ones with the flawed ideology, *they're* the ones making propagandistic claims, when they say something as simple as that it's not possible to change sex, or that sex matters politically. It's propaganda with a side of gaslighting.

The institutional enforcement of the language of one side distorts the ongoing argument by framing the entire issue as a conflict between women in which some are discriminating against others. But it isn't; it's a conflict between the sexes in which some are attempting to protect their sex-based rights. Dismissing women with legitimate political concerns as 'hateful', 'bigoted', 'racist', 'whorephobic', 'transphobic', and so on is just a convenient way to justify not listening to what they're actually saying, or having to engage with the substance of their arguments.[99]

6.5 Public Perception

The explanations presented in this chapter are not exhaustive, merely those I think are the most plausible and interesting. There is more to be said, in particular, about the way that attacks on radical and gender-critical feminists help to shore up in-group solidarity between feminists from different 'tribes'. The remaining challenge is for gender-critical feminists to find a way to show the public that these deeply emotional attacks are grounded in assumptions and values that are not widely shared, and that there is after all a conflict of interest between two social groups, which needs constructive public discussion and deliberation.

PART II

HARD QUESTIONS FOR GENDER-CRITICAL FEMINISM

7

Is Gender-Critical Feminism Intersectional?

Something strange happened to feminism during the later stages of the second wave. Instead of being focused on the rights, needs, and interests of female people as a class, 'feminism' became about all sorts of other issues not obviously connected to being female, or being female in a particular social and cultural context. Here's Phyllis Chesler, writing about Gloria Steinem: 'Over time, Gloria's brand of institutional and media iconic feminism was increasingly less about violence against women and more about racism, prison reform, climate change, foreign "occupations", and nuclear war—all important issues but not exactly "on message", or likely to appeal to women of all political persuasions.'[1] While this may have been unusual in the second wave, it is mainstream today. The @UN_Women Twitter account defined 'feminist' in January 2019 as 'a person who believes in & stands up for the political, economic, and social equality of human beings.'[2] This definition makes three amendments to the historical radical feminist line, where a feminist was *a woman* (men could only be allies) who stood up for the *liberation* (not merely equality with men on men's terms) of *women* (not of all human beings). On this modern retelling, feminism is for everybody and about social equality generally understood.

Is it a good thing that the definition of feminism has been transformed, from *a movement by women for the liberation of women* to *a movement by anyone for the equality of everyone*? That depends on whether the transformation is justified by good reasons. I suggested one explanation of the shift already in Chapter 6, Section 6.2, where I talked about the stream of accusations of 'exclusion' that made feminists less critical about what is and isn't a feminist issue, and relatedly, who is and isn't part of the constituency of feminism. But that explanation didn't amount to a justification, because it remains unclear whether the refusal to defer to sex workers about their preferred policy solutions and the refusal to accept transwomen as women and centre their issues are justified or unjustified.

Gender-Critical Feminism: Holly Lawford-Smith, Oxford University Press. © Holly Lawford-Smith 2022.
DOI: 10.1093/oso/9780198863885.003.0007

In this chapter, I'll suggest two further reasons to think the revised definition is a good thing. One is that the oppression of women is either caused by another, more fundamental, type of oppression or it is mixed together with another type of oppression at the foundations (Section 7.1). This means focusing on 'women's issues' is artificial, a kind of arbitrary privileging of one symptom out of many of a deeper disease. Redefining feminism as for everyone and about everything would then be a good thing, because it goes directly to the disease itself, the roots of all oppression that affect everyone.

The other reason to think the revised definition is a good thing is that feminism is about making women's lives better, not only *as women* but more generally *as people* (Section 7.2). This means we have a constituency of people we care about, but once we really consider what it would take to make the lives of those people better, we simply end up with a movement that is for (pretty much) everyone and about (pretty much) everything.

All of these ideas have something to do with the theory of 'intersectionality', which has become a key methodological commitment of *all* contemporary forms of feminism.[3] Disagreement about these three potential justifications—that feminism should be for everyone and about everything so as to avoid being exclusionary; that feminism should be for everyone and about everything so as to treat the root problem rather than a mere symptom of it; and that feminism should be for everyone and about everything because that's what it takes for it to do its job, which is to actually make women's lives better—is reasonable, in the technical sense sometimes used by philosophers to refer to disagreements in which two people can come to different conclusions even while both are competent and have engaged with the relevant considerations.[4] But I will argue that ultimately these justifications are mistaken. Considering them leaves us with a good understanding of *how we got to this point* in contemporary feminism, but they offer us no justification for thinking we got to the right point. On the contrary, they suggest that feminism has been undermined—by feminists themselves.

I will argue that women need to reclaim feminism, by refocusing on the idea of feminism as a movement for women *as women* (not *as people*) (Sections 7.3–7.4).[5] Gender-critical feminism is not inclusive (of men). It can be about women's oppression alone because it *is* possible to separate that from other forms of oppression. It is not intersectional in the sense of being interested in 'the whole person'. It is about *women's issues as women.* When gender-critical feminists talk about 'women', we certainly mean *all women*: black women, women of colour, women with disabilities, poor women, prostituted women, women exploited as surrogates, lesbian women, transmen, female nonbinary people. But the *as women* part is important too: for us, feminism is not concerned with the issues women with disabilities have in common with men with disabilities. Or so I shall argue.

Before I do that, a quick note of warning. The idea that feminism should be 'intersectional' has become virtually indistinguishable from the idea that feminism should be anti-racist. And because feminism (and every other social justice movement) should obviously be anti-racist, this makes it hard to escape the idea that it should be intersectional. As Jennifer Nash explains in *Black Feminism Reimagined*, 'debates about whether one is "for" or "against" intersectionality almost always seem to become referendums on whether one is "for" or "against" black feminism, and perhaps "for" or "against" black woman herself'.[6] So even if you are convinced by some of the ideas in this chapter, I wouldn't recommend simply announcing at the next meeting of your feminist activist group that you think the group should take the commitment to intersectionality out of its manifesto. Discussions on this topic will have to be approached with sensitivity about what they may be assumed to mean.

7.1 The Roots of Oppression

The concept of intersectionality, although it wasn't always referred to by that name, originated with black feminists.[7] Probably the first person to talk about it was Anna Julia Cooper in 1892.[8] Although it is commonly invoked across feminism today, it is rarely given a precise definition.[9] According to the International Women's Day Australia (IWDA) website, intersectional feminism is 'really just about acknowledging the interplay between gender and other forms of discrimination, like race, class, socioeconomic status, physical or mental ability, gender or sexual identity, religion, or ethnicity'. To make this point clearer, they explain 'the barriers faced by a middle-class woman living in Melbourne are not the same as those of a queer woman living in rural Fiji'.[10]

This makes sense: women experience inequality differently depending on the multiple and different ways in which they are discriminated against. But there's more packed into the word 'interplay' than you might glean from reading this sentence. After all, if it were merely that the queer woman living in rural Fiji also faces barriers as a result of homophobia or poverty, there would be absolutely no reason why feminism should be intersectional.

So long as there's a flourishing LGB (lesbian, gay, and bisexual) movement, and strong support for welfare provisions, we can expect such a woman to be served by independent social justice movements in a way that stands to represent all of her justice-related interests.

So what more might there be to the claim that there is an 'interplay' between different forms of discrimination? Cooper's claim was that race, class, gender, and region are *interdependent*.[11] The Combahee River Collective stated that 'the major systems of oppression are *interlocking*'.[12] Frances Beal and Deborah King thought the categories of gender, race, class, and sexuality were *mutually constitutive*.[13] Crenshaw claimed that 'the intersectional experience is *greater than the sum of* racism and sexism'.[14] Even the United Nations seems to have glommed on to this—the phrase 'multiple and intersecting forms of discrimination' is included four times in the agreed conclusions of the 61st Commission on the Status of Women.[15] All of these claims are slightly different, but together they get at something like the claim that sex discrimination cannot be considered on its own.

In her book *Feminist Theory*, bell hooks argues that 'all forms of oppression are linked in our society because they are supported by similar institutional and social structures, one system cannot be eradicated while the others remain intact'.[16] Taken literally, this means feminism as a movement for women's liberation is incoherent. You can't fight women's oppression alone, you can only fight the institutional and social structures that uphold all oppression. The conceptual point, that things which appear or are treated as distinct might all be connected, is true. For example, in *The Industrial Vagina*, Sheila Jeffreys notes that most of the academic and feminist literature on sexual exploitation which uses the term 'sex work', which signals ideological disagreement between feminists, tends to make distinctions between types of prostitution—e.g. child/adult, trafficking/prostitution, forced/free, legal/illegal, west/non-west.[17] But, she says, 'all these aspects of sexual exploitation depend upon and involve one another'. She establishes the case for that throughout the book. She is making the case that apparently distinct things are ultimately interdependent. The same could be true for all forms of oppression. The question is whether, in fact, it is.

Women's oppression is grounded in beliefs about natural female inferiority, and in expectations of femininity imposed upon female people. The idea that it is more worrying for a man with a family to lose his job than a woman with a family, because women are naturally better carers and men naturally better providers, is grounded in beliefs and expectations of this type. The content of these expectations is fairly specific: there is a whole set of norms of femininity, and a whole set of norms of masculinity, with not much overlap between them—and these can be articulated precisely enough to be the basis of psychological research.[18] What 'institutional and social structure' are these sets of norms linked into, and is it really *the same* as for racism, classism, and other forms of discrimination? This seems unlikely.

Some further insight can be gleaned from hooks' discussion of the family, which she thinks is the first site of domination for most people. Children witness the sexist domination of the mother by the father, and are thus 'primed to support other forms of oppression', including heterosexism (the domination of gay people by straight people).[19] Here, hooks seems only to be saying that sexism feeds into other modes of oppression, so that 'struggle to end sexist oppression that focuses on destroying the cultural basis for such domination strengthens other liberation struggles'.[20] But this doesn't sound any more like support for her claim that all forms of oppression are linked. It sounds like she thinks there's a sense in which sexism is *the first* form of oppression, and that getting rid of it would have positive implications for other forms of oppression. But this doesn't do anything to establish that all forms of oppression are supported by the same structures, or that one couldn't be eradicated without the others. Perhaps homophobia is partly supported by sexism, in that it is just another form of a social domination that was learned in the family home, but it still seems plausible that we could target homophobia directly and get rid of it without making a dent in sexism. That would be one being eradicated without the others.

When it comes to what the underlying structures are, hooks seems to have in mind 'the Western philosophical notion of hierarchical rule'.[21] She says that ideologies of group oppression 'can be eliminated only when this foundation is eliminated'.[22] But this is a rather extraordinary claim. Does hooks think there was no oppression prior to or outside of Western civilization? Surely not, given that women in ancient China clearly had a status subordinate to men's,[23] and that there was caste hierarchy in ancient India.[24] Perhaps she is not so much making a distinction between Western and non-Western societies, as maintaining that *all* societies have now integrated Western philosophical notions to do with hierarchy, and placing blame for domination at the feet of these notions. Again, this seems a little lavish: surely other traditions with their rich, long histories can lay claim to their own explanations of contemporary social injustice. Ultimately, the claim that there's a single unifying idea, 'the Western philosophical notion of hierarchical rule', and that this underpins *all oppression everywhere*, is an empirical one. hooks does not offer any evidence for it, beyond a citation to one philosopher.[25]

Without being able to resolve that empirical question here, a few comments from the armchair might still be helpful. Australia has made progress on workplace gender equality[26] and legalized gay marriage, but it still has not offered reparations to indigenous communities for stolen land or stolen generations. This looks like serious progress on the sex and sexual orientation systems of oppression, but not much progress on the race system. We can tell different stories about different countries, which are for various reasons better on some social justice issues and worse on others. Progress is not the same thing as eradication, so hooks may ultimately be right that we cannot *eradicate* one system of oppression without eradicating them all. But I am sceptical. If we can make serious differential progress, it would seem we can probably get rid of one and not others. So there is reason to think it's not true that all systems of oppression are linked.

If they *were*, we'd have a straightforward argument for intersectional feminism, understood as a theory which includes all the different ways that people can be oppressed. After all, if there's no separating one from the other we have no choice but to take them all if we want the one. The one we want is sexism, but the others would all come along with it. And if there's no eradicating one without the other, we have no choice but to work on them all by working on one. This seems to be hooks' understanding of, and vision for, feminism:

> To begin feminist struggle anew, to ensure that we are moving into feminist futures, we still need feminist theory that speaks to everyone, that lets everyone know that feminist movement can change their lives for the better... Feminist revolution is needed if we are to live in a world without sexism; where peace, freedom, and justice prevail; where there is no domination. If we follow a feminist path, this is where it leads.[27]

Gender-critical feminism denies virtually all of these claims. It might be true that feminism can change everyone's life for the better—I have said already that there will be *incidental* gains for other social groups. But it is not *feminism's* job to secure peace, freedom, justice, and no domination. These goals are too burdensome for a single social movement. Just as women do not have to be all things to all people, and are allowed to centre their own interests in their own lives, so too for their political movement. Feminism does not have to secure all goods for all people. It is allowed to centre the interests of its constituency, female people, in its own politics. Feminism is not for everybody and about everything, because the origins of patriarchal oppression are distinct from the roots of other kinds of oppression, and the mechanisms which sustain sexism and misogyny are different from those that sustain racism and ableism (e.g. norms of femininity applied to female people, like 'be warm, caring, nurturing, kind').

Not all gender-critical organizations *in fact* take this view. The radical feminist organization Women's Liberation Front (WoLF) in the United States, for example, seems to endorse bell hooks' understanding of the foundations of oppression. In their Statement of Principles from 2014, they give roughly the standard radical feminist line: female humans as a class are oppressed by male people as a class; patriarchy is organized around the extraction of resources from women by men; that gender is a hierarchical caste system and must be abolished. But they add a fourth point which is 'intersectional' in the way just described: 'we are enmeshed in overlapping systems of sadistic power built on misogyny, white privilege, stolen wealth, and human supremacism, and all of those must be dismantled'.[28] A radical feminist collective determined to abolish gender as a hierarchical caste system is going to struggle with that already momentous undertaking if it also sees as part of its remit racial equality, distributive justice, and animal liberation.

Among other things, WoLF also say they work to 'analyze and resist all systems of oppression, because until all women are free no woman is free'. That takes us into the next explanation, because it assumes that the project of feminism is to free women as people, rather than women as women.

7.2 Political Movement for Whole Persons

In a 1980 interview, black radical feminist Margo Jefferson made the following comment:

> I was worn out, I was exhausted, I seemed to have lost energy and interest in something called the black movement, in politics that means. And I began doing feminist theory and I said oh, it is possible for me to use every part of myself, and still be political. I don't have to say, well, that part of me is...is female and that's not important we don't have to talk about that. This part, as the exclusively black part, is fine; or this part, as the leftist part, you know and not the black part, is fine if I'm at a white leftist

> meeting. All of a sudden it was possible for me not to have to deny huge portions of myself to be politically active. And when I say 'me' you know I speak for—I suspect—most black women who encountered feminism.[29]

Jefferson's saying that feminism allowed her to be a 'whole person': she didn't have to separate the parts of herself into those that were relevant to these sorts of politics, and those that weren't; or to 'deny huge portions of' herself. Imagine how frustrating it would be, to be a black woman in the 1980s going to meetings of the black movement and being told that 'women's issues' weren't relevant, and going to meetings of the women's movement and being told that 'black issues' weren't relevant. It *would* be a relief to find a movement that accommodated both aspects of your experience.

This gives us a tempting reason to accept intersectional feminism, understood as a movement for women as 'whole persons'. This doesn't have to mean feminism is *for everyone*, it can still be for women, but it has to be for women in all their parts, not just women in some particular capacity, say *as women*, asking them to leave their race, their class, their disability, their religion, etc., at the door. On this view, feminism is a movement to make women's lives better. But there are lots of things that make women's lives go badly—not just women's issues, but all sorts of other issues too. So feminism is about much more than just women's issues in the narrow sense.

The problem with this is how it might change the scope of feminist activism. In Chapter 6 (Section 6.2), I made the distinction between the relations between women within feminist activism and the focus of feminist activism in terms of its goals, priorities, and projects. Certainly if most of the feminists in a particular activist group were middle-class and classist, this would create an obstacle to solidarity with working-class women in the group, and undermine effective working relationships between those sub-groups of women. But what if they weren't, or at least, everyone did the best they could and were receptive to criticism. Do feminists have reason to resist incorporating the goals, priorities, and projects of additional social groups that some of their constituency are members of? If feminism is a movement for women *as people* then the answer is 'no'. If feminism is a movement for women *as women* then the answer is 'yes'.

Here's the problem with answering 'no'. Suppose that we have a small group of women, and it's so diverse that it's almost like we designed it to showcase diversity (like the television show *Glee*). It contains only women, but it has a woman from every other socially, economically, or politically marginalized social group you can imagine. Some women are in only one other such group, others are in two, others are in three, and so on, for however many marginalized social groups we think there are. To give you a small selection, Adaeze is an international student in Australia from Nigeria, Hui-ju is a Taiwanese-Australian lesbian, Kirra is an Aboriginal Australian, Manaia is Maori with dual Australian and New Zealand citizenship and who is Christian, and Emma is a white Australian living with bipolar disorder. Now suppose that feminism is a movement for whole persons, and this means that all the issues that affect women are on the table as feminist issues.

That means all the following are feminist issues: *treatment/status of international students*, *immigration from Nigeria and New Zealand*, *religious rights and freedoms for Christians*, *treatment/status of lesbians*, *Taiwanese-Australian ethnicity*, *racism against Nigerian, Aboriginal, and Maori people*, *treatment/status of dual citizens*, and *treatment/status of those with bipolar disorder*. And the list goes on. For *every* woman in the group, added to the feminist agenda is *every* further marginalized social group membership she brings with her. This is enough of a problem when we're talking just about a particular feminist group in a particular city. Now imagine we're talking about feminism, the theory and the activism, globally understood. If this thing is a theory about all women and a movement for all women, and we understand this to mean women as persons rather than women as women, then suddenly virtually everything is a feminist issue. That's because for all the women that there are, they're going to be in virtually all of the further marginalized social groups. Notice that this also means that feminism is about an awful lot of men's issues too. There are autistic women. If feminism is about women as persons, then it's about autism. But if it's about autism, then it's about an issue that affects men too.

This helps to explain how we got not only to 'about everything' but also to 'for everyone'. If the only people left out of feminism are the small numbers of men who don't belong to any other marginalized social groups at all—the wealthy, white, heterosexual, middle-class, atheist, able-bodied, etc.—then it's barely worth making the distinction: 'feminism is for all women and most men but not all men!'. We could insist that feminism is only *for* women while being *good for* men, seeing the gains for autistic men, gay men, men with disabilities, black men, working-class men, religious men, etc., as incidental gains rather than the point and purpose of feminism. But this still leaves us with feminism being about virtually everything.

It's also not entirely clear why we'd call this thing 'feminism'. It doesn't, anymore, seem to have much to do with women, except that women were the starting point from which it collected all its issues. Given that such a social movement would be virtually indistinguishable from a generalized global justice movement, that would have the consequence of leaving a gap where a women's movement used to be. But women would still have all sorts of issues *as women* that deserved priority within a movement rather than just being one thing among many in a movement about everything. Women are one of the largest constituencies of marginalized people, within a country, and across the globe.

Reading 'women's liberation' or 'women's equality' to mean the liberation or equality of women as persons, rather than as women, gives us one explanation of how we might have ended up with a generalized social justice movement that, perplexingly, calls itself 'feminism'. If the explanation is right, then we still need a women's movement. This is not a merely verbal issue. It's not about what gets called 'feminism', it's that there needs to be *a theory and movement for women as a sex class.*

If we want to accommodate 'all the parts' of Jefferson, it seems we'll have to accommodate all the parts of all the other women too, and it's not clear how to stop this from over-burdening feminism with a million different issues. In the next section, I'll consider some ways that we might try to limit intersectionality in order to accomplish this.

7.3 Alternative Solutions: Limited Intersectionality

One way to try to retain the accommodation of 'whole persons' Jefferson spoke so enthusiastically about is to limit the social group memberships that are 'on the table' for addition to the feminist agenda. One obvious way to do that is to simply stipulate relevant groups. For example, bell hooks' early concern was with the intersection of race and sex,[30] as was Kimberlé Crenshaw's.[31] We could try to argue that this is the *only* relevant intersection, and so restrict intersectional feminism to race/sex. At least then it's only all the race issues, and all the women's issues, and all the issues where these two things meet, that are on the feminist agenda.

But what could the principled reason be to limit attention to the intersection of race and sex, when class is such a major system of oppression? Across different countries, race, sex, or class will be the major dividing line when it comes to disadvantage (arguably race in South Africa, sex in

Afghanistan, and class in the United Kingdom). Writing earlier than Crenshaw and hooks, Cooper talked about the interdependence of race, class, gender, and region;[32] and the Combahee River Collective talked about 'the major systems of oppression'.[33] Later, Spelman talked about race, sex, and class.[34] I can't see a way to justify the addition of the race/sex intersection without also defending the addition of the class/sex intersection. This might help a bit with the bloating of the feminist agenda, but *all* race and class issues (as they affect at least one woman) is still a massive addition.

Note also that both race and class have their own theory and movement: Marxism created theory and movement against class oppression (and determinedly refused to be hijacked by sex oppression),[35] and Critical Race Theory theorizes race oppression (as well as the more country-specific programmes like Black Studies, Indigenous Studies, etc.) while movements like Black Lives Matter advocate for social justice along racial lines. Why should feminism be any different? *Even if* there are 'intersections' between these major systems of oppression, we surely still need theory and movement of each major system, *and* we need to settle the question of how to accommodate their interactions too.

Another way to prevent bloating of the feminist agenda would be to think about the size of the social groups in question, and their proportion of the overall population of female people. While everything would technically be on the agenda, this would be a way to triage in order to get a narrower list of priorities. One of hooks' complaints against Betty Friedan's seminal text *The Feminine Mystique* was that she focused on bored housewives while 'more than one-third of all women were in the work force'.[36] If we cared about the size of the social groups, this would actually vindicate Friedan's approach: substantially many *more* women were affected by the predicament she outlined in her book. (This is compatible with hooks' main criticism, which is that she wrote in a way that suggested she was articulating the predicament of 'women' in general, rather than a specific group of women).

Let's think in more detail about how this would go. Take the group of all female people, then list separately all the social group memberships that are a source of disadvantage[37] for at least one such person, and then tally up how many members the group of female people with each such group membership has. Most women are women of colour. Most women are poor. Most women will not be able to protect themselves from the effects of climate change. Many women are uneducated. Some women are trafficked, or prostituted, or exploited in contract pregnancy. Some women are lesbians. And so on. Perhaps the 'intersections' that feminism should limit its attention to are just those that affect the largest numbers of women. That would seem like a reasonable approach—but what if it turned out that the issues affecting the largest numbers of women, e.g. the negative impacts of beauty norms, were less morally serious than those affecting much smaller numbers of significantly worse-off women, e.g. being exploited in contract pregnancy and prostitution? The number of women affected by different social issues is likely to work out quite differently in different places. Perhaps in a rich country the worst-off social group combinations will be women/cancer or women/infertility. In some countries, it will be a minority of women, not a majority, who have the woman/poor combination, and so this may not end up a priority.

An alternative, which solves that problem and still limits the feminist agenda, would be to think not about the size of the social groups but about how badly off they are. A 'prioritarian' (meaning priority-based) approach justifies focusing on the worst-off, so if a social group with a particular set of intersecting characteristics, for example poor/black/women were the worst-off then we could argue for giving them priority on those grounds. That would be true even if they were a very small proportion of the group of all women (although in this case they are not). Philosophers have tended to be sympathetic to prioritarian approaches, brought into prominence by John Rawls in *A Theory of Justice*,[38] and having particular uptake in the movement for 'effective altruism'. We can implement such an approach at the global level, in thinking about what the global priorities for feminist movement should be, and we can implement it at the national, state, and community levels too.

If we take this approach, questions about the fineness of description of social groups have to be addressed. 'Women' is a huge social group, making up half the population of the whole world. 'Black women' is a smaller social group, but it's still huge. 'Black lesbian women' is smaller, and 'black lesbian women with disabilities' even smaller than that. What is the right level of description when it comes to thinking about women's issues, and setting priorities for theory and activism? Many have pointed to 'fragmentation' as the death of social justice movements, including feminism,[39] so it's worth being wary about the possibility that with more complex social group descriptions we risk creating antagonism and in-fighting between sub-groups, over perceived difference, perceived status, and competition for resources. Uta Johansdottir put this point nicely: 'Intersectionality: A process of dividing ourselves by ever-more-parsed grievances, effacing our common humanity, until we are 7.6 billion factions-of-one calling each other toxic. It is the literal opposite of successful politics'.[40] To avoid that risk, we might choose to stay at very broad social groups, going only one or two levels deep (e.g. women; black women; women of colour; working-class women; poor women; disabled women; gay women; etc.).

One further problem with taking the approaches discussed so far is that we have only been thinking about the major and familiar social group memberships that bring disadvantage, like being gay or working-class. But what about all the other ways that women can be disadvantaged, for example by being: in a warzone; a refugee or migrant worker; unemployed; a survivor of childhood abuse; a survivor of sexual and/or domestic violence; prevented from unionizing in order to pursue her interests at work; adversely affected by health and safety issues at work; unable to afford the time off work she wants to spend post-pregnancy; unable to afford childcare when she wants to return to work; subject to discrimination on the basis of having a difference of sexual development (DSD); subject to risk of violence as a result of sex work; lacking opportunities in virtue of being uneducated; displaced as a victim of climate change harms?

These are not 'social groups' in the sense more familiar from what has come to be known as identity politics, but they *are* salient ways in which women can be made worse-off. Is there any reason to care about the groups we've talked about so far, and *not* these groups too? If not, we're back facing the problem of a hugely expanded feminist agenda.

The most serious problem with all of these ways of limiting the social groups in order to get a more manageable set of feminist issues is that we still haven't found a principled way to make sure feminism is focused on *women*. On the 'whole persons' approach it starts with women, but it soon ends up at (almost) everyone. We look at working-class women, we add class to the agenda, and then we end up working on lots of class issues that affect working-class *men* equally. We look at black women, and we add race to the agenda, and then we end up working on lots of race issues that affect black *men* equally. Feminism ends up 'doing the work' of both sex and class movement, or both sex and race movement, while class movement and race movement remain focused largely on class and race respectively.[41] Why should the women's movement allow itself to become diluted, to the advantage of other social justice issues? Why can't women do what the Marxists did, and say, firmly, *the women's movement is about women's issues—as* women*—and all these other things are just outside its scope*? In the next section, I explain one way that it can do exactly that.

7.4 Women as Women

A feminism centred on women as women is a feminism concerned with all of the ways in which women are oppressed or disadvantaged *in virtue of their sex-based rights and interests.* Some of these are grounded in the material facts about their bodies, while others are grounded less in bodies and more in the politics of how people with those types of bodies are treated. This will include issues relating to:

- Sex and sexual subordination
  (e.g. female genital mutilation (FGM), child brides, incest and abuse against girl children, rape, sexual assault, prostitution and pornography, trafficking into sexual slavery)
- The female reproductive role
  (e.g. period poverty, reproductive rights, breastfeeding in public, pregnancy and in/fertility healthcare, flexible work during pregnancy, maternity leave, non-discrimination against pregnant or breastfeeding employees)
- Female-specific medical conditions
  (e.g. cervical cancer, breast cancer, endometriosis, and comparative research funding for women's medical issues)
- Female sports
  (e.g. comparative speed, strength, agility, and the comparative underfunding of women's sports compared to men's)
- The way that product design caters to men's bodies not women's, including legislation for female-specific design where there is mortality risk
  (e.g. bullet-proof vests not fitting female police officers well,[42] airbags in cars being designed to protect male bodies,[43] personal protective equipment used by female healthcare workers treating COVID-19 fitting poorly because designed to fit men[44])

More generally such a feminism will be concerned with the norms, expectations, and stereotypes applied to women, which constrain their options and set the standard against which they are assessed (e.g. 'a gender non-conforming' woman is a woman who fails to realize the standards of femininity), and the treatment of women who violate those norms.

If we focus feminism in this way, we will have returned to the original insight of feminism, that 'Women are oppressed, *as women*', as Marilyn Frye says.[45] She elaborates as follows:

> One is marked for application of oppressive pressures by one's membership in some group or category. Much of one's suffering and frustration befalls one partly or largely because one is a member of that category. In the case at hand, it is the category, *woman*. Being a woman is a major factor in my not having a better job than I do; being a woman selects me as a likely victim of sexual assault or harassment; it is my being a woman that reduces the power of my anger to a proof of my insanity. If a woman has little of what she wants to achieve, a major causal factor in this is that she is a woman. For any woman of any race or economic class, being a woman is significantly attached to whatever disadvantages and deprivations she suffers, be they great or small.[46]

Or as Andrea Dworkin said: 'The nature of women's oppression is unique: women are oppressed as women, regardless of race or class'.[47] Dworkin acknowledged that this did not mean the 'primary state of emergency' for any given woman was *as a woman*. Jewish women in Nazi Germany would have experienced as their primary state of emergency being Jewish; many Native American and African American women at a particular time would have experienced it as being their race.[48]

This focus explains the priorities of the first and second waves of feminism in English-speaking countries. The first wave was focused almost exclusively on women's political enfranchisement. The second wave gave a great deal of attention to ending sexual violence against women, but also included issues like equal pay for women; abortion, contraception, and maternity rights; women's issues in the educational curriculum; women's economic independence and empowerment; women's workplace rights; sexist language; and police treatment of women victims and survivors.[49]

The easy test of whether something is an issue for women as women or women as persons is to ask whether the men of the further social group face the same issue. Take the sex/race combination. Black women involved in the civil rights movement in the United States talked about the sexual violence and harassment endemic in the movement, which was often suppressed as a matter of showing solidarity with, or not breaking rank with, black men.[50] The way that white people historically perpetrated racism against black people, especially under slavery, involved sexual violence against black women.[51] In both cases, we ask whether black men suffered the same issues. If they did, this was a race issue, not a feminist issue. But, in general, they didn't. Black women felt conflicted about revealing sexual violence in the civil rights movement, but black men were usually the perpetrators of that particular violence, not the equal victims of it.[52] White violence against black women under slavery was sexualized, but white violence against black men generally was not. So both of these are issues that should be part of feminism understood as being for women as women.

Similarly, women with intellectual disabilities are raped or sexually assaulted at a substantially higher rate than people without intellectual disabilities. We can ask whether men with intellectual disabilities face the same issue. If they do, this is a disability issue, not a feminist issue. But they don't—the rate is 7.3 per 1,000 for women, and 1.4 per 1,000 for men, with disabilities. The rate for men with intellectual disabilities is lower than the rate for women without. So this is a feminist issue, too. (And as per the discussion in Chapter 6, Section 6.2, the invisibility of butch and masculine women in discussions of workplace sexual harassment, and the Jewish religious law of *get*, are both feminist issues too.)

Consider also the cases where the same tests reveal the issue *not* to be a feminist one. Police violence against African American people in the United States affects black men more than black women; it is a race issue, not a feminist issue (although *sexualized* police violence affects black women more than black men, and so is a feminist issue).[53] Building access for people with physical disabilities affects men and women with physical disabilities equally, and so is a disability issue, not a feminist issue. HIV awareness and protection affects gay men more than gay women, so is an LGB issue, not a feminist issue. Kosher food requirements affect all Jewish people equally, so are a Jewish issue, not a feminist issue. And so on.

What if the issue doesn't clearly relate to women's sex-based rights and interests, but still affects more women than men? Because the world's poorest women are often restricted to their homes, they're more at risk from climate disasters (finding it harder to escape floods, and harder to access food and clean drinking water when there are droughts, for example).[54] If more women than men are the victims of climate injustice, even though climate injustice doesn't relate to the embodied or political aspects of women's sex-based oppression, should climate justice be on the feminist agenda?

More women than men will be adversely affected because more women than men are restricted to the home, in turn because there tend to be strong gender expectations in the world's poorest societies that lead to women being in that situation, e.g. expectations to raise children, care for the home, and prepare food. All of *these* things, relating centrally to women's reproductive role and gender expectations applied on the basis of her being female, will be on the feminist agenda as we've outlined it. But climate justice won't be. Climate justice is an everyone issue, not a feminist issue. And that's a good thing, because as I have been arguing, when it becomes feminism's job to *smash capitalism* and *fight climate change* there's a serious risk that feminism simply becomes debilitated by being stretched too thinly, by having too much asked of it.

A significant implication of this refocusing of feminist theory and activism is that it removes the automatic assumptions about hierarchy *within* feminist groups that contemporary identity politics has put in place. Women as women are all equal. It is perfectly likely that the most negatively affected person in the group is the woman who looks to have the most 'privilege' when all her social group memberships are taken into account. Middle-class white women may yet have suffered histories of childhood sexual abuse or been raped. Middle-class white women may have been bullied and harassed throughout their lives for not performing femininity in the right way. The number of marginalized social group memberships that a person has are no guide at all to the extent of her oppression as a woman.[55] This restores equality among women when it comes to feminist solidarity, and feminist projects. This doesn't mean such women don't need to be careful when it comes to the interpersonal relationships between the women in the group, which obviously can be disrupted by causal racism, ableism, homophobia, etc. But it means 'privileged' women don't need to spend all their time apologizing, and 'the most marginalized' women (according to identity politics) don't automatically deserve the deference of the other women in the group, or take priority when it comes to setting the group's goals and priorities.

This equality should help to restore the possibility of solidarity among women. The important questions for setting feminist goals and priorities are not what further marginalized social groups the women in the group belong to (which can lead to the unstable situation in which a new member joining means a complete rethinking of the group's aims, because the focus is always on 'the most marginalized' person whoever she happens to be), but which of the issues on the agenda deserve priority, which might be settled in different ways, e.g. issues that affect the greatest number of women; issues that affect women in the most morally serious way; issues that the group has the expertise to cover; issues delegated through a division of labour with other groups; and so on.

Opponents of gender-critical feminism are likely to say that this version of feminism works to the benefit of middle-class white women, because these are the women who are *only* oppressed as women, and so it is a feminism that therefore pursues their interests. This is false for two reasons. First, it is a version of feminism that works to the benefit of all women as women, even if it does not solve the further problems of all women as people. Any feminism that pursues the interests of all women as people will suffer from being impossibly broad, and there is no principled way to limit it. Second, many of the issues mentioned at the start of this section—FGM, child brides, period poverty, trafficking into sexual slavery, reproductive rights—are more likely to affect globally poor women and women of colour. Once we map out the feminist agenda for this version of feminism, gender-critical feminism, and we set priorities in the ways discussed above, it is highly unlikely that what we'll have is a movement to prioritize the interests of middle-class white women alone.

7.5 Intersectionality as Novel Forms of Oppression

It's time to take stock. We've considered several potential justifications of the fact that we've ended up with a feminism which is considered to be for everyone and about everything. All have to do with mistakes taking hold. The first was that feminism had better be for everyone otherwise it's excluding some people (from Chapter 6). The second was that feminism had better be about everything otherwise it's just putting band-aids over symptoms rather than getting to the root cause of oppression. The third was that feminism is for (almost) everyone and about (almost) everything, because it's about making women's lives better, and there are all sorts of things that make women's lives (as whole persons) go worse. I've rejected all of these justifications, and defended a narrower focus for feminism on women as women.

But where does this leave intersectionality? It wouldn't be quite right to equate these three explanations with intersectionality and leave things there, because there are many different theorists who give many different versions of intersectionality, some more plausible than others. In this final section of the chapter, I want to present Kimberlé Crenshaw's version, which I think is the most plausible, and argue that incorporating *this* into gender-critical feminism—or indeed, any version of feminism—would lead to significantly less bloating than the other versions discussed so far.[56] But, ultimately, there is still a question about whether it is *feminism's* job to account for the forms of oppression that this version of the theory identifies.

In Crenshaw's presentation, intersectionality is not just about membership in two or more marginalized social groups. If that were all there was to it, we wouldn't need movements to be intersectional. One movement could address race oppression, and another could cover sex oppression, and between them they'd have black women covered. But this won't do, Crenshaw argues, because there is discrimination that occurs specifically at the *intersection* of blackness and femaleness (hence the term, '*intersection*ality'). Crenshaw thought this intersectional discrimination was greater than the sum of its parts, and that its discovery had implications for both the feminist movement *and* the anti-racism movement.[57] One example she gave was of a case in which a company had laid off all its black women employees, and yet couldn't be prosecuted for employment discrimination because it had both black employees (men) and women employees (white). The court said it was reluctant to 'creat[e]... new classes of protected minorities... by... combination'.[58] The court wanted to leave discrimination at race and sex, not create a further minority class out of race *and* sex.

This suggests there are four ways that a black woman may face discrimination: as a woman, as black, as black *and* as a woman, and *as a black woman*, the latter being understood as its own particular thing. It is perfectly possible that a black woman could face discrimination and know that it is related to one of her social group memberships rather than another. Most obviously, if this discrimination involves slurs or insulting comments, it is easy to identify what they relate to. Shirley Chisholm, the first woman and first African American to run for president of the United States, said she faced much more discrimination during her time in politics as a matter of her sex than her race. In her words: 'I had met far more discrimination because I am a woman than because I am black'.[59] It's the last category, *as a black woman*, that is most interesting to us here.

Crenshaw was specifically interested in race and sex, although as discussed earlier, there's no principled reason to limit our attention to only this intersection. The logic of the idea extends naturally to other marginalized social group memberships. But I'll stick with race and sex here just to keep the discussion simple. If discrimination *as a black woman* is something entirely new, then it's not clear that it fits into the method outlined in Section 7.4. There we talked about starting with all women, then looking at further social group memberships like being black, and then for any given issue asking whether it is held in common with black men, or uniquely faced by black women. But how would that go with this unique form of discrimination *as a black woman*? There's no comparison class that contains men that will let us ascertain whether this is a feminist issue or another movement's issue. Because the issue is novel, it's not obvious whose jurisdiction it falls into. Crenshaw clearly thought it belongs to *both*. The anti-racism movement should care about discrimination as black women, and the feminist movement should care about discrimination as black women. If that means some doubling up, so what? Maybe the issue will be solved more quickly.

Perhaps Crenshaw is right. But it's worth pointing out that this is not the only answer. Once we consider that this is also true for other intersections, we'll notice that it's a lot of additional content for each movement to take on. And it is not the only option that all existing movements with a single social group focus (sex, race, class, disability, sexual orientation, etc.) incorporate all intersectional issues where those groups are part of what's intersecting. That would mean instead of disability rights activism being about e.g. building accessibility, it would need to also be about all of the issues occurring at the intersections of female/disabled, black/disabled, working-class/disabled, gay/disabled, black/female/disabled, working-class/gay/disabled, and so on, and so on. There is a risk of fragmentation and a risk of over-burdening the group so that its energies are spread too thinly and it can accomplish nothing.

There are three alternatives, at least in theory, which leave the intersections out of the existing movements with a single social group focus. One is the creation of additional social justice movements for intersectional groups, e.g. a movement for black women *as black women* specifically. Audre Lorde appears to take this view, when she says 'As Black women, we must deal with all the realities of our lives which place us at risk as Black women',[60] and 'Black women have particular and legitimate issues which affect our lives as Black women'.[61] She goes on, 'As Black women we have the right and responsibility to define ourselves and to seek our allies in common cause: with Black men against racism, and with each other and white women against sexism'.[62] Black women here are conceived as a distinct social group that has common cause with other social groups, black men, and white women. On this alternative, gender-critical feminism is a theory and movement for *all* women, including, obviously, black women as women—which, as discussed earlier, includes racial issues with a differential impact on women, but excludes racial issues impacting the sexes equally. But there would also be an independent theory and movement for black women as black women (as there already is). And so too for all the other social groups that describe novel forms of oppression.

A risk of this first alternative is fragmentation. There is no guarantee that women will have the energy to participate in two or more distinct movements (the feminist movement and a specific intersectional movement), and if the consequence is that any woman dealing with novel forms of oppression (arising from her multiple social group memberships) *leaves the feminist movement* then this is bad news for the feminist movement. Perhaps this is the ultimate explanation of why the feminist movement has simply embraced the intersections, and so become for (almost) everyone and about (almost) everything: in a choice between having a small and non-diverse movement with a clear, narrow focus, and having a large and diverse movement with an impossibly broad focus, the latter is more appealing.

Another alternative is a division of labour *between* the existing movements to avoid doubling-up on issues and to keep the agenda manageable. For example, black women's intersectional issues might be incorporated into feminism, but women with disabilities' intersectional issues might be incorporated into the disability rights movement. The problem with this alternative is that social movements are 'bottom-up', meaning they emerge from grassroots activism in sometimes spontaneous or chaotic ways, rather than being carefully organized or orchestrated 'top-down'. A division of labour like this would require careful top-down organization, or at the very least, a lot of mutual responsiveness between movements.

Finally, it could be that instead a new, comprehensive 'intersectional social justice' movement should rise up to claim the novel forms of oppression at *all* the intersections. Indeed, I think what has actually happened is a version of this alternative. As described in Section 7.2, feminism has been reconceived as a movement for women as whole persons. Then, that movement has also claimed the novel forms of oppression at all the intersections. The feminist movement has become an intersectional global justice movement. The problem is not that there is such a movement. Such a movement is a good thing. The problem is rather that this new movement still calls itself 'feminism'. This gives the impression that it is a women's movement, focused on women as women, comparable to movements focused on race, class, disability, sexual orientation, and so on.

While there are pockets of holdouts, most notably the radical and gender-critical feminists, the culturally dominant form of feminism is not a movement focused on women as women. (It is not clear that it is even a movement focused on women as people; it may be closer to a movement focused on people as people). But this leaves a serious gap in the social justice landscape. We need a women's movement. Even if there is loads of intersectional discrimination, there is still, *also*, just good old plain vanilla discrimination against women, for being women.[63]

8
Is Gender-Critical Feminism Feasible?

> ...there are no precedents in history for feminist revolution—there have been women revolutionaries, certainly, but they have been used by male revolutionaries, who seldom gave even lip service to equality for women, let alone to a radical feminist restructuring of society.
>
> (Shulamith Firestone, *The Dialectic of Sex*)[1]

The gender-critical feminist utopia is characterized by liberation for all female people from patriarchal oppression. For gender-critical feminists, this means no more gender norms, either masculine or feminine. This in turn means no more patterned male violence against women and girls (rape, domestic violence, sexual assault, child abuse), no more sex industry (no more trafficking, no more prostitution, no more pornography), no more sexual objectification of women and girls—whether by individuals or through cultural institutions like the media and advertising, no more sexual coercion, no more discrimination against women and girls (whether the result of individual attitudes or of institutionalized biases). It means no more self-destructive behaviour by women and girls as a result of having internalized standards of femininity that they feel themselves not to be meeting. So no more cutting, no more anorexia or bulimia, no more sex asymmetry in the suffering of depression,[2] no more elective double mastectomies (breast removal) or phalloplasties (neopenises, sometimes created out of women's forearm flesh) inspired by ideas about gender identities, or caused by feelings of inadequacy relative to gender norms.[3]

People have written about utopias of many different kinds: 'there are socialist, capitalist, monarchical, democratic, anarchist, ecological, feminist, patriarchal, egalitarian, hierarchical, racist, left-wing, reformist, free love, nuclear family, extended family, gay, lesbian, and many more utopias'.[4] A utopia need not be perfect in *all* respects. If there is more than one value it is seeking to maximize then it will often be the case that it *cannot* be:

Gender-Critical Feminism: Holly Lawford-Smith, Oxford University Press. © Holly Lawford-Smith 2022.
DOI: 10.1093/oso/9780198863885.003.0008

sometimes values are linked, so that more of one means less of another, for example freedom and security. Citizens in a democracy may reasonably disagree about the correct balance of different values, and end up choosing perfection in some at the expense of imperfection in others. In fiction, utopias often contain serious injustice. In Naomi Alderman's *The Power*, female empowerment comes with a lot of electrocuting of men (although to be fair, it is often in retribution for injustice).[5] In Kurt Vonnegut's *Harrison Bergeron*, an egalitarian utopia is accomplished by 'levelling down' (handicapping the clever, talented, and beautiful).[6] Thomas More's 1516 *Utopia* contained patriarchy, slavery, and restricted freedom.[7] The gender-critical utopia is perfect only in the respect of having eliminated sex oppression. This follows from its being exclusively about women's liberation, rather than combining multiple movements, or incorporating the intersections of multiple movements (see also discussion in Chapter 7).

In the gender-critical feminist utopia, sex is likely to be acknowledged, because the pathways taking us there will have required anti-discrimination protections that tracked sex. But it is not something that people will use as a basis for making predictions about people's personalities or preferences (except, most likely, when it comes to preferences about sexual and romantic partners). While there will still be the same *people* who think of themselves as 'transmen', 'transwomen', or 'nonbinary' today, they will not use those labels, because 'feminine' will be a way that males can be, 'masculine' will be a way that women can be, and 'androgynous' will be a way that anyone can be. The idea of being 'gender non-conforming' won't make sense to anyone in the utopia, because gender will be a system of oppressive norms that people living there have long-since gotten rid of, so there will be nothing left to conform *to*. When we get to the utopia, there will be no more need for a feminist movement—except as a matter of protection against backsliding.

The realization of these feminist goals might also come with incidental gains for other social justice projects. For example, if freeing women from patriarchal oppression means eliminating systematic male dominance entirely, and systematic male dominance was a common cause of both widespread female subordination *and* the failure to take radical action against climate change, then female liberation could end up a major catalyst for climate justice. The large-scale social changes involved in realizing gender-critical feminist goals, and the potential incidental gains involved, are difficult to fully anticipate. Because the same mechanisms that oppress women have also involved collateral damage to gay people, non-masculine men, non-feminine women, trans people, and fun people (by which I mean people—especially men—who like to exercise a little creativity over their presentation), it is likely that none of these groups of people will still be oppressed in the gender-critical feminist utopia. Some of these people are male, so their liberation was not the point of the feminist theory and movement that achieved the utopia, but is an incidental gain of female liberation.

For any major social shift to overturn injustice, there's usually an opponent in the wings waiting to accuse the reformers of having a vision the implementation of which is infeasible. Those working against the institution of slavery were told that people wouldn't produce more than they needed for subsistence if they weren't forced.[8] Those working for women's suffrage were told that women didn't want the vote.[9] Advocates for marriage equality in the early days were told there wasn't the political will to support it.[10] It's important to note that for all the social justice movements that have succeeded, there are many more that didn't. But the fact that some did establishes that the opponents were not always right.[11]

We can assume the same criticism will be made against the gender-critical feminist movement, and also, independently, against its major commitments, for example to the asymmetric criminalization of the sex industry (criminalization of punters, pimps, pornographers, and other third parties);[12] and to its stubborn insistence that gender is *harmful norms* rather than *identity*, given how much uptake the ideology of gender identity has already had. So let's get on with figuring out what that criticism means, and what it would take to show that it's unwarranted.

8.1 What Does It Take for Something to be Feasible/Infeasible?

Suppose the accusation of infeasibility is made in a general way, without any further specification of the aspects in which this is supposed to be the case. Suppose someone just proclaims that 'what gender-critical feminists want isn't feasible'. Perhaps, if pushed, they will insist that the exchange of sexual intercourse for money is like alcohol or marijuana in that appetites are not much suppressed by illegality, and where there is appetite there will be provision, so abolition of the sex industry is infeasible. Or perhaps they have a story to tell about *what men are like* (there seem to be an infinite supply of these stories) which would make it infeasible to get rid of sexual assault or domestic violence or even just sexual objectification.

In a 2017 *TEDx* talk in Canberra, Australia, Nicholas Southwood offered the following set of dangers that come along with the 'just not feasible' conversational device (which he says is 'utterly ubiquitous'):

1. *Self-fulfilling prophesies*: 'we may reject as infeasible an idea that is only infeasible insofar as and because we judge it to be infeasible'.
2. *Conflation*: 'we may reject as infeasible an idea that is merely unlikely to happen because we are unlikely to try to make it happen'.
3. *Implicit constraints*: 'we may reject as infeasible an idea that is perfectly feasible within a broader temporal horizon and given a more permissive understanding of the ways it might be brought about'.
4. *Loss of symbolic value*: 'we may reject altogether an idea—even if it *is* really infeasible—that nonetheless has value and should somehow be kept alive'.[13]

Let's take abolition of the sex industry as an example to explain each of these dangers, because it's simpler to talk about one component of the gender-critical utopia than all of it at once, and because this is an absolutely key component.

If we decide that getting rid of the sex industry, either in one country or globally, is infeasible, then we won't be motivated to try to get rid of it. Why would we waste our energy on something hopeless, when we could be doing something more constructive with our time? This makes infeasibility a self-fulfilling prophesy, because it's the very fact that we *declare* abolition of the sex industry infeasible that it *becomes* infeasible. It is infeasible because we won't, not because we can't.

Or alternatively, we may judge that abolition is not that likely to succeed even if we try, or that it will be costly to try, or that it will be really difficult to pull off. Sometimes 'infeasibility' is confused with nearby notions like this. But it's important to get clear on what's really being said, because they raise different follow-up questions. *Why* is it not that likely to succeed, and is there anything we can do to make it more likely? *How* costly will it be, and what kinds of costs will it involve? Is that a price worth paying given what we stand to gain? *How* difficult will it be? Lots of things are difficult, but worth doing. Because claims about infeasibility often involve conflation with other concepts, it is important to find out what is meant.

The third 'danger' was that when people dismiss something as infeasible they're sometimes making particular assumptions that aren't made fully available for inspection. Imagine someone says to me that asymmetric criminalization of prostitution is infeasible in my home state, Victoria, but when I press them their reason is that 'the Labor government has already thrown its weight behind decriminalisation'. It turns out they're assuming a timeframe of *this year*, or *before the next election*, and our conversation might go differently with a longer timeframe in mind.

These assumptions can also be moral: we may disagree about what is feasible because we disagree about what is morally permissible (and therefore 'on the table'). Juno Mac & Molly Smith think that reducing harm to prostituted women *by* introducing asymmetric criminalization is infeasible.[14] One of the reasons seems to be that they consider it morally repugnant to select a policy that would put already vulnerable women at even more risk. Making men scared of arrest means prostituted women having to go to more secluded locations with punters. So for Mac & Smith, criminalization is 'off the table' as an option. If we don't have a basic income or a decent welfare provision in place, and don't commit to offering support like retraining to women exiting prostitution, then they may be right that it should be off the table.

Because our assumptions might not be shared, it's good to get them made explicit so that they can be assessed. Not all projects for the public good can be done in a way that involves gains for some without any losses to others, and in those cases it *should be* on the table whether these losses can be justified by potential gains. Perhaps increased risk to prostituted women in the short-term, and fewer punters, is worth it if it means those women end up moving out of sex work and the sex industry is eventually squashed.

Finally, the last danger was that in dismissing something as infeasible—*even if it actually is*—we lose something important. Suppose we'll never quite fully get rid of the sex industry, we'll only manage to reduce its size a bit while driving it underground. Still, given all its manifold harms, and given the massive roadblock it throws up for sex equality, we should maintain its abolition as an ideal, and do the best we can to get close to it. *Even if* infeasible, abolition can function as an endpoint against which we measure our success.

Out of these four, I suspect that much of the disagreement between feminists over the abolition of the sex industry is a version of *self-fulfilling prophesies* and *implicit constraints*, and that the implicit constraints are moral rather than empirical. In the next two sections, I'll make the case for that in more detail. There is also room for a disagreement about the feasibility of realizing the gender-critical feminist utopia even without any of these mistakes. Feasibility is not easy to establish (although the converse is also true, and this should give us pause whenever we hear anyone throw 'that's infeasible!' around as a conversation-stopper). So in Section 8.4, I'll sketch out some of the considerations that go into a judgement about whether the gender-critical feminist utopia, or specific components of it, are feasible or not. Then in the final section, Section 8.5, I'll make a point about pathways to utopia which shows that there need not be any disagreement between higher and lower ambition—reformist and revolutionary!—feminist proposals, at least in terms of first steps.

8.2 Self-Fulfilling Prophesies

It is possible to be so cynical about the chances of change that we don't even try. Some people defend a market in organs on the grounds that for some very poor people, selling their organs is a way to make some money, which will make them a little better off. Similar arguments are made about surrogacy ('reproductive prostitution', Ekman calls it)[15] and about prostitution. Destitute and desperate women are very badly off, but at least if they can sell their organs, sell sex, or sell their capacity to reproduce, then they can improve their situation a little, for at least a little while. That's better than the alternative, surely.

The argument seems to be that there are *only* these two choices, and so ruling one of the choices out means condemning poor people to a very bad situation. We can either leave the desperately poor to their poverty, or we can allow wealthier people to exploit them in a way that makes them marginally better off for a short while. If that's what someone thinks about what is possible, then it's hardly surprising that she would defend to the death the continued existence of the surrogacy, organs, and prostitution industries. One would have to be entirely lacking in compassion to argue to take away the slightly better options that very poor people have available.

This kind of argument showed up in *Revolting Prostitutes*, discussed in Chapter 4. Mac & Smith assume that if we try to criminalize part or all of the sex industry it will just be run illegally, but in a way that is worse for women. There is almost no discussion, anywhere in the book, of a deterrence effect from any policy proposal, even though the whole book is about comparing and contrasting policy proposals. The assumption seems to be that *there will always be a sex industry*, or even that *these particular women will always work as prostitutes*, so the only question is about the conditions in that industry, and of that work. Sheila Jeffreys reports another example of this reasoning, namely Diane Otto's argument against the United Nations prohibiting its staff from having sex with anyone under 18, where she reconceives child prostitution as 'survival sex' and focuses on the child's exercise of agency in making trades that protect her from the starvation that poverty would otherwise make inevitable.[16]

There might really be some cases where there are only two very bad options. If all the street prostitutes in a specific area are drug- or alcohol-dependent, and the social services to transition them into other kinds of work are not particularly good, and don't include drug and alcohol rehabilitation, then it's fairly likely an abolitionist campaign won't succeed in transitioning those women out of the sex industry, and that (so long as there remains some demand, even when buying sex is made illegal) they will keep selling sex. After all, they have no other means to survive, and most people do what they need to do in order to survive.

But it is unlikely that for all the cases where exploitative industries are defended on the grounds that they make the exploited better off, exploitation really is the only alternative. Usually there is enough latitude in a budget that local governments *could* decide to put more resources into policing and prosecuting men who buy sex, and into the social services to help prostituted women exit the industry. They could also put more money into training programmes so that women have better options than prostitution. Women who are exploited in these ways are some of the most vulnerable women in any society, who have a very strong claim to being prioritized.

The same is true, at a conceptual level, for gender as identity versus gender as norms. Gender as identity is a *low ambition* project. It seems to suppose that we can't make things much better for all the people who are hurt by the policing of gender norms. Instead of thinking about how to change the social structures that cause some people to identify as trans, it focuses on the individual solutions of transition and medicalization. It doesn't worry about the fact that it is entrenching gender norms, by signalling that 'feminine' is not a way to be a man, and 'masculine' is not a way to be a woman. It is as though the gender as identity crowd think the choice is between just two options, one being to carry on with roughly the gender binary we have now, the other being to free up some people to opt out of one side of the binary and into the other, or to opt out of both and into a third category (nonbinary).[17] But where is the justification for thinking that these are our only choices?

In both of these cases, it is possible that feminists are *creating* the infeasibility of ending women's exploitation, and the infeasibility of securing women's liberation from gender norms, by taking the cynical view that very little is possible in the way of reform, and so justifying a 'second-worst' solution as being equivalent to the practical 'best' solution. But the burden of proof should be on those who defend these reforms, who seem to be assuming that we can only make things a bit better, to prove that this is the case. If they can't, then we have no reason to limit ourselves to just the options they have bothered to consider.

One shortcut to defeating a claim about infeasibility that smuggles in a self-fulfilling prophesy is to show that better options are *actual* in some places.[18] The Nordic Model (also known as asymmetric criminalization) for prostitution *is* actual in a number of countries—although not for pornography, somewhat inconsistently.[19] These include Sweden, Norway, Iceland, Canada, Northern Ireland, France, Ireland, and Israel. (There are a few countries where pornography is illegal, but these tend to be countries that are socially repressive for women.)

Domestic violence and sexual violence are illegal in many countries, although in many where that is the case the crimes are not particularly well-policed or prosecuted. There is much less sexual objectification of women in some countries, to the point that men and women are comfortable sharing saunas (where there is full nudity) and changing rooms. No country is a gender-critical feminist utopia, but some—like Sweden—show how much progress it is realistically possible to make.

At the opposite extreme from self-fulfilling prophesies—being so cynical about the possibility of change that you talk yourself out of trying to achieve it—is caring so much about ideals that we insist something is feasible when it isn't, in a way that causes more harm. Another way to refer to this is as 'ideological puritanism'. Mac & Smith complained about this when they talked about radical feminists worrying about the symbolic nature of prostitution, rather than about real harms to sex workers.

I said at the end of Chapter 4 that gender-critical feminists mustn't let the 'perfect' be the enemy of the 'good'. Perhaps what is perfect is no exploitation, and that means no sex industry. Still, what is good is less suffering, rather than more. We shouldn't let the one become the enemy of the other by being so immovable on our commitment to *no exploitation, therefore make the sex industry illegal!* that we end up licensing more, rather than less, real harm to women, even when we shift to thinking about all women. That would be ideological puritanism, because it puts the symbolic value of the commitment above the pragmatic value of compromising where necessary to make gains for women. (This issue is especially salient among radical and gender-critical feminists over questions about political alliances.)[20]

Of course it is not clear-cut when and where we should compromise, not least because sometimes the long-game commitment to 'the perfect' will bring greater benefits that are not comparable to the smaller benefits achieved by a pragmatic acquiescence to 'the good'. If MacKinnon is right about it being a pervasive gender expectation of women that they are *for men to fuck*, then allowing the sex industry to go on, just with better working conditions for the women in it, is incompatible with dissolving pernicious gender expectations, and so capitulation in the name of the good is only going to make things worse for a greater number of women for longer. There is no option but to simply put all these considerations out on the table and do the work in thinking them through.

8.3 Implicit Moral Constraints

The idea behind *implicit constraints* was that we can disagree about what is feasible because we have different ideas about what the constraints are that we're working within. One specific form this can take is that we disagree about what is morally permissible, and that leads us to have different things on the table.

Mac & Smith were doing something like this when they argued against making things any worse for sex workers.[21] The moral constraint is something like *it is impermissible to make things any worse for groups that are already very badly off*. When law-makers talk about developing their legislation by 'listening to sex workers themselves' they are also employing this kind of constraint.[22] But both the constraint and whether the constraint applies in the case of prostitution may be questioned.

First of all, while it's true that asymmetric criminalization may make some prostituted women worse off in the short-term, in the sense that they will lose punters and may be pushed into accepting riskier jobs, it is not clear whether this makes them worse off in the longer term. There is a risk here of assuming *implicit constraints* about time periods, and being cynical about how things will go. But why should we only be interested in the very short-term? (One obvious answer is that we can be more confident about being able to accomplish short-term plans; another is that restricting our plans to time periods that fit between elections mean a particular government can enact them. But this does not suffice to establish that we *cannot* pull off longer-term plans, and the length of time between elections does not rationalize planning to an even shorter term.) Why should we assume that asymmetric criminalization is paired with poor policing, so that there will still be punters, they'll just be scared of being arrested and so take prostitutes to more secluded locations where they are more at risk? If policed properly, the result is simply no more punters, and if paired with adequate welfare support, healthcare, and retraining, there's no reason at all to think that this would make prostituted women worse off rather than better off.

Second, even if it was the case that such policy reform would make prostituted women worse off, it's open to us to push back on the moral constraint. Obviously we should try very hard not to make things any worse for groups that are very badly off. Ideally, we would make improvements for some groups without making any other groups or individuals worse off. Where that isn't possible, it would be good to design improvements so that if they had to make anyone worse off, it would be those who are already very advantaged. But as I said in Chapter 4, the existence of the sex industry has implications for all women. And when we consider which policy makes women better and worse off, it is no longer completely straightforward whether it is impermissible to make things worse for groups that are already badly off. There's no easy answer to how the goods of a gain to a social group must be distributed among its members. We would clearly have a problem if reforms made things better for the best-off and worse for the worst-off, but what about in all the other cases?

Moral disagreements, smuggled in as implicit constraints on what can be done and how, are likely to be behind much of the critics' objections that the gender-critical feminist utopia, or particular of its components, are infeasible. For example, (real) liberal feminists place a heavy emphasis on the importance of freedom from state interference, and on the importance of the freedom to make choices—for people to pursue their own good in their own way, as it is usually stated. They reject paternalism over adults. Even if a person is clearly making a mistake, they argue that it's her life to make mistakes in. Radical and gender-critical feminists are generally happy with the idea that state interference can be used to secure non-domination, and with the idea that the set of choices available to people should exclude those which are incompatible with women's full humanity (e.g. men's 'choice' to buy the use of women's bodies, whether for reproduction or prostitution). This is a moral disagreement between liberal and radical feminists, and one that can mean they will impose a different set of constraints on the 'available options'.

8.4 What Does It Take for a Political Proposal to be Feasible?

Suppose two feminists are sitting down for a coffee together and disagreeing about their respective visions for women's liberation, but that neither are making any of the mistakes just discussed. Both are aware that cynicism can lead to a lack of motivation that actually creates infeasibility; neither confuse 'infeasible' with 'unlikely'; they've established common ground in what the constraints are and what's morally off the table; and they both agree that sometimes infeasible ideas have symbolic value and so should be held onto as ideals. But they still want to establish whether it is *really possible* to get rid of all pornography;[23] to eliminate prostitution, and surrogacy, and trafficking, and forced marriage, and rape, and sexual assault, and domestic violence; to completely change the way women are viewed, from aesthetic and instrumental (sexual, service) objects to full human persons; to end all forms of discrimination against women.

We can advocate for all of these things at once, but the different components are separate projects. They will require different types of legal reforms and reforms to policing, different types of public information campaigns, different measures for changing how women are represented. For example, there is a campaign underway at the moment to have Pornhub shut down, initiated by Laila Mickelwait and having attracted nearly 2.2 million signatures.[24] Shutting down Pornhub would be a huge victory in the feminist fight against pornography. It is the website with the tenth highest internet traffic in the world, and the second biggest pornography website.[25] Gail Dines writes for the campaign to shut it down:

> For too long pornography has been framed as a moral issue, but from over forty years of empirical research, we know that it is an issue of harm. Pornhub is in the business of commodifying and monetizing violence against women and children. There is no place for Pornhub in a world committed to sexual equality, dignity, and social justice.[26]

Still, even without pornography, long-standing cultural ideas about what women are *for*, cemented by the existence of pornography—even when it has become just an embarrassment of the past, a historical injustice against women whose many reparations cases have begun weaving their way through the courts of countries all around the world—will take some undoing. A separate but complementary project is to increase and improve the representation of women characters in entertainment media, in order to provide depictions of women as full human persons, and create a challenge to the perception of women as objects. In her book *Norms in the Wild*, Cristina Bicchieri draws on evidence showing that television and radio soap operas can have a huge influence in shifting social norms, including gender norms.[27] In Brazil, soap operas have been credited with reducing the number of children women have from an average of seven to an average of two.[28]

The point is that when feminists want to explore questions about feasibility, it will be more tractable to consider these distinct components separately, than to try to account for everything all at once. This is compatible with acknowledging that it is likely that as more progress is made on separate components there will be a kind of 'snowball' effect where it becomes easier to implement components that have a similar underlying rationale or justification. In what follows, I'll talk about a few different specific components of the gender-critical feminist utopia in order to explain some of the considerations that need to go into making a judgement about feasibility.

Here's one way of thinking about feasibility: something is feasible if we'd be reasonably likely to succeed in bringing it about if we tried.[29] This is a useful way of thinking about feasibility because it means something can be feasible even when we won't try to do it: even if we *won't* try to eliminate the sex industry, it would be feasible to do so, because *if* we were to try, we'd likely succeed. If people object to the gender-critical feminist utopia by claiming that it's infeasible (rather than that it's immoral, which I talked about in Chapter 6),[30] and we can show that we could bring it about if we tried, it's only that we won't try, then we have defeated the objection. Suppose I tell you 'you should stop commenting on your female colleagues' appearance', and you say 'but I won't'. Neither of us would think that was equivalent to saying it's infeasible for you to stop.

Securing more convictions against domestic violence, and thus creating a deterrent for perpetrators, is feasible in this way. Domestic violence is already illegal. More resources could easily be put into policing it, and more could be done to combat the androcentrism in policing that causes under-policing and under-prosecution. Jess Hill's book *See What You Made Me Do* discusses domestic violence in Australia, and contains two examples of policing that have been effective in reducing domestic violence against women.[31]

This way of thinking about feasibility is all or nothing: something either is or isn't feasible, and whether it is or isn't depends on what counts as a 'reasonable' likelihood. A way to complicate this idea and make it more useful for political decision-making is to make it a matter of degrees instead: something is *more* or *less* feasible, depending on how likely success would be, given trying.

What does this likelihood depend on, though? A lot of things are relevant here: economic, institutional, and cultural facts, and facts about people's incentives, psychologies, and motivations.[32] Take the gender-critical insistence that gender is harmful norms, and resistance to the idea that gender is identity. Bringing a legal case to challenge the use by transwomen of women-only spaces (as a way of defending women's sex-based rights) will cost money. In the UK, cases like these have generally been crowdfunded. If the people who support the case don't have much money to donate, it will be less likely to succeed.

Many institutions have already adopted gender identity ideology into the way they operate, either through infrastructure like gender-neutral bathrooms; signalling like pronouns in email signatures; or policy like diversity quotas including 'gender minorities'. The more institutionalized gender identity has become, the harder it will be to unwind. People can gain social status from signalling their allegiance to ostensibly 'progressive' norms, like using preferred pronouns, and espousing pseudo-science about sex and sex differences; and conversely, they risk social sanctions by failing to signal that allegiance, or by actively speaking out against these things. These incentives all make resistance harder to accomplish. People like to think of 'inclusion' as a positive value, and may not think to question the use of 'inclusive' to describe a policy of opening women-only spaces up to transwomen. This makes it psychologically difficult to get the gender-critical feminist argument across, which depends on the right of oppressed groups to exclude.

One more factor that determines the likelihood of success is that many people have a lot going on, and may be already committed to alternative social justice causes. So even if there are a lot of motivated, passionate, gender-critical women advocating for change (and resisting alternative proposals for change), people just may not have the capacity to support them.

These are all things that can make achieving the specific commitments of gender-critical feminism *less feasible.* Thinking about it this way, we don't use 'that's infeasible!' as a way to dismiss ideas, taking only the 'feasible' ones forward in deciding which to really work for. Rather, we use information about *how feasible* an idea is, together with other information like how risky it is, and how desirable it is, to make informed decisions about what to do.

Some have worried about thinking of infeasibility in this way, because of cases involving individuals where it looks like someone can't *try*, say because they have a serious phobia, addiction, compulsion, or something like that tied to their capacity to follow through on their intentions or desires (Southwood 2018). Suppose for the sake of argument that the only way to get rid of pornography is through a consumer boycott, which means people—predominantly men—stopping watching it, and especially stopping paying for it. Then we ask for each porn consumer whether it's feasible for him to stop. What establishes that, in turn, is how likely he is to stop if he tries. But for the men with porn addictions, it may well be that even when they try to stop, they fail. It looks like we end up in a situation in which we have to declare something to be feasible when we know it won't happen, because addiction will interfere with the relevant men's ability to try.

This objection isn't obviously important for the kinds of legal and political reforms we'll largely be interested in.[33] No one has a phobia against asymmetric criminalization policy. It's clearly true that some men have addictions, compulsions, and serious weaknesses of will when it comes to sexual gratification. But as anyone who has tried to eat healthily will know, one of the best ways to manage weakness of will is to scaffold our immediate environments in ways that help us to get what we ultimately want, namely to not have junk food in the house. The same is true for prostitution and pornography. If it's not available, then weakness of will can't be what its consumption depends on. The existence of addictions and compulsions might at best give us reasons to offer mental health care to men along with the reforms as they happen. The objection also tells us that we should not approach the abolition of pornography and prostitution *solely* through consumer boycott strategies. But that's not how boycotts generally function anyway. Usually the idea is to get a groundswell of social support that forces the targeted companies to change their practices. This can happen without all consumers being on board, and generally does.

Another problem with thinking about infeasibility in this way is that it creates issues with who the 'we' is supposed to be, when we figure out the likelihood of succeeding if we try. If *who* tries? In earlier work, I suggested that claims about what is feasible must always be made relative to agents, whether those agents are individual humans, or organized groups like corporations and states.[34] Being an 'agent' means being the kind of thing that is in control of what it does, that can make decisions on the basis of evidence about how to act. This doesn't mean their 'trying' is limited to mobilizing their members—it might mean mobilizing a whole lot of people who aren't members, but who they merely have influence over. What this means is that when we assess a claim like 'asymmetric criminalization of the sex industry in Victoria is infeasible!', we have to think about *who* would be trying to bring it about, who *they* have influence over, and how likely they are to succeed when they try. There might be a number of different agents all of whom could try and each of whom would have different probabilities of success.

Let's take the question 'what is the likelihood of CATWA (the Australian branch of the Coalition Against Trafficking in Women) stopping decriminalization and gaining support for asymmetric decriminalization in Victoria, assuming that the organization tries its best?' Answering this question involves thinking about everything it would take to succeed, and how likely that is given all the various constraints and variables. This includes the stability of the relationships between members; how well-organized they are; how well-resourced they are (money, research assistants, resources for staging political actions and running campaigns); how motivated they are; how many setbacks they can endure without losing hope; and what position all their prospective supporters are in when it comes to donating money, adding real names to public statements, lobbying members of parliament (MPs), volunteering in campaigns, and so on. And even allowing that CATWA would be fairly likely to succeed if it tried, there is still a further question when it comes to *whether* it should try, which is how those costs trade off against the desirability of the outcome and the risks incurred by pursuing it or securing it, given the opportunity costs, which means, other things they could be doing.

Still, it can't be just *any* agent who could try. Transgender Victoria, an organization utterly committed to gender as identity, *could* try to implement the gender-critical commitment to gender as harmful norms, and if it did it would probably succeed. Still, it is not going to try, because that is something entirely outside the remit of what the organization is set up to do and what its members want it to do.[35] For some agents, there is just no realistic sense in which it is an option for them to try to do particular things, not because they're lazy or unmotivated, but because they are constituted so as to do otherwise (in the case of corporations and organizations) or because of their most fundamental value commitments and ideological beliefs (in the case of individuals). So we should consider the best-placed agent, understood as an agent who has it as a realistic option to try to bring about a specific gender-critical commitment, or indeed the whole gender-critical feminist utopia, and think about what the chances of success are if it tries.

The Victorian parliament wouldn't even have to try very hard to introduce asymmetric criminalization of the sex industry. If they wanted to do it, they could. But CATWA is less likely to succeed, because their success would depend on mobilizing a large segment of Victorian society, and not facing significant opposition, which is unlikely when it is large numbers of paid sex lobby activists against small numbers of grassroots feminists, and when group polarization has led to large numbers of *women* supporting the sex industry, as discussed in Chapter 4. The lowest chances come when there's no organized group yet, so we're starting with just one motivated individual hoping to bring people together and start a social movement. This has been incredibly successful in some times and places on some issues, and incredibly unsuccessful in other times and places, on other issues. The more that other people have been independently concerned about something, the easier it will be for a single activist to unite them into action. The less, the harder. All of these things affect the likelihood of success.

I had experience of this in 2019, when the slow-paced organizing of a new radical feminist group, Feminist Action Melbourne, was interrupted and a breakaway group formed specifically to address a bill before parliament attempting to make sex in Victoria a matter of statutorily declared self-identification. We called ourselves the Victorian Women's Guild. Immediately we began a campaign of sending letters out to MPs, organizing meetings with MPs, sharing information via a new website and social media page, writing for the media and giving interviews, and running a public event to raise awareness of the bill and voice opposition to it. These are all long-established tactics.[36] If someone had asked, 'how feasible is stopping sex self-identification in Victoria?' we probably would have been the best agent they could base their assessment on. As far as I'm aware, we were the only group formally opposing the bill. I'm sure they would have assigned us a fairly low probability of success. We were highly motivated, but we were few, and we only had a couple of months' notice. We also faced extensive opposition from those convinced that kindness and inclusion meant supporting the idea that gender identity should determine which legal sex category one belongs to. In the end the bill went through, and sex became a matter of statutorily declared self-identification on the 1st of May 2020 (while I was still writing this book).

8.5 Compatible Pathways

It seems that at least some of the disagreement gender-critical feminists have with other types of feminists comes down to a disagreement over what is feasible. The gender-critical feminist's vision for women's liberation is more ambitious than the vision for women's equality that many feminists today seem to have as their ideal. But this need not mean that they disagree about what needs to be done, at least when it comes to the first steps along the pathway from this world to the worlds they each desire. I talked in Chapter 1 about the many things that these feminists actually agree about, agreement which tends to be overshadowed by the heatedness of their disagreements over the sex industry and transgenderism. Here I want to re-emphasize that point, but not in terms of issues, rather in terms of overlap in pathways.

Take the example of women and work, for example. Gender-critical feminists can agree with other types of feminists about the importance of women having equal access to meaningful work, even if they disagree about *why* this is important. Betty Friedan, the liberal feminist whose 1963 book *The Feminine Mystique* kicked off the second wave in the United States, argued for the importance of women being in meaningful work on the grounds that it was important for women to have something for themselves. She thought the social status and confidence that would come along with having this kind of challenging and meaningful project would be a remedy for the malaise of the large segment of the population who were housewives at the time, and bored out of their minds. Some of her reasons for wanting women to work are a little odd, looking back; one is that women are too domineering over their husbands and children. Because she has nothing for herself, the woman as mother and housewife rests all of her self-conception on her husband and children, and this makes her overbearing. This seems to be an argument *from the point of view of men who want their wives to get off their backs*, not an argument from the point of view of the women who have been forced into this unbearable situation. Radical feminists might prefer to argue for women in work by talking about women's financial independence from men, and how that facilitates non-domination.

But the fact that they want the same thing, or at least that there is some overlap in what they each want, gives them common cause. Gender-critical feminists might be able to agree with other types of feminists that a basic income is desirable. Liberal feminists may desire a basic income because they care so much about autonomy, and autonomy is increased when women have more choices (see also the discussion in Chapter 9). Gender-critical feminists may desire a basic income because they care so much about ending the domination of women by men in the surrogacy, prostitution, and pornography industries, and financial independence is a good mechanism for protecting against domination. A basic income removes the possibility of arguing that there are only two choices when it comes to work that is exploitative and degrading and we must preserve a woman's right to choices that make her better off, even if not by much. It expands the range of choices, removing the objection that 'the choice for some women is prostitution or starvation, and if you make prostitution illegal you're condemning them to starve!'.

In addition to fighting for the implementation of a basic income, all types of feminists might be able to agree that it is good to work to close the gender pay gap, achieve more equality between the sexes in leadership positions, and achieve more equality between the sexes in industries that have been typically dominated by one sex (e.g. women in education, men in engineering). This is compatible with some thinking that is *all* they want to work for, perhaps because they think that women's liberation simply requires the removal of formal obstacles, and that sex equality signals that those obstacles have been removed; and others thinking there is much more to be done. Feminists with more positive welfare commitments and gender-critical feminists might be able to go further together, fighting for flexible work, carer's leave, alignment of the work and school day, matched paternity leave, and the realigning of salaries to address the differential social value attached to what has typically been considered 'women's work' and 'men's work'. Perhaps the pathways to liberation for each type of feminism overlap at the start, on exactly these measures, and then depart, with gender-critical feminists going on to do more work against the social structure in which these incremental reforms are made possible.

This common cause won't exist when incremental reforms start us down a pathway (or worse, lock us into a pathway) that makes it very hard to achieve the more radical reforms. This point is commonly made about the design of the common keyboard: QWERTY is not the most efficient system, but almost everyone who types in English has learned it, and it would be massively inefficient for everyone to relearn typing just so that the typing they do afterwards can be done more efficiently.[37] The decriminalization of prostitution might be like this. It shifts prostitution as an industry out of the criminal law and into labour law. Doing this may shift social perceptions about the moral legitimacy of the industry, further encouraging the sex-industry-supporting feminists' refrain that 'sex work is work!'. It may be harder to roll back from decriminalization to asymmetric criminalization, than it would be from alternative policies like full criminalization. So this is not a case where gender-critical feminists can find common cause with other types of feminists in measures to make things a bit better and a bit safer for prostituted women. Making things a bit better and a bit safer for prostituted women *means* ensuring that they won't be made *much* better and *much* safer for all women.

9
Is Gender-Critical Feminism Liberal?

What I have been referring to as the socially or culturally dominant form of feminism throughout this book is generally referred to as 'liberal feminism' by other radical and gender-critical feminists. Vaishnavi Sundar, for example, writes 'It was when I began voicing my opinion on the perils of liberal feminism that cancel culture started making sense to me. I could see that women were being banned for speaking against patriarchy'.[1] Or Jindi Mehat writes 'Liberal feminists stop debate by crying "choice" when radical feminists unpack the context and impact of choices—especially choices that reinforce male supremacy'.[2] Raquel Rosario Sánchez wrote a piece for *Feminist Current* in 2017 titled 'Liberal Feminists Ushered Ivanka Trump into the White House', criticizing among others those 'leading the charge' of 'liberal feminism' in the US, particularly Jessica Valenti and Andi Zeisler.[3]

If the dominant form of feminism is liberal feminism, and gender-critical feminism is opposed to that form of feminism, it would seem that gender-critical feminism is not liberal. But that would surely be a bad thing, given the important values that liberalism protects, chief among them freedom and autonomy (on which more below). There is some reason to think that gender-critical feminism is at least not fully liberal. The radical feminists deliberately gave up existing, male-authored theory and worked to build a new theory of their own. So it would be surprising if that theory fully coincided with liberalism. Gender-critical feminism is continuous with radical feminism, so the same is true of it. But there is also some reason to think gender-critical feminism *is* fully liberal. Just because an influential set of ideas is casually referred to as 'liberal feminism' by its detractors is no reason to think it has any genuine theoretical connection to liberalism. In turn, then, there's no reason to think that opposing that set of ideas means opposing liberalism. I said in Chapter 1 that the culturally dominant form of feminism seems to be influenced in a loose sense by academic feminism, mostly postmodern feminism, but in a more distorted way also liberal and intersectional feminism. The distortion could account for a lot of the

Gender-Critical Feminism: Holly Lawford-Smith, Oxford University Press. © Holly Lawford-Smith 2022.
DOI: 10.1093/oso/9780198863885.003.0009

disagreement between gender-critical and the dominant form of feminism, and in the end we might all be liberals.[4]

Before we look more closely at the relation between gender-critical feminism and liberalism, it's worth noting that the explanation of why there is this heated disagreement between gender-critical and other types of feminists today might not in fact have much to do with the underlying theory at all. Perhaps there is no more to it than that some influential women in the past disagreed with each other, and further women tended to side with one or the other of them, and these groups turned into factions and the factions splintered off and feminism turned into a war among competing tribes—liberal v. radical—and here we are. Perhaps it is entirely contingent that some issues got grouped together with others, like support for sex work with self-identification for sex, and it could easily have been otherwise. Perhaps there is no deeper explanation of why some feminists tend to bang on about choice and autonomy, and other feminists (including radical and gender-critical) tend to bang on about unjust social structures. The more that these things are true, the more that this chapter will be an imposition of method onto madness, rather than a revealing of the method that was always there.

9.1 Liberalism

There's no single understanding of what 'liberalism' is. Russell Blackford in *The Tyranny of Opinion*, for example, variously distinguishes 'so-called liberalism' (for US-style liberalism), 'classical liberalism', 'Enlightenment liberalism', 'revisionist liberalism', and 'identity liberalism' (these last two are roughly synonymous).[5] The traditional form of liberalism he refers to as Enlightenment liberalism, which held firm to 'such Enlightenment and post-Enlightenment liberal values as reason, liberty, free inquiry, individuality, originality, spontaneity, and creativity'.[6] For the purposes of understanding the relation of gender-critical feminism to liberalism, which will help us to understand the differences between it and the dominant form of feminism, a brief survey of traditional liberal values will do.

Limitation of state power. One of the earliest liberal philosophers was John Locke. In *A Letter Concerning Toleration*, written in 1689, Locke argued for the separation of church and state, with the church having domain over the personal and the state having domain over the protection and promotion of life, liberty, and welfare. As he put it (although in Latin), 'I esteem it above all things necessary to distinguish exactly the business of civil government from that of religion and to settle the just bounds that lie between the one and the other'.[7] Locke saw the state as a society of men (and he really meant *men*) created to secure, protect, and advance their civil interests, which he understood as life, liberty, health, and absence of pain; and possessions such as land, money, etc.[8]

Locke argued for impartial laws securing these things, and not doing any *more* than that, in particular, not concerning itself with 'the salvation of souls'.[9] While it was more significant at his time of writing to clearly demarcate the business of the state from the business of the church, the precedent for limiting the domain of the state's actions was very important for subsequent liberal philosophy. It tracks through to some of the disagreements between liberals even today, for example between what we now call 'libertarians' on the right who prefer less state intervention and what we now call 'liberals' on the left who prefer more state intervention, even while both appeal to liberty as a justification.

Toleration. Locke also argued for religious toleration, an early version of 'live and let live' (which for Locke at the time did not extend to atheists). He wrote,

> The toleration of those that differ from others in matters of religion is so agreeable to the Gospel of Jesus Christ, and to the genuine reason of mankind, that it seems monstrous for men to be so blind as not to perceive the necessity and advantage of it in so clear a light.[10]

He argued that no one had the right to discriminate against someone in a way that affected his civil interests (listed above) on the basis of that person's church or religion.[11] Locke's idea of 'the mutual toleration of private persons' is the beginning of the mutual toleration we see in secular states today, where people of different religions, cultural backgrounds, and opinions are able to live and work side by side in relative harmony.

Individuality. Liberalism is individualistic, in the sense that it takes human individuals to be the fundamental unit of importance, rather than, say, communities or societies or nations. In this respect it has a dispute with all communitarian modes of social organization, which sacrifice the individual good to the good of the group. Note that this does not mean that theories with their roots in liberal values cannot be *collectivist*, it just means that the individual is the entity that has rights and entitlements. Individuals may come together with others to pursue common interests, and in association. But this does not change where the rights and entitlements sit.

Reason. The liberal tradition takes human mental capacities, particularly the capacity for reason and rationality, to be central to human nature. This is generally understood as a matter of the means taken to given ends, and not of ends ('ends' are thing like projects and aspirations, while 'means' are the routes to achieving them). For example, here's the prominent liberal philosopher John Rawls: 'the concept of rationality must be interpreted as far as possible in the narrow sense, standard in economic theory, of taking the most effective means to given ends'.[12] The value of reason is clearly related to the value of individuality. It is individuals that have the capacity to be rational, and all individuals have that capacity in equal measure. (Historically, this meant that *men* were assumed to have this capacity in equal measure.) Liberals tend to see reason as working in the service of more fundamental values, either autonomy or self-fulfilment.

Liberty. Perhaps the best-known liberal defence of the value of liberty was given by John Stuart Mill, who was himself both a liberal and a feminist ally. In *On Liberty*, written in 1859, one of the ways that Mill defended the liberty of the individual was by arguing for limitations to the power of society over the individual. Where Locke before him had argued to limit the power of the *state* over the individual, Mill was more concerned with the power of public opinion (Blackford's title, *The Tyranny of Opinion*, is a hat tip to Mill's idea). Mill agreed that a person's actions could be hurtful or injurious to others, and in that case could justifiably be limited. This included both violations of other people's rights, and failures to do a fair share of collective labour, e.g. for the defence of the country or other persons.[13] But 'when a person's conduct affects the interests of no person besides himself', he said, the person should be legally and socially free to do what he likes and accept the consequences.[14]

Mill justified this by pointing out that each of us is the person most interested in our own well-being, and therefore best-placed to advance it.[15] He thought the best argument for limiting the authority of society over a person's conduct was the likelihood 'that it interferes wrongly and in the wrong place',[16] meaning that majority opinion is just as likely to be wrong as right. People have different tastes and preferences, and some feel strongly about what others do (Mill proceeds, in the relevant chapter, to give several colourful examples).[17] But that does not give them any right to control what those others do.

There has been much philosophical debate over liberty, particularly over whether the best understanding is 'negative liberty', being free from certain things, like physical violence,[18] or having more than one option to choose between;[19] 'positive liberty', in fact having shaped your own life,[20] or being provided with certain things, like healthcare or education;[21] or 'republican liberty', being free from domination, understood as *possible* violation of negative liberty.[22]

These different approaches to liberty have become the basis of distinct positions in political theory: libertarianism, emphasizing negative freedom; contemporary liberalism, emphasizing positive freedom; and republicanism, emphasizing non-domination (although republicanism can be traced back to a much earlier time, as Philip Pettit discusses).[23] Liberty probably became the distinguishing value because there is widespread agreement on most of the others, in particular toleration, individuality, and reason, which means the locus of disagreement has shifted—from liberalism itself as an alternative to other kinds of social arrangements, like theocracy or feudalism—to the finer points of liberalism. Libertarianism is what we think of as the 'conservative' or right-wing position in many liberal democratic countries today, and contemporary liberalism is what we think of as the 'progressive' or left-wing position. It is not clear whether republicanism is really represented within contemporary politics.

Because there has been the greatest amount of disagreement between theorists of *all* types over limitation of state power and over the correct understanding of liberty, we can expect these two values to have also produced divisions between feminists.

9.2 Liberal Feminism

Liberal feminism has aimed at ensuring women are fully included within the liberal view, which meant historically that women were considered to have the same capacity for reason as men, and so were deserving of all the same rights and liberties that men had as a result. (Note that here I mean *real* liberal feminism, as theorized by academic feminists, as opposed to what gets dismissively called 'liberal feminism' today by disenchanted feminist activists). Liberal feminism emphasizes liberal values: autonomy, self-determination, self-fulfilment. A woman must be able to decide on her own good in her own way, and she should not be obstructed in the pursuit of her interests as she defines them. Insofar as it stays close to traditional liberalism, the scope liberal feminism has to criticize a woman's choices is limited to cases where (i) she did not take the relevant means to her ends (and is therefore criticizable against reason/rationality) or (ii) it is possible to demonstrate that there has been an interference with autonomy, for example that a woman has been coerced or indoctrinated. So the liberal feminist can criticize a wife's 'choice' to remain in a marriage when she is subject to coercive control, but cannot criticize a sex worker's 'choice' to engage in sex work (unless, for example, she was trafficked or otherwise forced).

Some notable liberal feminists were Mary Wollstonecraft, John Stuart Mill,[24] Harriet Taylor Mill, and Betty Friedan,[25] as well as the leaders and members of the National Organization for Women (NOW) and the Women's Equity Action League (WEAL) in the United States.[26] Wollstonecraft in particular emphasized women's capacity for rationality as being equal to men's. Wollstonecraft, Mill, Taylor, and Friedan were all concerned with the formal and informal obstacles that prevented women from obtaining an education equal to men, or the opportunity to access paid work in the way that men could. Rosemary Tong writes 'We owe to liberal feminists many, if not most, of the educational and legal reforms that have improved the quality of life for women'.[27] Friedan was probably the most prominent liberal feminist of the second wave.[28]

Janet Radcliffe Richards is an influential liberal feminist philosopher who wrote a book called *The Sceptical Feminist* in 1980. In Chapter 3, 'Enquiries for Liberators', she took up the question of exactly what the *liberation* of the women's liberation (and more generally feminist) movement was meant to be. She says 'Freedom is a central issue in feminism, since even in those parts of the movement which do not actually call themselves "Women's Liberation" it is generally agreed that freedom for women is one of the things that must be achieved'.[29] However, this word has created a lot of confusion; she says '"freedom" is like "natural" in having such good connotations that people are only too delighted to take advantage of any confusion to juggle with half a dozen meanings of the word at once in order to confuse their opponents and win political points'.[30]

Radcliffe Richards thinks the best account of freedom is being in control of one's own destiny, and not being controlled by other people or other 'alien forces'.[31] And, she says, freedom on this understanding is generally considered to be more important than happiness, as evidenced by the fact that many people would refuse interventions that would improve happiness at a cost to freedom (her examples are a miserable artist being offered drugs that would make them happy but cause a loss of artistic ability, and a political dissident living under an oppressive regime being offered 're-education').[32] It's easy to see the liberal values here: a heavy emphasis on negative freedom and the exercise of personal autonomy. What's most interesting is that Radcliffe-Richards uses these commitments to raise questions about the feminist commitment to 'liberating' women.

One point she makes is that if feminists are committed to women being in control of their own destinies, we might expect to see them helping women to get what they want. But, she says, we often see just the opposite. Women who happily choose a traditional division of labour within marriage are criticized, not celebrated, as are women participating in beauty pageants, or working as strippers or prostitutes. She comments

> the true liberator can always be recognized by her wanting to *increase* the options open to the people who are to be liberated, and there is never any justification for taking a choice away from a group you want to liberate unless it is demonstrable beyond all reasonable doubt that removing it will bring other, more important, options into existence.[33]

Still, the feminist who wants to reduce a woman's options has one available justification. She can show that the woman's choice to take a particular option is conditioned, which means something like, created through the process of her socialization. The best way to understand such conditioning is as either ignorance or bad habits that themselves intervene on a woman being able to get what she desires. But interference on this basis must meet a high bar. Radcliffe Richards says 'the only case in which it would be reasonable to override a woman's wishes in the name of her freedom would be where it was absolutely certain that she was conditioned, and equally certain what she really wanted and how it could be brought about'.[34]

We cannot simply tell by looking at the *content* of a woman's preferences, she thinks, that the woman's choice was 'conditioned'. If we get things wrong, then we are acting paternalistically by attempting to impose our own ideas about what other people should want onto them. And given the importance of autonomy in the liberal vision, this would be a very serious violation. For this reason, Radcliffe Richards argues that feminists should limit themselves to two kinds of general interventions: alleviate ignorance by increasing women's understanding of how things came to be as they are; and offer help and support to women who decide on the basis of this new understanding that they want to change their habits, because these are getting in the way of their new desires.[35]

Her conclusion was that as long as people are in a position to choose, then we should prioritize their freedom to do so. When they are not, then we should prioritize the minimization of suffering (and *not*, contrary to some utilitarian liberals, the maximization of happiness).[36]

9.3 Liberal Feminism and Autonomy

If we stopped here, then it would be possible to offer an explanation of the disagreement between gender-critical feminists and other feminists. Those who subscribe to the dominant feminist perspective tend not to criticize women's choices. Stay at home with the kids; put the kids in childcare and go back to work. Shave your legs and wear makeup; grow out your body hair and don't wear makeup. Wear almost nothing; completely cover up. Post streams of selfies and nudes to Instagram; eschew social media all together. Whatever she chooses is a feminist choice *because it is what she has chosen*. This is a way in which the dominant feminist perspective is liberal. The role of the state, they maintain, is to remain neutral between women's competing conceptions of what a good life looks like, and simply protect their ongoing capacity to choose from a broad range of options. They maintain that because the state should remain neutral and not interfere, it is inappropriate for it to be banning industries like prostitution or pornography, which women have chosen to work in, or regulating access to 'sex reassignment' or other body-modifying medicines or surgeries, which women have chosen to have. These, they claim, are all just conceptions of the good and it is disrespectful to women's autonomy to presume to know better than her what is good for her.

Because this liberal respect for choice tracks the dominant feminist position so well, it is plausible to think that this is roughly the version of liberal feminism that has trickled down from academia and into popular culture. If this *is* liberal feminism, then it is true that gender-critical feminism is not liberal, and neither was the radical feminism before it. Both want to criticize the background conditions against which women's choices are made, the reasons why she comes to make the choices she does, the incentives that push her to choose one way or the other. But it's not clear that this is where liberal feminism stops.

Mary Gibson challenged the liberal view that every individual is an authority on her own interests, and reason/rationality is a matter only of assessing the way that she pursues those interests. She gives two examples that she thinks we should obviously be uncomfortable with, the first a voluntary master-slave society,[37] the second a voluntary sadist-masochist society.[38]

She objected to the fact that even if particular ends are 'inegalitarian, exploitative, or otherwise morally repugnant', liberals have no grounds for criticism.[39] Her particular target in the paper was the liberal philosopher John Rawls. She said liberal theory 'provides no basis for criticizing a society whose institutions systematically promote, and whose members acquire and act upon, objectionable desires and ends, including some that would, on a less neutral conception of rationality, be termed irrational'.[40] But surely we want to be able to criticize societies like these, which means either that liberalism will need to gain the ability to criticize some voluntarily chosen ends or that we should not, after all, be liberals.

This brings us back to a point from Section 9.1. Reason works in the service of a more fundamental value, autonomy or self-fulfilment. There is disagreement over the correct interpretation of liberty, with some taking it to mean we have in fact shaped our own lives. There seems to be a question of what exactly liberals mean by 'autonomy', and whether their conception of autonomy gives them any way to criticize some of the choices people make. If it doesn't then Gibson is right, and moreover, there is room for an alternative theory that *does* allow criticism of choices. Perhaps radical feminism is that theory, at least in the domain of sex oppression.

But let's give liberalism a chance. Clare Chambers argues that liberalism, and so liberal feminism, does after all have the ability to criticize some choices. She distinguishes two 'levels' of autonomy, the first over big decisions about what kinds of lives we want to lead, the second over more everyday decisions about what we want to do (including, in particular, about whether to follow particular social rules and norms). This helps to show that there are four possible ways to have (and lack) autonomy. We can have autonomy over the big and the small decisions, e.g. we make an autonomous choice to be a philosopher, and in being a philosopher we constantly question the social norms. We can have autonomy over the big but not the small, e.g. we make an autonomous choice to be in the army, or to become a nun. We can have autonomy over the small but not the big, e.g. a child sent to a progressive school who didn't get a say in which school she went to, but once at the school was taught to routinely question social norms. And finally, we can have neither kind of autonomy, e.g. we can have the misfortune to live under a fundamentalist religious dictatorship, which we didn't choose but were born into, and can't leave, and which restricts what it is possible for us to do on a daily basis.[41]

Liberals care about people being able to pursue their own conceptions of the good life. Some liberal feminists have thought that only autonomy over big decisions, but not over small ones, matters.[42] In other words, autonomy matters only at the level of choosing what kind of life you want to lead. Someone should not be born into or pushed into a religious life where they lack daily autonomy, but if they choose that life for themselves, then it would be paternalistic to insist that it is not an acceptable conception of the good life. It's not that autonomy is so good that people need to be exercising it absolutely all the time.

Chambers' view, however, is that liberals have the grounds to criticize decisions that forego everyday autonomy when they are substantially harmful, when they depend only on a social norm, and when using the state to ban or regulate them wouldn't be a disproportionate interference. Take breast implants, for example. Breast implants are chosen under patriarchy, a social context of inequality between the sexes. Many women feel that breast implants are necessary for career success.[43] But there is nothing about breast implants themselves that brings benefits to women; it is only that there is a pernicious social norm regulating how women should look, particularly that women should be sexually attractive to men and that this involves having large breasts. Chambers writes 'The answer, then, is not to educate women but to alter the social circumstances that justify the harmful practice, and banning the practice is a good way to do this'.[44] Bans solve situations in which social norms are just going to keep producing harm unless nearly everyone stops complying at once; they are a way to *ensure* widespread non-compliance. On Chambers' view, 'nobody should have to harm themselves to receive benefits that are only contingently related to that harm, and where the contingency is a social one'.[45]

This is presented as a *liberal* view that nonetheless allows us to look at background social structures, social inequalities between groups like men and women, and social norms that have grown up over time to create incentives that may lead to one group taking on substantial and harmful costs in order to secure particular benefits. If Chambers is right, and we take her more sophisticated understanding of autonomy into account, then we are likely to be in a better position to accommodate the concerns of the gender-critical feminists under the umbrella of liberal feminism.

Furthermore, we are also in a better position to criticize the feminism that has become so widespread today. In operating with a limited version of liberal feminism, this feminism has found itself largely unable to criticize women's choices, and this means its hands are tied even when it is revealed that *hundreds of thousands* of women are making the same choices in a way that fit into patterns of unjust relations between the sexes. The dominant form of feminism is thus status-quo biased. It has ended up propping up the interests of the male-run and male-profiting sex industry,[46] by supporting the 'autonomous choice' of women to sell men the right to use their bodies, even when those choices are made by women whose only other option is destitution. It has ended up cheerleading for women's self-objectification, standing by while huge numbers of women turn to surgery in order to 'perfect' their bodies according to unrealistic beauty standards. And it has ended up supporting the claims of young gender non-conforming girls that they need medical or surgical interventions to make their bodies more like the opposite sex.

9.4 Gender-Critical Feminism

What was the core insight of radical feminism, that has been picked up and continued by gender-critical feminism? If we can answer this question then we will be in a position to work out whether gender-critical feminism is liberal, and can be fully accommodated within the framework of liberalism.

Radical feminists talked about *unfreedom*, for example in Frye's metaphor of the cage or the idea of women being in a double bind,[47] and in MacKinnon's discussion of psychological unfreedom.[48] They talked about objectification and 'thingification',[49] exploitation,[50] and domination.[51] There was discussion of the role of fear of male violence.[52] There was discussion of the importance of recovering women's lost history.[53] They were centrally concerned with the social inequality between the sexes, with men's control of women (including through institutions), with women's internalization of sexist ideas about herself. They talked about the appropriation of women's labour, both physical and mental.[54] Atkinson wrote

> we are so violated by another group/groups as to deprive us of our humanity. Our mental processes are absorbed, so that choice and evolution are denied us. We are not discrete. We are not unique. Our time and activities are used, not to the end of each of our unique constructions, but as parts and additions to other individual's ends.[55]

Radical feminists also made frequent reference to *liberation* as opposed to 'mere' equality. Germaine Greer, for example, positioned women's liberation in opposition to women's equality saying that the former rejects the possibility of equality with men on men's terms.[56] Gerda Lerner made a similar point, describing patriarchy through a metaphor of a theatre, in which 'the stage set is conceived, painted, defined by men. Men have written the play, have directed the show, interpreted the meanings of the action. They have assigned themselves the most interesting, most heroic parts, giving women the supporting roles'.[57] She says

> What women must do, what feminists are now doing is to point to that stage, its sets, its props, its director, and its scriptwriter, as did the child in the fairy tale who discovered that the emperor was naked, and say, the basic inequality between us lies within this framework. And then they must tear it down.[58]

Liberalism can account for some of this. Arguably even libertarianism, the most minimal version of liberalism, can care about sexist social norms, insofar as they constitute a violation of individual liberty by treating people according to group traits rather than as individuals. Liberalism permits 'paternalistic' interference in childhood, to protect a child's future options, so they have scope to interfere with particular choices made there (this is relevant to the issues of Chapter 5, but also makes room for a feminist education, including the teaching of women's history, as a way to increase options). And as we have seen, liberals can criticize and even ban some choices, particularly ones that are caused by sexist social norms and are substantially harmful. In this way they can go a long way to making sure that women have independence from men, and are not controlled by men either at the level of decisions about how they want their lives to go or in the more banal everyday choices they make.

Still; it is not clear that gender-critical feminism can be fully accommodated within the framework of liberalism. This is for four reasons.

First, liberalism is for and about *everyone*. Liberal feminism works to make sure women are part of that 'everyone'. But gender-critical feminism is not for or about everyone, as I have already argued. And it is not satisfied to merely achieve equality with men, according to male standards for what that means. Gender-critical feminism is for and about female people (women and girls). It thinks *feminism* should be for and about female people. It wants female liberation. On this understanding, feminism cannot give us advice about legal, social, political, and economic reform that is *decisive*. I don't think it's feminism's job (or indeed, the job of any social justice movement) to present demands that are decisive. Suppose that gender-critical feminists demand six months of mandatory paid parental leave, taken by both parents, in order to correct for hiring and advancement discrimination in the workplace. This proposal might secure gains for women and be neutral for other social groups, or secure gains for women and come with some costs to other social groups that are justifiable, or secure gains for women at a cost to other social groups that is unjustifiable. It is too much to ask all social justice movements to formulate their demands with a perfect awareness of what every other group needs and is demanding. It's enough to stay on top of what your own group needs, especially when that group is women—half of the whole human population. Governments and policy-makers, and where appropriate the people through democratic mechanisms, must decide between competing demands in the final instance, and make evidence-based decisions about costs and trade-offs.

Second, liberalism is intended as a comprehensive theory, which means, a total theory, of social and political justice. Liberal feminism works to make sure women are fully included in that theory. Gender-critical feminism is not intended as a comprehensive theory. I don't think feminism should be thought of as a comprehensive theory—although some people have tried to make it so, e.g. by claiming that sex oppression is the root of all other oppression, or by going 'intersectional' in a way that brings in all other causes. We could accomplish gender-critical goals and still be in a world with a lot of injustice in it. In my view, social justice movements cannot do everything, and so they should remain focused on a single axis of oppression until their goals are substantially accomplished. That does not prevent alliances and strategic coalitions where those will produce mutual gains for all parties.[59] This is not motivated by a failure to care enough about social groups other than women, or a failure to care about social justice more generally. I think oppressed communities are better served by having social justice movements focused on their interests, than by movements for which they are just one part of a much broader set of concerns. I also worry about the instability caused by a constant shifting of priorities when those with authority over agenda-setting inside movements are concerned to focus on the least well-off, because as noble a goal as this is, *who* is least well-off can change rapidly.

Third, radical feminism was the first type of feminism to assert that women are oppressed as women, and deserve a theory and movement in their own right. Gender-critical feminism inherits this commitment. This sets gender-critical feminism apart from other feminist theories that originated with men. It would be somewhat perverse given this historical achievement of radical feminist theory to then attempt to argue that it is, after all, merely a version of an older, male-authored political theory, namely classical liberalism, revised and updated over time. If gender-critical feminism fit perfectly within the liberal framework then this perversity wouldn't be a reason to resist the classification of gender-critical feminism *as* liberal, but it doesn't fit perfectly, and the fourth reason may be the most decisive in establishing this.

The fourth reason is that liberalism is centrally concerned with autonomy. This captures something of what gender-critical feminists have been worried about. But it does not capture it all. I have said at multiple points in this book that feminism is a political movement for women's self-determination. I think it is crucially important that the androcentrism of human history, at least since the beginning of patriarchy some three and a half thousand years ago, has so deeply shaped the world we live in. Particularly, I am concerned with how men have created ideas about what a woman is, and what women are for, and how these ideas have served men's needs particularly well by providing them with sexual and domestic service. Perhaps more than any oppressed group throughout history, women have *internalized* their oppressors' ideas about themselves. Women's liberation is not possible without women being able to get free of these ideas. It is not clear that autonomy, even on Chambers' more sophisticated conception, gets to the heart of this point. A woman whose desires have been thoroughly 'constructed' under patriarchy may choose, both at the level of big decisions and at the more everyday level, in ways that nonetheless work to the advantage of men. Self-objectification, a willingness to sell sex, and the view that one is 'not a woman' (or girl) may all be explained in this way.

What is the 'self' when it has been so thoroughly constructed, by others, to be *for* others? Lerner wrote:

> Women's lack of knowledge of our own history of struggle and achievement has been one of the major means of keeping us subordinate. But even those of us already defining ourselves as feminist thinkers and engaged in the process of critiquing traditional systems of ideas are still held back by unacknowledged restraints embedded deeply within our psyches. Emergent woman faces a challenge to her very definition of self. How can her daring thought—naming the hitherto unnamed, asking the questions defined by all authorities as 'non-existent'—how can such thought coexist within her life as woman? In stepping out of the constructs of patriarchal thought, she faces, as Mary Daly put it, 'existential nothingness.'[60]

Women in the 1960s who threw absolutely all of their energies into their husbands and children, and were then told by Betty Friedan to get into paid work so that they had something for themselves, must have struggled to know what this would even mean. What did they want, in and of themselves? What did they like? If you haven't had a chance to find these things out, then you may have no idea at all. When women join together in political associations they can begin to discuss these things, and work out ways to reject men's ideas about women, and work out what they want to be, as women and as individuals. (These kinds of discussions started in the women's consciousness-raising groups of the second wave.) Although Friedan herself is usually considered a liberal feminist, she seems to agree that there is the problem I'm pointing to here. She said 'a woman could only exist by pleasing a man. She was wholly dependent on his protection in a world that she had no share in making: a man's world. She could never grow up to ask the simple human question, "Who am I? What do I want?"'.[61]

This issue cannot be captured in the usual way, as a lack of negative freedom, or a constraint upon autonomy. It is not that men are stopping women from doing something in particular, the problem comes earlier than that. And it is not that if only women had more resources, or more information, or were less in the grip of social norms, they could do the things they knew they wanted to do. They may not know what they want to do, and this is part of the problem. There is a problem in the very construction of the 'self'. Atkinson wrote in 1970 'It is one of the many nightmares of feminism, that to even conceive of what could count as significant changes for women, one must begin by jumping off one cliff after another'.[62]

The disagreement between gender-critical and the culturally dominant liberal-*ish* feminism is *not* a disagreement over whether to be liberals. Broadly speaking, we are all liberals. It is a disagreement over how deep the lack of (the possibility of) autonomy goes, and where it is permissible for the state to intervene to take certain choices off the table for everyone.

9.5 Feminism with Teeth

The gender-critical feminist is not concerned to avoid the 'paternalism' of interference with choices that are rational responses to sexist social norms. She's concerned with building a world in which women are not dominated by men, in which there is not social inequality between the sexes. If she can build a strong case that there is domination or inequality, and that some women's 'choices' are caused by it, or reinforce it, then she will be critical of those choices. She may even think it appropriate that the law be utilized in a way that will ultimately take those choices off the table. But her motivation is to take away *men's* choices to treat women in particular ways. The gender-critical feminist is fundamentally opposed to women's slavery, subjection, domination, exploitation, and vulnerability. Her vision of women's liberation is a society in which the law gives women robust protection from all of these things. Worrying about how this interferes with women's choices is like worrying about the abolition of slavery on the grounds that some slaves enjoyed the work. Gender-critical feminism is uniquely positioned to take patterns of domination seriously, because it looks at women as a class, and so social *patterns*, rather than at individual women. And it is uniquely positioned to criticize the status quo. It is feminism with teeth.

CODA

10
A Gender-Critical Manifesto

10.1 Feminism as a Movement for Women as Women

As I hope this book has shown, it's far from obvious that feminism should be 'inclusive'. We should be particularly cautious about inclusiveness in response to men's needs. One of the commitments of feminism is to resisting feminine gender stereotypes, and one prevalent feminine gender stereotype is that women need to focus on men's needs. It is also far from obvious that feminism should be 'intersectional', at least when that means ceding ground to other movements or combining together with them. It's not obvious that we get a better, more coherent, or more effective social justice movement out of focusing on women *as people* rather than on women *as women*. The former loses sight of the original source of women's oppression, and overburdens feminist activists and theorists with more content than they can possibly manage. This is all a way of imploding feminism from the inside, making it hopelessly broad and unfocused.

Being female is a discrete source of oppression, and *all* women, as women, need a theory and movement to tackle that oppression. Women need to work to reclaim a coherent and effective version of feminism, one that is focused on the oppression of all women as women. Below is a female-focused list of demands, formed in consultation with gender-critical women across multiple social media sites in 2019.[1] It's not meant to be the final say, not least because there is still work to be done in applying the test suggested in Chapter 7 to figure out which of the further social group issues has a sex-differentiated element. But it is an indication of the seriousness of the difference from the list many feminists today seem to be working to, of which the International Women's Day (IWD) Melbourne Collective's was an example (see Chapter 1).

Because it refuses to combine multiple movements, it does not include issues that affect women in virtue of other aspects of their identities, *unless* the impacts on women are disproportionate in a way that is ultimately explained by sex and the treatment of the sexes. Because its constituency is

Gender-Critical Feminism: Holly Lawford-Smith, Oxford University Press.
DOI: 10.1093/oso/9780198863885.003.0010

female people, it does not include any issues that impact male people, *unless* those issues impact female people and mitigating them will merely bring side benefits for men. Because it is about all women, and it aims at women's liberation in the long-term, it is opposed to prostitution and pornography, which feed the sexual objectification of women in general and enact violence against women, both those working in the sex industry and likely those outside of it.

Many of the items in the list are about women's specific physiology (especially in sections I, III, and V). That is a reassertion of the importance of women's bodies in feminism (as opposed to, say, 'gender identities' or 'femininity' regardless of body). The list includes protection from discrimination for women's lesbian and bisexual sexual orientations, which can't be a priority for a feminism that has replaced sexual orientations with attractions between gender identities.[2] It includes protection for feminist speech, which won't be secured by a feminism busy cancelling its detractors for 'whorephobia', 'transphobia', or 'white feminism'.

The list is a starting point, not the end point, for a refocusing of feminist priorities. It may be most useful inside gender-critical feminist collectives, newly formed and deciding where to channel their energies. Feminists who have a clear sense of their constituency, of what women's subordination consists in, and of which issues affect the greatest number of women and which issues affect women the worst, will be in the position to stand firm against accusations of 'exclusion' when they are not justified, will refuse to cede ground to other movements, and will centre women and advance women's interests in all their work.

10.2 The List

*I. **An end to male violence against women and girls***

1. An end to female genital mutilation (FGM)
2. An end to female infanticide
3. An end to child brides
4. An end to forced marriage
5. An end to rape and other forms of sexual violence
6. An end to domestic violence
7. Criminalization of intimate partner strangulation as a separate offence
8. No 'sex games gone wrong' defence for men's killing of female sexual partners

9. Criminalization of the purchase of sex (the Nordic Model)
10. Criminalization of the making of professional pornography[3]
11. Freedom from violence for female intersex people
12. Freedom from sexual violence for women with disabilities
13. Freedom from sexual violence for women living in refugee camps
14. Recognition of torture and slavery as domestic (non-state) offences
15. Criminalization of all forms of paid surrogacy
16. An end to all forms of male violence against women and girls

II. ***Addressing contributors to male violence against women and girls***

1. An end to the sexual objectification of women in advertising
2. Portrayal of women as whole persons in film and television
3. An end to the hypersexualization of black women
4. Education on the tactics used by domestic abusers, to aid in the prevention of women and girls becoming victims of domestic violence
5. An end to all enforced modesty of women and girls
6. Legal reform to enable police to bring domestic family violence and sexual offence criminal charges without complainants, to alleviate pressure on survivors

III. ***Protecting women's health and bodily autonomy***

1. Adequate healthcare to prevent deaths in childbirth
2. An end to period poverty
3. Increased funding for research into women's health
4. A call for all new pharmaceuticals and medical devices to have their effects on women evaluated
5. An end to the 'default male' assumption in healthcare research
6. Support for the health and safety of prostituted and exited women
7. Full reproductive rights for all women, including free and accessible abortions[4]
8. Reassertion of the importance of female-only spaces (bathrooms, changing rooms, prisons, etc.)
9. Free, accessible vaccination for women and girls against human papillomavirus (HPV) strains 16 and 17 (which cause the bulk of cervical cancer)
10. Reassertion of the right of women and girls to request female doctors and healthcare professionals for all intimate examinations and procedures

11. More research into the causes of the rise in teenage girls reporting to gender clinics
12. In order to avoid creating a market for women's organs, zero funding for research into womb transplants into male bodies
13. Support for female survivors of male violence, in particular in housing and mental health services
14. Access to midwives for high quality maternity care
15. Intrapartum and postpartum healthcare to prevent postpartum depression, postpartum psychosis, post-traumatic stress disorder (PTSD), and maternal suicide
16. An end to obstetric violence

IV. *Protecting women's freedom of conscience and freedom of thought*

1. Women-only shortlists to secure the increased participation of women in politics
2. Demand for women's equal participation in politics
3. Rejection of transwomen acting as women's officers for any party (regardless of their gender identity)
4. Reassertion of the importance of female-only spaces (political groups, women's festivals, etc.)
5. A reassertion of the importance of language that refers to female people and articulates political problems affecting female people, including the terms 'woman', 'female', 'lesbian', 'mother', and 'wife'
6. Acceptance of the political choice some women make to refuse to extend female pronouns (she/her/hers) to transwomen, particularly in cases where those people have engaged in or threatened violence against women and girls, or exemplified toxic masculinity
7. Reaffirmation of the sex/gender distinction
8. Rejection of concept creep from 'accurately referring to sex' to 'misgendering'
9. A rejection of all forms of misogyny perpetrated in the name of religion, in particular against Muslim women
10. Reassertion of women's right to organize politically to pursue their interests
11. Rejection of all pressure on women to include other causes in their feminism or to prioritize male interests in their feminism
12. Education on patriarchal domination, and rejection of all social conditioning that tells women and girls to put boys' and men's needs before their own

13. In order to avoid violations of women's bodily autonomy (specifically their reproductive choices) premised on poor science understanding, universal education on pregnancy and the process of gestation

V. *Women's access to and full participation in public life*

1. An end to pregnancy discrimination
2. An end to breastfeeding discrimination
3. Reassertion of the importance of women's sex-based rights
4. Protection from discrimination for lesbian and bisexual women
5. Protection from discrimination for gender non-conforming women
6. Protection from discrimination for transmen
7. Increased incentives for women to enter science, technology, engineering, and maths (STEM) subjects
8. A living wage for all women in all industries
9. Generous paid parental leave and affordable childcare
10. Generous welfare support for parents who wish to care full-time for children with special needs
11. Women's equal pay for equal work
12. An end to the 'default male' assumption in product design
13. Better education about sexual orientation in teenage years, in particular lesbian and bisexual orientations
14. Better support for women's pursuit of criminal proceedings against fathers who fail to pay child maintenance
15. Flexible work and paid leave for women in the workplace going through menopause, difficult pregnancies, and painful menstruation
16. Preservation of female sporting categories
17. Increased recognition and respect for professions dominated by women
18. Respect for women's human rights
19. Consultation with women on all matters that affect them, including reform to laws for who will be housed in the female prison estate, and reform of laws determining who may access single-sex services more generally

Afterword

I've always been fascinated by the people we might think of as 'moral prophets', the people who lived amidst terrible injustice that was at the same time completely ordinary and accepted, and yet *saw it* for what it was. There are many celebrated examples—some of my favourites are in Adam Hochschild's account of the early movers in the abolition of slavery in the British Empire[1]—although for all the examples that we celebrate, there are surely many more that are lost to history.

The early feminists were moral prophets in this sense. It is hard now, looking back, not to underestimate the magnitude of the accomplishment that feminism is.[2] We know so much about what women are capable of that we cannot fully inhabit a mindset in which they are virtually another species than man, and thought to be capable of so much less. But that was the mindset of almost everyone in the period when feminism first emerged.

Imagine being such a woman, at various points over the last several thousand years: looking around and seeing enormous differences between men and women, not just in terms of dress, mannerisms, and behaviour, but in terms of opportunities and probable life outcomes too. Women and men look different, behave differently, and seem to be good at different things. Where there is religion, that religion generally reinforces those differences as good; where there is science, that science generally explains those differences as natural. Almost everyone accepts the situation. Women themselves are not railing against it; many seem quite happy with it.

It would be enormously tempting for a woman who noticed something amiss at one such point in history to make an exception of herself, rather than to reach a conclusion about *all* women. She might think, well, *women* are indeed different from men, and inferior to men, but I am not like them, I am more like a man. And perhaps she would dress up as a man, or take the pseudonym of a man, to access men's opportunities. The early feminists did not make exceptions of themselves, however. They did something much more ambitious.

They argued that *women* as a group were being limited in ways that at least partly created their inequality with men. This was a class analysis—not in the technical Marxist sense, but in the colloquial sense that they saw themselves as part of a bigger social group impacted by a common set of circumstances. Because they saw a common problem for women, they began to work to convince women that this problem existed, that as women they were capable of much more than they had been led to believe.

What an uphill battle this must have been! Some women would have found the whole idea absurd; other women might have believed it, ultimately, but just not been up for the lifelong struggle that comes when the scales fall from your eyes and you see injustice clearly. After all, we only get one life, and we might rationally choose to spend it on other projects than a potentially futile struggle for equality, or liberation, or both.

Nothing has ever seized my attention and refused to relax its grip like feminism has. I have cared about social justice issues, most significantly in recent years climate justice, but I have never been consumed by them. With feminism, in particular with feminist thinkers, I can't get enough. I want to read everything, although even working on this project virtually full-time for several years, there is much more to read than I could possibly get through.

My respect and admiration for the earliest feminists, who had the conviction that woman was more than she appeared to be, and imagined a future in which she could realize her full potential, is limitless. I wish that we all knew more about the first wave feminists' struggle to get women the vote, and the second wavers' struggles for the many legal reforms that have greatly advanced women's equality with men, so that we would not take those gains so much for granted. But what I am most fascinated by is the radical feminist strand of feminist theory, the intellectual work women had to do to imagine woman differently, to see a path to liberation, to articulate a sex-equal future, to uncover all the insidious ways that women had been made to believe (and act) as though they were lesser than men.

I hope that this book has made you just as excited about feminism as I am, and that knowing more about feminist ideas from the period at which feminism re-emerged as a movement and became a full-blown theory will help to provide an antidote to some of the less exciting ideas of the contemporary feminist movement.

Notes

Preliminary material

1. 'there is no "objective" or natural sex...it is performatively constructed' (Morgenroth & Ryan 2018, p. 40); 'perhaps this construct called "sex" is as culturally constructed as gender; indeed, perhaps it was always already gender with the consequence that the distinction between sex and gender turns out to be no distinction at all' (Butler 1990, pp. 9–10); 'sex is, then, a cultural thing posing as a natural one. Sex, which feminists have taught us to distinguish from gender, is itself already gender in disguise' (Srinivasan 2021, p. xii).
2. 'Two sexes have never been enough to describe human variety' (Fausto-Sterling 2018); 'sex and gender are best conceptualized as points in a multidimensional space' (Fausto-Sterling 2000, p. 22); 'I suggest that the three intersexes...deserve to be considered additional sexes each in its own right. Indeed, I would argue further that sex is a vast, infinitely malleable continuum that defies the constraints of even five categories' (Fausto-Sterling 1993)'; 'we now know that sex is complicated enough that we have to admit, nature doesn't draw the line for us between male and female, or between male and intersex and female and intersex, we actually draw that line on nature (Dreger 2011, 06:15–06:30).
3. Riley Dennis is a transwoman and gender identity activist who creates content for YouTube (as of September 2021 Dennis had 111K subscribers). In a video from 2017, Dennis argues that it's 'cissexist' to 'only be attracted to people with one kind of genitals'. Sexual orientations are described as 'preferences' and these 'preferences' are claimed to be shaped by 'implicit biases'. The video has since been deleted (it got a *lot* of backlash), but there's a transcript at (Dennis 2017), and parts of the video are still available as part of a response video by gender-critical feminist activist Magdalen Berns (Berns 2017). For a more recent and milder version of this claim, the Oxford philosopher Amia Srinivasan wrote in the *London Review of Books* that 'Trans women often face sexual exclusion from lesbian cis women who at the same time claim to take them seriously as women', and mused about 'whether there is a duty to transfigure, as best we can, our desires' (the last bit comes from reflecting on the many social groups marginalized in sex and dating, including but not limited to transwomen) (Srinivasan 2018).
4. Lauren Dinour writes about breastfeeding that 'By using gendered terms like woman and mother when conducting and reporting lactation research, making infant feeding recommendations, or implementing breastfeeding policies, we

risk alienating an already marginalized population' (Dinour 2019, p. 524). She goes on, 'several studies have reported how using heterosexual and woman-focused lactation language in obstetric and pediatric practice settings can misgender, isolate, and harm transmasculine parents and non-heteronormative families' (p. 524), and recommends replacing female-specific language with 'breast/chest feeding', and 'human/parent's milk' (p. 527). About pregnancy and birth, she recommends that 'gestational parent' or 'birthing parent' replace 'mother' (p. 527). There is also a useful table in the paper identifying all the peer-reviewed journals publishing breastfeeding-related articles that mandate 'inclusive' language (p. 528). A number of organizations have now made a move towards 'inclusive' language for female-specific issues. For example, in 2017 the British Medical Association circulated an internal document to staff advising on terminology to avoid offence, including the replacement of 'expectant mothers' with 'pregnant people'. They said this terminology was a way to 'include intersex men and transmen who may get pregnant' (Donnelly 2017). More recently, in Australia, there were divisions within the Australian Breastfeeding Association after a new transgender-inclusive guide was released which referred to 'chest-feeding' and described how lactation could be induced in males (Lane 2019).

5. A nonbinary author wrote for *Seventeen* magazine 'for a group of activists who cite "inclusion" and "intersectionality" on the signs that they carry and the chants that they shout, they should reconsider whether donning a pussy hat is actually in alignment with what they preach...the idea that biological sex determines gender proves itself time and time again to be outdated and transphobic. When it comes down to it, not all women have vaginas and not all people with vaginas are women' (Mandler 2019).
6. This is just one example where there are many. In the book, I'll talk about two more. I'll talk about the socialization of women into the sexual service of men, as a perspective on the prostitution and pornography industries (Chapter 4). And I'll talk about the construction of what it means to be a woman, in addition to merely being female (Chapters 2 and 3).
7. Firestone (1970, p. 15).

Chapter 1

1. For discussion of various plausible views of biological sex, see discussion in (Stock 2021, ch. 2).
2. Re. the heading of this section, cf. hooks' subtitle 'From Margin to Centre' (hooks [1984] 2000).
3. See internationalwomensday.com accessed 20th March 2020. This website, the first Google search result for 'international women's day', is run by a private company that does 'gender capital management' (The Minefield 2020).

4. The list was posted in the 'About' section of their public Facebook event page. Online at https://www.facebook.com/events/381589392387395/?active_tab=about accessed 28th December 2019.
5. https://www.and.org.au/pages/disability-statistics.html
6. For various examples, search 'women + centre themselves + movement' in Twitter, sorted by 'Latest'.
7. https://youtu.be/7Yu9enVjNs8
8. Kaplan et al. (2003).
9. http://sydney.edu.au/handbooks/arts/subject_areas_eh/gender_studies.shtml
10. According to the *Times Higher Education*'s World University Rankings data from 2019. Online at https://www.timeshighereducation.com/student/best-universities/best-universities-australia accessed 20th March 2020.
11. https://www.arts.unsw.edu.au/hal/study-us/subject-areas/womens-gender-studies
12. The 'waves' model of feminist history is not universal, but specific to the United States, the United Kingdom, Australia, New Zealand, Canada, France, and Germany.
13. Chesler (2018).
14. Jaschick (2009).
15. Ginsberg in Jaschick (2009).
16. Ginsberg in Jaschick (2009).
17. See e.g. https://www.auckland.ac.nz/en/study/study-options/find-a-study-option/maori-studies.html
18. This is the date of the first women's suffrage petition in the UK, presented to Henry Hunt MP by Mary Smith from Yorkshire. See https://www.bl.uk/votes-for-women/articles/womens-suffrage-timeline
19. See e.g. https://www.girlsnotbrides.org/themes/health/and https://iwhc.org/resources/facts-child-marriage/
20. Chesler (2018, p. 43).
21. Taddeo (2019, p. 2).
22. Fine et al. (2020).
23. Cf. Pinker (2002), who argues that some of the sex inequality across industries can be explained by average differences in male and female preferences (stemming from average differences in natural aptitudes that have a biological basis).
24. See also Radcliffe Richards (1980, pp. 392–393).
25. Greer (2018).
26. Bolinger (2019).
27. Kipnis (2017).
28. A good example of positive education for women's sexual pleasure is OMGYES, a website that surveyed 20,000 women between 18 and 95 years old, in partnership with researchers from Indiana University and the Kinsey Institute. See https://www.omgyes.com accessed 7th June 2020.

29. Bindel (2018).
30. O. Jones (2015).
31. Bindel (2018).
32. hooks (2000).
33. Mackay (2017).
34. Second-wave feminism was determinedly women centred, while third-wave pushback began opening the movement up to men. On the second-wavers, see discussion in Chapter 2; for one prominent version of the third-wave 'feminism is for everybody' (meaning, is also for men) line, see hooks (2000).
35. I'll say 'caste/class' in Chapters 1–3, rather than 'class' alone, to avoid confusion with Marxism. Neither term is perfect; the important point is that 'women' is a social group with political interests, parallel to groups like 'New Zealand Maori', or 'the working class'. Shulamith Firestone uses both 'class' and 'caste' (Firestone 1970). For a defence of the term 'caste' being used in connection with women, see Daly (1973, pp. 2–3). In the rest of the book, I'll use 'class' alone, for simplicity.
36. There is further discussion of the place of men in gender-critical feminism in Chapter 3, Section 3.4.
37. Mackay (2015).
38. For the origin of this section's title, see n. 36 to Chapter 9.
39. Chesler (2018, p. 3).
40. Freeman (1976). See also discussion in Lawford-Smith (forthcoming).
41. Norma (2018).
42. Norma (2015).
43. https://hmaustralasia.files.wordpress.com/2019/12/schedule-hm-2-dec-19.pdf
44. Norma (2018).
45. Lori Watson is an academic feminist who holds the latter combination of views, see e.g. Watson (2016) and Watson & Flanigan (2020).
46. See further discussion in Chapter 3, Section 3.3.
47. Women started calling themselves 'gender critical' around 2014. This coincided with increased disagreement about trans/gender issues, but was explained by radical feminist commitments. An article at Bitch Media in 2014 commented on 'modern-day feminists [who] continue to actively question the inclusion of trans people in women's spaces', and said 'These feminists refer to themselves as "radical feminists" or "gender critical feminists"' (Vasquez 2014). This is the same year that the Reddit feminist community r/GenderCritical (now banned) was created. From its inception to mid-2017, it had less than 10K subscribers. As of late May 2020 it had 60.4K members, and its top two keywords, at more than double the frequency of the next, were 'womanhood' and 'radfem'. ('Radfem' is the colloquial term for 'radical feminist'). Its description began 'Feminism is the movement to liberate women from patriarchy', and while it placed an emphasis on resistance to gender identity ideology, it also cited

radical feminist concerns like respect for lesbian sexuality, reproductive freedom, and opposition to the exploitation of women by men in prostitution and pornography. (These details were accurate as of 22nd May 2020, and can currently still be viewed at https://subredditstats.com/r/gendercritical. By the 30th of June 2020, r/GenderCritical had been banned from Reddit for 'violating Reddit's rule against promoting hate'. See the notice at https://www.reddit.com/r/GenderCritical/.) A 2015 article in *Slate* reported on two transwomen, Helen Highwater and Miranda Yardley, as 'part of ... a dissenting faction of trans people, one that's often described as "gender-critical"'. The author goes on to write that 'To be gender-critical is to doubt the belief, which its critics call "genderism", that gender is some sort of irreducible essence, wholly distinct from biological sex or socialization' (Goldberg 2015). Perhaps the best-known gender-critical feminist in the world (her own choice of labels aside) is the British feminist activist Kellie-Jay Keen-Minshull. Keen-Minshull, better known by the alias Posie Parker, has a YouTube channel with 38.6K subscribers (as of mid-September 2021). In one of her videos, released just before the UK consultation over the Gender Recognition Act (GRA) opened, she articulated concerns with the proposed reforms to the law including that it would mean an end to all women-only space; the legal category of sex becoming a matter of mere self-identification; a shift from 'gender reassignment' to 'gender identity' as a requirement for a man to demand social treatment as a woman (with no definition of gender identity given); impacts on women's ability to request same-sex service providers; and impacts on women's sports given that men would be able to compete against women merely by identifying as them (Keen-Minshull 2018). These reasons are all about how proposed legal changes designed to advance the interests of trans people work to set back the interests of women. The rationale for opposition to the reforms is a specific set of feminist commitments.

48. Pettit (1993, p. 163). In-text citation removed.
49. https://www.womensdeclaration.com/country-info/ accessed 15th May 2020.
50. Lori Watson, for example, uses 'self-identified feminists' to refer to feminists who don't share her view on trans issues (Watson 2016, p. 246); Jennifer Saul says she 'hesitate[s] to attach the label feminist' to the gender-critical position on trans issues (Saul 2020).
51. Morley (1999).
52. Firestone's proposal was complete freedom from reproduction and child-rearing, and political autonomy based on economic independence, integration, and sexual freedom (Firestone 1970, pp. 184–187). We'll talk about her more later in the book.
53. Firestone (1970, p. 189).
54. Firestone (1970, p. 191).
55. Firestone (1970, p. 197).
56. Perry (2019).

Chapter 2

1. Catharine MacKinnon, probably the best known of the radical feminists, understands radical feminism much more narrowly than I do. In a 1983 paper, she said that radical feminism was methodologically post-Marxist, could not rest on a naturalist understanding of gender, and could not be classically liberal. She said that Andrea Dworkin and Adrienne Rich were good examples of radical feminists in this sense; Mary Daly, Shulamith Firestone, and Susan Griffin (normally thought of as radical feminists) were not (MacKinnon 1983, p. 639, fn. 8).
2. There were also prominent Australian, British, and French radical feminists, not least Germaine Greer, Sheila Jeffreys, and Monique Wittig, but the earliest essays do seem to be exclusively by the Americans. Interestingly, the splintering off of the radicals from the reformers seems to have happened the other way around in Australia; first came the women's liberationists, inspired by the American radical feminist movement, then came the Women's Electoral Lobby, who considered themselves reformers rather than liberationists (and in that regard were a correlate of the NOW). See further detail in the documentary *Brazen Hussies* (2020), see https://documentaryaustralia.com.au/project/brazen-hussies/
3. Greer (1970, pp. 334–335).
4. See n. 58, this chapter.
5. Atkinson (1974*a*, p. 41).
6. Insofar as liberal feminism had disagreements with liberalism and began to critique it, it has some claim to being somewhat female-authored, but it still owes a great intellectual debt to the classical liberals, who were mostly men. See discussion in Wendell (1987).
7. Lerner (1986, pp. 12–13). The full quote is in Chapter 9.
8. Lorde ([1984] 2007, p. 64). From the essay 'Sexism: An American Disease in Blackface', first published as 'The Great American Disease' in 1979.
9. MacKinnon (1983, p. 639).
10. Atkinson (1974*a*, p. 41).
11. Atkinson (1974*a*, p. 52).
12. Firestone (1970, p. 3).
13. Millett (1970, pp. 24–25).
14. MacKinnon (1982, p. 515).
15. Lerner (1986).
16. Dworkin (1974, p. 130). Dworkin says that the ratio of women to men burned has been estimated as being between 20:1 and 100:1, so that 'Witchcraft was a woman's crime'. A paper in the *American Journal of Sociology* puts the number of people executed as witches in continental Europe between the early 14th century and 1650 at between 200,000 and 500,000, 85 per cent or more of these executions being of women (Ben-Yehuda 1980, p. 1). A more recent economic

study collected data on 'more than 43,000 people prosecuted for witchcraft across 21 European countries between 1300 and 1850' (Leeson & Russ 2018, p. 2067). The country with the highest number of persons tried for witchcraft in this period was Germany, with 16,474 persons (p. 2078).

17. Dworkin (1974).
18. Brownmiller (1976).
19. Firestone (1970).
20. Atkinson (1974*a*).
21. Millett (1970).
22. E.g. Dworkin (1974); MacKinnon (1991*b*, 1993).
23. Atkinson (1974*a*); Frye (1983).
24. MacKinnon (1989).
25. For an early discussion on this point, see Hacker (1951).
26. The Leeds Revolutionary Feminist Group wrote 'We do think that all feminists can and should be political lesbians. Our definition of a political lesbian is a woman-identified woman who does not fuck men. It does not mean compulsory sexual activity with women...we think serious feminists have no choice but to abandon heterosexuality' (1981, p. 5).
27. For a contemporary statement of this view, see Julie Bindel's video for *The Guardian*, 'I'm a lesbian, but I wasn't born this way', 22nd April 2015. Bindel asks 'are we born gay, or is it possible to make a positive choice to reject heterosexuality, and decide to switch sides? Of course it is. Sexual attraction normally comes about as a result of opportunity, luck, or curiosity'. She says her view of sexual orientation came from the feminists she met in the 1970s, 'who helped me understand that loving women can be truly liberatory'. Online at https://www.youtube.com/watch?v=PDKwYbV1jQs
28. Pateman (1988).
29. These are nearly Kate Phelan's words: in a forthcoming paper she talks about 'the magnitude of the achievement that feminism is'. See Phelan (forthcoming).
30. Other interesting ideas I don't have the space to discuss in this section can be found in Pizan (1405); Gouges (1791); Taylor Mill (1851); and (Mill 1869).
31. Wollstonecraft ([1792] 2017, ch. IV). Wollstonecraft is generally thought of as a liberal feminist, as a result of her views about the equality of men and women in terms of rational personhood, and the importance of equal education for women (see e.g. Tong 1989, pp. 13–17). Here I'm tracking a specific point she made, and the way it anticipates (and surely influenced) the later development of radical feminism.
32. Wollstonecraft talks about women in general; here, in thinking about how the differences between men and women must have seemed at the time, I'm making a more limited claim about the men and women of Wollstonecraft's class.
33. Wollstonecraft ([1792] 2017, p. 76). A notable exception to this 'choice' was Anne Lister, dubbed the first modern lesbian, who lived in the late 1700s to the early

1800s, and was gender non-conforming in presentation, a lesbian, self-educated, and engaged in business and travel highly atypical for women at the time.

34. Simone de Beauvoir makes a similar point about the role of physicality in *The Second Sex* (1949, Volume II, Part I, ch. 1, esp. pp. 311, 320, 354–358).
35. Wollstonecraft ([1792] 2017, p. 87).
36. Wollstonecraft ([1792] 2017, pp. 102–103).
37. Wollstonecraft ([1792] 2017, p. 104).
38. Or, in the theistic worldview of the time, the result of their having different types of 'souls'—or perhaps of women not having 'souls' at all.
39. Wollstonecraft ([1792] 2017, p. 80).
40. Aristotle, for example, thought that people had different souls, and that these were distinguished by their proportions of rationality/irrationality (alternatively intellect/appetite). Slaves of either sex were virtually all appetite/irrationality, women (free females) were a little rationality/intellect and a lot irrationality/appetite, and men (free males) were all or mostly rationality/intellect, none or only a little irrationality/appetite (Spelman 1988).
41. While both Alison Jaggar (1983) and Rosemary Tong (1989) classify Beauvoir as an existentialist feminist rather than a radical feminist, there is so much in her book that looks like early radicalism, which can be taken up quite independently of her existentialism, that I will tend to talk about her together with the radicals in this book.
42. Beauvoir ([1949] 2011, p. 15).
43. Beauvoir ([1949] 2011, p. 13).
44. Volume I, Part I, ch. 1.
45. Volume I, Part I, ch. 2.
46. Volume I, Parts II and III.
47. Volume II.
48. Beauvoir ([1949] 2011, p. 433).
49. See discussion in Volume I, Part II, ch. 5.
50. In a 2014 piece for *New Statesman*, Helen Lewis wrote 'As an intellectual movement, Second Wave feminism has suffered more than most by being ground down into soundbites, its leaders flattened into caricatures. It is nothing less than an outrage that so little should remain of, say, Andrea Dworkin's legacy that her most famous utterance is something that she never actually wrote or argued. Her peers have similarly been crushed by a feminist movement whose primary method of moving forward often seems to be kicking against its foremothers' (Lewis 2014).
51. Beauvoir ([1949] 2011, p. 293).
52. See e.g. Butler (1986). Butler begins the paper by quoting Beauvoir, but then goes on to say 'Beauvoir's formulation…suggests that gender is an aspect of identity gradually acquired', and then moves to decouple sex and gender so-understood (as an identity): 'The presumption of a causal or mimetic relation

between sex and gender is undermined. If being a woman is one cultural interpretation of being female, and if that interpretation is in no way necessitated by being female, then it appears that the female body is the arbitrary locus of the gender "woman", and there is no reason to preclude the possibility of that body becoming the locus of other constructions of gender' (Butler 1986, p. 35). Where Beauvoir was making a point about *what is done to female people*, Butler is reifying what is done into an 'identity' that people of either sex can take up. Butler does not own up to this innovation, but rather declares that it was Beauvoir's all along: '"being" female and "being" a woman are two very different sorts of being. This last insight, I would suggest, is the distinguished contribution of Simone de Beauvoir's formulation "one is not born, but rather becomes, a woman"' (Butler 1986, p. 35).

53. Volume II, Part I, ch. 1.
54. Volume II, Part I, ch. 2.
55. Volume II, Part I, ch. 3.
56. MacKinnon put it like this: 'Where liberal feminism sees sexism primarily as an illusion or myth to be dispelled, an inaccuracy to be corrected, true feminism sees the male point of view as fundamental to the male power to create the world in its own image, the image of its desires, not just as its delusory end product. Feminism distinctively as such comprehends that what counts as truth is produced in the interest of those with power to shape reality, and that this process is as pervasive as it is necessary as it is changeable' (MacKinnon 1983, p. 640).
57. Most of these women were Americans. The emergence of radical feminism in the UK is a little more complicated. In 1977, Sheila Jeffreys published a short article defending the idea of 'revolutionary feminism', which was, just like radical feminism, a reaction against socialist feminism and an articulation of a theory of women's oppression as a distinct phenomenon. Jeffreys acknowledged radical feminism but said that it seemed to have gone into hibernation. Revolutionary feminism was also more centrally separatist, seeing the source of woman's oppression in her reproductive labour, and a solution in her complete withdrawal from men and refusal to perform this labour. Revolutionary feminists advocated for political lesbianism. One way to understand it is that radical feminism emerged at different times under different names in the United States and the United Kingdom. But this can't be entirely accurate, given what Jeffreys said about radical feminism, and given that in 1970 several key radical feminist books were published and available in both countries, including Shulamith Firestone's *The Dialectic of Sex*, Kate Millett's *Sexual Politics*, and Germaine Greer's *The Female Eunuch*. So, more accurate might be to simply say that radical feminism really only caught on in the UK in/after 1977, with Jeffreys as the catalyst. See Jeffreys (1977) and Jeffreys' answer at ~01.26.00 here: https://www.youtube.com/watch?v=PDHq4WJKsNM

58. At least, Atkinson seems to have the published piece with the earliest date on it; the paper 'Abortion' published in her collection *Amazon Odyssey* (1974*a*) is recorded in a footnote as having been given at the National Conference of the NOW in November 1967. Another piece, 'Vaginal Orgasm as a Mass Hysterical Survival Response', is recorded as having been given in April 1968 at the National Conference of the Medical Committee for Human Rights. The next radical feminist papers to appear after that seem to have been in the magazine *Notes from the First Year*, published by New York Radical Women in June 1968, and featuring contributions from Shulamith Firestone, Anne Koedt, Jennifer Gardner, and Kathy Amatniek.
59. As indeed Alison Jaggar does, see esp. Jaggar (1983, chs. 5 and 9).
60. Chesler (2018, p. 3).
61. Prior to the innovation of agriculture, skilled labour was generally sex-differentiated (e.g. male large-game hunters and female small-game hunters and foragers), but contributions were thought to be valued equally, and females are thought to have had control over choices about sexual partners. See discussion in Kelly (2000); Marlowe (2010).
62. Sherfey (1970).
63. Brownmiller (1976, pp. 4–5).
64. Firestone (1970).
65. Daly (1978).
66. Griffin (1980). All of these examples are discussed in Jaggar (1983, pp. 88–98).
67. Jaggar (1983, pp. 106–113).
68. Stoljar (1995, p. 261). She cites Fuss (1989, p. xi) and Schor (1994, p. 42) saying something very similar.
69. Natalie Stoljar refers to these as the 'naturalizing argument' and the 'diversity argument' against essentialism. On the first, she cites Elizabeth Grosz's discussion of 'naturalism' (as opposed to 'biologism'), which 'analyzes woman's essence in terms of "natural" characteristics which may be biological but need not be—characteristics such as being emotional, irrational, passive, etc.' (Stoljar 1995, p. 288, fn. 5). On the second, she cites Spelman (1988). Stoljar herself makes a version of the diversity argument, after defending essentialism against the naturalizing argument. She rejects the idea of there being 'a natural and intrinsic property constituting universal womanness' on the grounds that 'the only genuine candidate' for this property is the type 'female human being', and this type excludes what she calls 'sexually indeterminate people', as well as 'transvestites…as well as transsexuals' (Stoljar 1995, p. 273).
70. She writes, '[i]n the past, when it was a question of carrying heavy clubs and of keeping wild beasts at bay, woman's physical weakness constituted a flagrant inferiority: if the instrument requires slightly more strength than the woman can muster, it is enough to make her seem radically powerless' (Beauvoir [1949) 2011, Volume I, ch 3, p. 63).

71. Criado-Perez (2019).
72. Whether Beauvoir understood her own explanation as contingent is slightly confused by the fact that she says later in the book 'The devaluation of women represents a necessary stage in the history of humanity' (Beauvoir 1949, p. 86). But this may be a reference to Hegel's similar claim about the master/slave dialectic, and mean only that this stage was necessary *in order to produce human development as we currently know it*, rather than necessary in a strict sense (true in all possible worlds).
73. Lerner (1986).
74. Engels (1891).
75. Beauvoir (1949, Volume I, Part I, ch. 3, p. 64).
76. Beauvoir (1949, Volume I, Part I, ch. 3, p. 65).
77. Lerner (1986, p. 46).
78. Lerner (1986, p. 47).
79. Lerner (1986, p. 52; her emphasis).
80. Lerner (1986, p. 10; see also p. 220).
81. Beauvoir (1949, p. 67).
82. O'Connor (2019).
83. See e.g. Wollstonecraft (1792); Beauvoir (1949); Firestone (1970); Millett (1973); Frye (1983).
84. Atkinson ([1970] 1974*d*, p. 49).
85. Frye (1983); this metaphor of the cage was also pre-empted in Wollstonecraft ([1792] 2017, p. 77); and later Firestone (1970, p. 25).
86. Frye (1983, pp. 9–10).
87. Other groups have been pressed into service, but none have been so co-opted as to internalize—as a class—this service role as their self-conception as woman have. There is still much work to be done in articulating what 'woman' is when she is not pressed into the service of men. That is why self-determination must remain an important goal of feminism.
88. Frye (1983, p. 36).
89. MacKinnon (1989, p. 112).
90. MacKinnon (1989, p. 111).
91. MacKinnon (1989, pp. 111–112).
92. Atkinson (1974*a*, pp. 41–45).
93. Atkinson (1974*a*, p. 43).
94. Firestone (1970, p. 125).
95. Firestone (1970, p. 116).
96. Wittig (1976, p. 64).
97. Wittig (1976, p. 67).
98. Dworkin (1974, p. 174); quoted in Jaggar (1983, p. 99).
99. Atkinson (1974*a*, p. 48–49).

100. Kreps (1973, p. 234).
101. Kreps (1973, p. 239).
102. Millett (1973).
103. Frye (1983).
104. Firestone (1970).
105. Atkinson (1969).
106. The Feminists (1973). The Feminists were also known as 'The Feminists—A Political Organization to Annihilate Sex Roles.' They split from the NOW in 1968, and were active in New York from 1968 to 1973. Their most prominent member was Ti-Grace Atkinson; their membership also included Anne Koedt (until 1969 when there was another split), Sheila Michaels, Barbara Mehrhof, Pamela Kearon, and Sheila Cronan. The Feminists believed that women were subject to false consciousness as a result of their internalization of oppressive sex roles. They were separatists, who advocated for the development of women's culture.
107. New York Radical Feminists (1973). The New York Radical Feminists (not to be confused with The Feminists or New York Radical Women) was founded in 1969 by Shulamith Firestone (having left the Redstockings) and Anne Koedt (having left The Feminists). Both Firestone and Koedt left the group in 1970, but it carried on until the mid-1970s.
108. See discussion in Lerner (1986, p. 27).
109. Gilligan (1982); Gilligan (2018).
110. E.g. Noddings (1984). I'm not sure whether Gilligan, Noddings, and other women advocating an ethics of care thought of themselves as radical feminists. But the ethics of care tradition is clearly related to maternalism, and Lerner identifies Dorothy Dinnerstein, Mary O'Brien, and Adrienne Rich as maternalists. Rich, at least, was a radical feminist. See discussion in Lerner (1986, p. 28 and fn. 38, p. 248).
111. Difference feminist reasoning shows up in an influential strand of transgender theory. Julia Serano writes in *Whipping Girl* (2007) 'because anti-trans discrimination is steeped in traditional sexism ... we must also challenge the idea that femininity is inferior to masculinity and that femaleness is inferior to maleness' (p. 16); and 'until feminists work to empower femininity and pry it away from the insipid, inferior meanings that plague it—weakness, helplessness, fragility, passivity, frivolity, and artificiality—those meanings will continue to haunt every person who is female and/or feminine' (p. 341).
112. MacKinnnon (1987, p. 37).
113. Collins (2015, pp. 7–9).
114. Budapest (1980, pp. xi–xii).
115. Budapest (1980, p. xiii).
116. Budapest (1980, p. xiii).
117. Budapest (1980, p. xiii).
118. Budapest (1980, p. xvii).

119. Budapest (1980, p. xviii).
120. Budapest (1980, p. 2).
121. The Pussy Church of Modern Witchcraft is a church founded in the United States in 2018, and follows in this tradition—Budapest's book is listed as one of their Tenets of Faith. See https://pussychurchofmodernwitchcraft.com/about/ and discussion at Reilly (2018).
122. Firestone (1970, ch. 10).
123. See discussion in Shiffrin (1999).
124. Dworkin (1974, p. 191).
125. Daly (1987, p. 112).
126. 'Bio-logical' is defined as 'characterized by Life-loving wisdom and logic' (Daly 1987, p. 108).
127. Daly (1987, p. 77).
128. For more detailed criticism of the contemporary version of this project, which is known as 'conceptual engineering', see Sankaran (2020).
129. Rowling (2020, p. 492).
130. MacKinnon (1982, p. 520). MacKinnon goes on in the same paragraph to acknowledge that this psychological aspect can be difficult for those who are (only) materially deprived to *see* as a form of oppression, including 'women whom no man has ever put on a pedestal'.
131. MacKinnon (1982, pp. 519–520).
132. MacKinnon (1982, p. 515).
133. Frye (1983, p. 38).
134. Frye (1983, p. 38).
135. Frye (1983, p. 29).
136. Frye (1983, p. 33).
137. Frye (1983, p. 33; my emphasis).
138. Dembroff & Wodak (2018*a*, 2018*b*).
139. Butler (1990), see also discussion in Morgenroth & Ryan (2018, pp. 240–241).
140. Fausto-Sterling (1993, 2000, pp. 19–22, 2018).
141. For sex to be a 'spectrum' we'd have to be able to start with a male-typical set of sex characteristics at one end of a line and a female-typical set of sex characteristics at the other, and then show that there were fine gradations of those characteristics occupying all of the space in between. That is *not* what is established by Differences of Sexual Development (DSDs) / intersex variations. Fausto-Sterling (together with several co-authors) estimated the percentage of intersex people at 1.7 per cent (Blackless et al. 2000). The philosopher Carrie Hull corrects several mistakes in their analysis, bringing the figure down to 0.37 per cent (Hull 2003). Leonard Sax gives an even lower estimate, at around 0.018 per cent (Sax 2002), which Alex Byrne puts together with Hull's corrections to reach an *even* lower estimate of 0.015 per cent (Byrne 2018). Why does the percentage matter? Because the higher the number, the easier it is to make the

case that there are no clear boundaries between male and female, so even if sex is not a 'spectrum' it is at least a conceptual space with a large, blurry middle area. If 1.7 per cent of all humans are in this blurry area this puts a lot of pressure on the idea of sex as a binary, at least. But if only 0.015 per cent of people are in this blurry area, it seems more plausible to say that sex is roughly what we thought it was, but that there are some outlier cases.

142. Frye (1983, p. 25).
143. MacKinnon (1987, p. 44).
144. Wittig ([1976] 1982), p. 68). Shulamith Firestone also wrote of eliminating sex: 'the end goal of feminist revolution must be, unlike that of the first feminist movement, not just the elimination of male *privilege* but of the sex *distinction* itself: genital differences between human beings would no longer matter culturally' (Firestone 1970, p. 11).
145. See e.g. Searle (1995, 2005); Hindriks (2012).
146. There is reasonable disagreement over the extent to which sex differences would create/attract social meaning in any possible world, and thus produce a limited form of gender (albeit different in content from gender as we know it). See discussion from 29.40 in 'Gender-critical Philosophers | Kathleen Stock & Holly Lawford-Smith' at https://www.youtube.com/watch?v=CjXshdq4ZlQ&
147. Beauvoir (1949).
148. See nn. 1 and 2 to the Preface; and n. 2 to Chapter 3.
149. Mill (1869).
150. Beauvoir (1949).
151. Frye (1983).
152. Mill (1869); see also discussion in Beauvoir (1949), Frye (1983), Burgess-Jackson (1995), and Chapter 4.
153. Kate Millett wrote of the socialization of the sexes, including 'the concept of sex role, which assigns domestic service and attendance upon infants to all females and the rest of human interest, achievement, and ambition to the male; the charge of leader at all times and places to the male, and the duty of follower, with equal uniformity, to the female'. She advocated for a 'sexual revolution' that would bring about 'the end of separatist character-structure, temperament, and behaviour, so that each individual may develop an entire—rather than a partial, limited, and conformist—personality', and 'the end of sex role and sex status' (Millett [1968] 1973, in Koedt et al. (Eds.) 1973, pp. 366–367). She talks in more detail about the sex role system in *Sexual Politics*, ch. 2 (Millett 1970). Ti-Grace Atkinson wrote 'The class of women is formed by positing another class in opposition: the class of men, or the male role. Women exist as the corollaries of men, and exist as human beings only insofar as they are those corollaries' (Atkinson 1969, in Atkinson 1974*a*, pp. 41–42). The Feminists (a collective) wrote 'all those institutions which were designed on the assumption and for the

reinforcement of the male and female role system such as the family (and its sub-institution, marriage), sex, and love must be destroyed' (The Feminists 1973, p. 370). The subtitle of their essay, also the longer version of their name, was 'A Political Organization to Annihilate Sex Roles'. The New York Radical Feminists (another collective) wrote 'Radical feminism recognizes the oppression of women as a fundamental political oppression wherein women are categorized as an inferior class based upon their sex. It is the aim of radical feminism to organize politically to destroy this sex class system' (New York Radical Feminists 1973, p. 379). Naomi Weisstein wrote 'I don't know what immutable differences exist between men and women apart from differences in their genitals; perhaps there are some other unchangeable differences; probably there are a number of irrelevant differences. But it is clear that until social expectations for men and women are equal, until we provide equal respect for both men and women, our answers to this question will simply reflect our prejudices' (Weisstein 1973, p. 196). Andrea Dworkin wrote, at the end of *Woman Hating*, 'We must make a total commitment...no longer to play the male-female roles we have been taught...We must refuse to submit to all forms of behaviour and relationship which reinforce male-female polarity, which nourish basic patterns of male dominance and female submission' (Dworkin 1974, pp. 192–193). Shulamith Firestone proposed a dramatic solution for ending sex roles, namely 'The freeing of women from the tyranny of reproduction by every means possible, and the diffusion of the child-rearing role to the society as a whole, men as well as women' (Firestone 1970, p. 185). She talked about artificial reproduction as allowing this freedom (p. 185).

154. Atkinson (1974*a*, pp. 42–43).
155. Firestone (1970, ch. 9).
156. Heilburn (1973, p. xv), quoted in Raymond (1975).
157. Roszak (1969, p. 304), quoted in Raymond (1975).
158. Woolf (1929, p. 102), quoted in Raymond (1975).
159. Raymond (1975); Daly (1975); Allen ([1986] 2001). Alison Jaggar attributes the criticism that androgyny 'fails in the naming of difference' to Adrienne Rich (Jaggar 1983, p. 88), but provides no reference. As far as I have been able to find, this line is actually from Jeffner Allen's ([1986] 2001).
160. Raymond (1975); discussed in Jaggar (1983, p. 88).
161. Frye (1983, p. 36).
162. See e.g. Joel (2015); Fine (2017); Joel & Vikhanski (2019).
163. These haven't changed so much over the years. A 1912 text describing British stereotypes of *France*—the whole country!—as feminine included traits like being charming; having graceful manners, a lack of strong-will; being under-ambitious, frugal, delicate, a perfectionist, precise; lacking in emotional discipline; and being exuberant (de Pratz 1912, pp. 8–9). Mary Wollstonecraft (1792)

mentions as feminine virtues those of patience, docility, good-humour, and flexibility (she comments, 'virtues incompatible with any vigorous exertion of intellect'—Wollstonecraft [1792] 2017, p. 80).

Chapter 3

1. Reilly-Cooper (2016).
2. See nn. 1 and 2 to the Preface. It is straightforward to state the gender-critical project in terms that feminists who think sex is a social construct can accept. Money is a paradigmatic social construct. But now that it *has been constructed*, it is real. We can point to the fact of its social construction to highlight that it is contingent, not necessary, that we have it; and to inspire thinking about how we might organize society without it. But once we have decided that we want to dismantle ('deconstruct') it, simply acting like it doesn't exist seems like a poor strategy, given that some people have a lot of money, and some people have almost no money, and in the short-term having money still makes a huge difference to how people's lives go. Similarly for sex. Even if Judith Butler and those who follow them (Butler has recently announced a nonbinary gender identity) are right that sex is socially constructed out of arbitrary physical differences—some bodies have one kind of reproductive anatomy, other bodies have another, and on this view that is about as significant as having big or small earlobes, or being tall or short (see also discussion in Ásta 2018)—once sex assignments are in fact made, children are subject to different treatment on that basis. There are significant average differences between men and women, not least when it comes to the perpetration of violent crimes. The 'sex as a social construction' line rules out a biologistic explanation of those differences, but it does not rule out a socialized one. Once we have socially constructed sex, sex is real. It may be contingent, and we may be able to eliminate it, but we're stuck with it for now, just like money. And that means we're stuck with the *effects* of it for now, which include the way that these 'arbitrary' assignments of bodies to categories have in fact *shaped* the individuals in each category. We can accept that those persons *could have been otherwise*—a boy baby instead assigned 'girl' and raised 'girl' could have become 'girl-like'—without believing that they are not *now* the way that they have been shaped to be. Thus feminists following Butler can accept that the best route to dismantling the system of sex/gender is, in the short-term, to pay attention to the way persons have been shaped on the basis of (constructed) sex/gender, in particular to make sure that the category constructed as inferior/subordinate, namely those 'assigned female at birth', has equal opportunities with the category constructed as superior/dominant.
3. http://worldpopulationreview.com/countries/countries-where-abortion-is-illegal/

4. https://www.humanrights.gov.au/education/students/hot-topics/womens-rights
5. Chambers, manuscript.
6. Chambers, manuscript.
7. By 'women-only spaces', I have in mind sex-separated prisons, changing rooms, fitting rooms, bathrooms, homeless and drug and alcohol shelters, rape and domestic violence refuges, gyms, spas, sports, schools, accommodations, shortlists, prizes, quotas, political groups, clubs, events, festivals, and teams.
8. Jaggar (1983, pp. 41–42).
9. See examples in n. 4 to the Preface.
10. Christina Hoff Sommers, a vocal critic of a number of prominent feminists and feminist ideas, has criticized the idea of women as a caste for allowing privileged women to claim that they are hurt whenever a disadvantaged woman is hurt. She writes: 'you need not have harmed me personally, but if I identify with someone you *have* harmed, I may resent you... Having demarcated a victimized "us" with whom I now feel solidarity, I can point to one victim and say, "In wronging her, he has betrayed his contempt for us all", or "Anyone who harms a woman harms us all", or simply "What he did to her, he did to all of us"' (Sommers 1994, p. 42). We can imagine a world in which Sommers is quite right. Suppose that every country except one has securely achieved the real social, political, legal, and economic equality of the sexes; women's liberation is won. These aren't necessarily 'privileged' women, but they are women who don't have a complaint when it comes to sexism. But in the one remaining country, there is still systematic discrimination against girls and women. It might seem a stretch, then, for women in the other countries to say that they are hurt when those women are hurt. In our world, however, rather than the world we have to imagine to make Sommers' criticism reasonable, there is enough of a pattern that it is reasonable for women to consider some harms to specific women as harms to all women. The existence of prostitution and pornography are good examples of this. Even though it is the women working in those industries who are most harmed, it is also true that *all women* are negatively impacted by the fact that it is possible for men to buy the use of women's bodies, or watch other men have the bought use of women's bodies (more in Chapter 4). No matter how privileged, a woman can point to the degradation of women in pornography and truly say 'in wronging her, he has betrayed his contempt for us all'. This is partly because in using her as an object, he regards her as interchangeable with other 'objects' relevantly like her. Sommers' claim also puts her in a tricky position relative to other social groups. Would she deny that it can be true for Jewish people that when one is subject to anti-Semitism, contempt has been betrayed for all Jewish people? Or that it can be true for all Aboriginal Australians, that what was done to one (at least when motivated by racism) was done, symbolically, to all? There is simply too much evidence of group-based discrimination or hatred for it to be plausible to deny

it, and if Sommers doesn't deny that it exists in general, then she owes us an explanation for why it should exist in the case of social group characteristics like race and religion, but *not* sex/gender.

11. The hard questions that do exist relate to specific and rare intersex variations, not to gender identities.
12. See discussion in Barker (1997).
13. Frye (1983, p. 36).
14. Reilly-Cooper (2016).
15. Reilly-Cooper (2016).
16. (Reilly-Cooper (2016).
17. Bicchieri (2017, p. 35).
18. Rachelle (2019).
19. Rachelle (2019).
20. For a discussion of beauty norms as ethical norms, see Widdows (2018).
21. For further discussion on norm change, see Bicchieri (2017, chs. 3–5); for an alternative account of norms, see Brennan et al. (2013).
22. There's an interesting discussion of moral norm change, focused specifically on norms about *honour*, in Appiah (2010).
23. Dickinson & Bismark (2016).
24. Aubusson (2019).
25. Jenkins (2018, p. 728; see also pp. 728–736).
26. Jenkins (2018, p. 729).
27. The exact details of what this means can be filled in more precisely and may be somewhat context-dependent.
28. *R.G. & G.R Harris Funeral Homes v EEOC & Aimee Stevens.*
29. Hungerford (2019). What she means is that anyone gender non-conforming, such as an effeminate boy or a tomboy girl, can be burdened by the social enforcement of gender roles, not just trans people.
30. There is commentary on stone butch lesbians who passed as men in the 1950s United States in Feinberg (1993).
31. Watson (2016, p. 247).
32. Haslanger (2000, p. 39).
33. Haslanger (2000, p. 38).
34. An Egyptian zoo actually did this—see https://www.youtube.com/watch?v=cnqa9Ma5CXY accessed 23rd May 2020. A similar example (put to the use of ruling out relevant alternatives when making claims to knowledge) appears in Dretske (1970, pp. 1015–1016).
35. She wrote, 'The claim for tolerance, based on the notion that transgenderism in all its forms is a form of gender resistance, is alluring but false. Instead, transgenderism reduces gender resistance to wardrobes, hormones, surgery, and posturing—anything but real sexual equality. A real sexual politics says yes to a view and reality of transgender that transforms, instead of conforms to,

gender' (Raymond 1979, p. xxxv). Her discussion in chapter 5 is particularly interesting. She says that trans people are in a unique position to turn their gender dissatisfaction into rage against the society that creates it (p. 124); that there is more freedom in feminism, as a liberation project, than in conformity through surgery (p. 127); and that one cannot give truly informed consent when one hasn't even considered the role that a sex-stereotyping and homophobic society has played in the creation of the desire to change sex.

36. Reilly-Cooper (2016). For further criticism of gender identity ideology as an unambitious solution to the social problem of gender norms, see Lawford-Smith (2020*a*).
37. See especially Budapest (1980).
38. hooks ([1984] 2000, ch. 11).
39. I don't know of any articles covering the recent controversy on this topic, which has regularly blown up on Twitter in the last few years. But Julie Bindel talks about political lesbianism in a few places, and describes the 'born this way' view as the alternative. See e.g. Bindel (2009) and her video for *The Guardian* 'I'm a lesbian, but I wasn't born this way', 22nd April 2015. Online at https://www.youtube.com/watch?v=PDKwYbV1jQs
40. hooks ([1984] 2000, ch. 5).
41. It might focus on a limited set of intersections; see further discussion in Chapter 7.
42. Landrine (1985, p. 73).
43. For more discussion of both allyship and deference in matters of social groups, see discussion in Lawford-Smith & Tuckwell, manuscript. On speaking on behalf of social groups, see Lawford-Smith (2018).
44. The definition has been defended at length by philosopher Alex Byrne (2020).
45. BBC (2018). See also n. 47 to Chapter 1.
46. I say 'most' rather than 'all' because there are some exceptions. In some cases, other axes of privilege/oppression will trump: the Queen might not have been socialized into femininity because her socialization as sovereign took priority (see also Stoljar 1995). In other cases, the socialization will not have been lifelong: transmen who pass as men, or butch lesbians who are sometimes mis-sexed, may escape it earlier or in part. In yet other cases, it may be possible to escape it: e.g. daughters raised by fathers as sons (and in social isolation, as in the wild) (there are some accounts of this in de Beauvoir 1949).
47. Greer (1970, p. 335).
48. Firestone (1970).
49. See discussion in Mehat (2015).
50. Journalist Helen Joyce writes 'Until the past decade, hardly any teenage girls sought treatment for gender dysphoria; now, they predominate in clinics around the world. British figures are typical. In 1989, when the Tavistock clinic opened, there were two referrals, both young boys. By 2020, there were 2,378

referrals, almost three-quarters of them girls, and most of those teenagers' (Joyce 2021, p. 91). *The Economist* reports an increase from 41 per cent of adolescents referred to the UK's Gender Identity Development Service (GIDS) being female in 2009, to 69 per cent being female in 2017 (*The Economist* 2018).

51. See discussion in Littman (2021). Littman surveys a hundred detransitioners, with 69 per cent of participants being female and 31 per cent male. She notes that 'Only 24.0% of participants had informed the doctor or clinic that facilitated their transitions that they had detransitioned' (p. 11), which may help to explain previous assumptions that rates of detransition are extremely low.
52. Cameron (2019, p. 2).
53. Mackay (2015).
54. Frye (1983, p. 127).
55. Frye (1983, p. 127).
56. For some ideas coming from men, see Jensen (2017) and Pease (2019).
57. Redstockings (1969).
58. Firestone (1970, p. 37).
59. hooks (1984).
60. Freeman (1976).
61. Chesler (2018, p. 140). The Robin she refers to here is Robin Morgan.
62. Sommers (1994, pp. 212, 218–222).
63. Twitter @janeclarejones 'I'm also going to disagree with Rosa on something here...(We can do this...Because we're not a frickin cult)', 15th November 2018 at 7.45 p.m. See also Twitter @janeclarejones 'We're not a cult, we not all singing from the same sheet' [*sic*], 2nd December 2018, 1.48am.

Chapter 4

1. Ekman ([2010] 2013, p. 111).
2. Houston, in Wagoner (2012).
3. Moran (2013, p. 5).
4. Bisch (1999); Pennyworth (2003).
5. Chesler (2018, p. 149).
6. There is no evidence that this is true, and some evidence that it is not, see e.g. Cho (2018).
7. Chesler (2018, p. 149).
8. Cameron (2018, p. 32).
9. Cameron (2018, p. 32).
10. For one recent discussion using this broader notion of sex, see Danaher (forthcoming).
11. Frederick et al. (2018).

12. Chesler (2018, p. 229).
13. See e.g. Grant (2014); Mofokeng (2019).
14. See e.g. Jeffreys (2009*a*), Dines (2010), Tyler (2011), Ekman ([2010] 2013), Moran (2013), Bindel (2017); cf. Mac & Smith (2018), Watson & Flanigan (2020).
15. Some feminists prefer 'contract pregnancy' as the more accurate term, given that the gestational mother is a real, not a substitute, mother. See e.g. Satz (1992, p. 107, fn. 2); Finn (2018).
16. Chesler (2018, pp. 246–7).
17. Ekman ([2010] 2013, ch. 1).
18. Murphy (2020*b*). Rachel Moran, a woman exited from prostitution in Ireland, says much the same thing in her memoir *Paid For* (2013): 'this really is one of the cornerstones that support the sex industry—the male insistence on offloading onto another class of women perversions they cannot reasonably expect to present to the women in their lives' (pp. 85–86). An empirical study of 103 London men who buy sex found that for 20 per cent of the men, their reason for buying sex was that they couldn't get what they wanted from their current relationship (Farley et al. 2009).
19. Fickling (2006); BBC (2015). A less extreme example, discussed in Chapter 5, is legislation that bans practices aimed at the 'change or suppression' of a person's sexual orientation or gender identity, even when an adult consents to that practice and has good reasons for desiring it (relating for example to religion, culture, or family).
20. There is documentation of cases in which 'rough sex' was used as a defence here: https://wecantconsenttothis.uk/
21. MacLennan (2018); McCulloch (2018).
22. I include being subject to advertisements on free porn sites under this description.
23. Thornton (1991).
24. Campbell (2016, pp. 167–168).
25. Campbell (2016, p. 168).
26. Some feminists attempt to draw a bright line between trafficking into sexual slavery and commercial prostitution. There are certainly some differences, relating to the degree of coercion exercised and the amount of freedom the victim / sex worker has. Juno Mac & Molly Smith argue that, however, on the pro- sex industry side, this bright line is illusory because attempts to migrate using people smugglers can turn into trafficking when debts accumulate or there is deception about the work available upon arrival (Mac & Smith 2018, ch. 3).
27. Campbell (2016, pp. 165).
28. Campbell (2016, p. 172), citing Dehghan (2012).
29. Campbell (2016, p. 171).
30. Moran (2013, p. 96).

31. See also Pateman (1988, 2002); Ekman ([2010] 2013, ch. 1–3); and discussion in Chapter 6, Section 6.2 of this book.
32. I take this description from the Netflix documentary *After Porn Ends*, where one of the male porn actors—Randy West—said 'I used to say it's like borrowing somebody's body to masturbate with. Excuse me, if you're not busy, you mind if I jerk off into your pussy with my dick? Ah, it's kind of like that…which is not bad, I mean, you know, better than real jerking off' (Wagoner 2012, 19.01–19.31).
33. Project Respect make this point well in arguing against the National Disability Insurance Scheme in Australia funding the use of sex workers. See their position statement: https://d3n8a8pro7vhmx.cloudfront.net/projectrespect/pages/15/attachments/original/1526432652/Position_Statement_sexual_services_on_NDIS_FINAL.pdf?1526432652 accessed 24th May 2020.
34. Dixon (2001).
35. Mike Robillard & BJ Strawser (2016) make a similar point about recruits to the army.
36. Dixon (2001, p. 326).
37. Dixon (2001, p. 327).
38. 'Molly Smith' is a pseudonym. See https://www.theguardian.com/profile/molly-smith accessed 10th April 2020.
39. Mac & Smith (2018, e.g. pp. 49, 50, 115, 215).
40. Dixon (2001, p. 324).
41. Moran (2013, p. 5).
42. Farley et al. (2004); Ekman ([2010] 2013). See also discussion in Chapter 6, Section 6.4.
43. Goodin & Barry (2014, p. 373).
44. Murphy (2020*a*).
45. For simplicity, and because the parallel to prostitution and pornography is what matters here rather than university admissions in their own right, I'm ignoring complications to do with when structural obstacles have affected who meets the entry requirements or is in the pool of well-qualified applicants. There is no good parallel to this when it comes to sex, because sex is not a distributive good, and no one has a right to it.
46. See discussion in Greer (2018); Gavey (2019).
47. Bisch (1999, p. 5).
48. Bisch (1999, p. 4).
49. Shamsian & McLaughlin (2020); McLaughlin (2020).
50. Pateman (1988); Frye (1983).
51. I feel compelled to add a #notallmen here, because clearly not all men need to reconceptualize their ideas about sex and sexual pleasure. But those who do are not limited to those who buy sex. There are plenty of men who don't pay for sex, and yet who do not bother to ensure that sex is mutually pleasurable, and who

feel entitled to sex from their partners. There are also plenty of men who don't pay for sex in the strict sense, but in another sense do, e.g. by granting wealth and resources (often in the context of a marriage) in exchange for sex.

52. In this section, I deliberately take up Debra Satz's directive, that 'if we are troubled by prostitution…we should direct much of our energy to putting forward alternative models of egalitarian relations between men and women' (Satz 2010, p. 154).
53. Satz (2010, p. 96).
54. Satz (2010, p. 148).
55. Schulze et al. (2014, p. 6).
56. Schulze et al. (2014, p. 10).
57. Cf. n. 26 to this chapter.
58. Schulze et al. (2014, p. 10).
59. Schulze et al. (2014, p. 7).
60. Schulze et al. (2014, p. 10).
61. Schulze et al. (2014, p. 6).
62. Schulze et al. (2014, p. 6). The authors of the report distinguish sexual exploitation from prostitution according to whether sex is sold 'under conditions of coercion or force'. If it is, then it's sexual exploitation, and if it isn't, then it's prostitution, according to them.
63. UNODC (2009).
64. Bindel & Kelly (2003).
65. Farley et al. (2004).
66. These were 2 per cent from the South Pacific; 6 per cent from Scandinavia; 5 per cent from the Indian Subcontinent; 1 per cent from the Middle East; 1 per cent from North America; 6 per cent from South America; 3 per cent from the Caribbean; 2 per cent from Africa; and another 5 per cent with ethnicities not recognized in the study (Dickson 2004, p. 21, table 3).
67. Dickson (2004, pp. 10, 27).
68. See discussion in Moran (2013).
69. Reeve et al. (2009, pp. 6–7).
70. Reeve et al. (2009, p. 7).
71. Reeve et al. (2009, p. 7).
72. Reeve et al. (2009, p. 9).
73. Bindel & Kelly (2003, p. 16).
74. Bindel & Kelly (2003, p. 48).
75. Bindel & Kelly (2003, p. 50).
76. Bindel & Kelly (2003, p. 43).
77. Dickson (2004, p. 11).
78. Two to Tangle Productions, at ~59.58–1.00.58.
79. See discussion in Alarcón et al. (2019).

80. E.g. Rosewarne (2017).
81. See e.g. the Woman's Place UK Manifesto (2019), which demands that we 'Recognize prostitution as sexually abusive exploitation which is harmful to all women and girls', and 'Implement the abolitionist model, criminalising those who exploit prostituted people (including pimps and sex buyers) and decriminalising the prostituted, providing practical and psychological exiting support'. Online at https://womansplaceuk.org/wp-content/uploads/2019/09/Printable-manifesto.pdf accessed 24th May 2020.
82. Mac & Smith (2018).
83. See discussion in Mac & Smith (2018, chs. 4–8).
84. Mac & Smith (2018, p. 215). On the same page, they talk about 'the humane abolition of sex work', saying that this 'can only happen when marginalised people no longer have to sustain themselves through the sex industry; when it is no longer necessary for their survival' (Mac & Smith 2018, p. 215).
85. Amia Srinivasan (2021) does the same thing in her essay 'Talking to My Students about Porn', focusing on the harms to women in porn rather than the harms to all women affected by porn (arguably, all women). She does this even while reporting on conversations she has had with her students, and groups of high school students, *about* porn, which suggests this is a conscious decision to focus on those she considers to be the worst-off (or perhaps, the most-affected). But it is a decision that is not made explicit, or defended.
86. Ekman ([2010] 2013, p. 115).
87. Mac & Smith (2018, see e.g. pp. 2–3).
88. Fisher (2019).
89. Langton (1993).
90. Tong (1982, p. 14).
91. nordicmodelnow.org, n.d.
92. Mac & Smith (2018).
93. Quoted in Zeller (2006).
94. Anderson (2003).
95. Wright & Tokunaga (2016, p. 955).
96. Wright & Tokunaga (2016, p. 960).
97. Wright & Tokunaga (2016, p. 955).
98. Hald, Malamuth, & Yuen (2010, p. 17).
99. Hald, Malamuth, & Yuen (2010, p. 18).
100. Cho (2018, p. 13).
101. Cho (2018, p. 13).
102. As they understand it, violent pornography depicts sex without consent, with coercion or aggression, while non-violent pornography depicts consensual sex, without coercion or aggression (Wright et al. 2015, pp. 8–9).
103. Wright et al. (2015; my emphasis).
104. E.g. Moran (2013).

Chapter 5

1. Ekman ([2010] 2013, pp. 39–40).
2. On the terminology of class/caste, see n. 35 to Chapter 1.
3. Butler (1990, p. 522). Gender-critical feminists need not deny that there is performance. What is important is that we lay the blame for that performance elsewhere. We focus on what causes the performance, e.g. the socially imposed constraints, rather than on the performance itself. Focusing on the performance itself might count as 'victim-blaming' insofar as it suggests that women could simply choose to *perform differently*. Butler talks of a 'collective agreement to perform, produce, and sustain discrete and polar genders', and comments that 'The authors of gender become entranced by their own fictions' (Butler 1990, p. 522; quoted in Morgenroth & Ryan 2018, p. 241). But this ignores the social costs to women of violating gender expectations and the social rewards for conforming, which some women cannot afford to forego.
4. Bettcher (2009).
5. Inside academic philosophy, the proposed reform to the UK's Gender Recognition Act was what brought gender-critical feminism to widespread awareness. The philosopher Kathleen Stock wrote an essay titled 'Academic Philosophy and the UK Gender Recognition Act', noting that while there was a 'huge and impassioned discussion' going on outside the academy over the proposed reforms, 'nearly all academic philosophers—including, surprisingly, feminist philosophers—are ignoring it' (Stock 2018). She proposed calling the position that transwomen shouldn't be counted as women under the law, and therefore that the proposed reform should be rejected, 'the gender-critical position'. Gender-critical feminists do indeed oppose moving to sex self-identification (which we think conflates sex with gender identity), but there is more to gender-critical feminism than its position on sex self-identification, and that position follows from its more general view on what feminism is and who it is for.
6. The Cambridge University Student Union Women's Campaign released a brochure 'How to Spot TERF Ideology' ('TERF' stands for 'trans-exclusionary radical feminist') which included the claim 'Terf ideology fails to recognise that women are not homogeneous, and face many different kinds of intersecting oppressions; Black "womanhood" and white "womanhood" are not the same, just as trans "womanhood" and queer "womanhood" are not the same' (online at https://www.womens.cusu.cam.ac.uk/how-to-spot-terf-ideology/). Academic Alison Phipps spoke about 'TERFs' and 'SWERFs' (sex-worker-exclusionary radical feminists) to *Pink News*, commenting 'It's rooted in disgust…It's a white bourgeois disgust in bodies that are unnatural, or bodies that are not respectable enough, and not wanting those bodies to be part of our feminism. It's a disgust at difference, which is really deeply bourgeois' (Parsons 2020). For a radical feminist commentary on the concept of white feminism, see the excellent (MacKinnon 1991*a*).

7. Katelyn Burns, writing in *Vox* about what she terms 'anti-trans "radical" feminists', described '80-plus replies to a tweet…by prominent feminist writer Sady Doyle promoting a piece she wrote denouncing TERFs', and said 'some accused Doyle of being a handmaid of the patriarchy' (Burns 2019).
8. To give just a couple of examples (there are more in Chapter 6), division between feminists over this issue lead to the collapse of the Michigan Womyn's Music Festival (Michfest), a women's music festival that had run for forty years (McConnell et al. 2016). Women who run female-only services and stand their ground against the inclusion of transwomen have been targeted. In one recent case, a transwoman in Vancouver managed to have the city funding withdrawn from Vancouver Rape Relief, which is Canada's oldest rape crisis centre (Murphy 2019*a*). The centre has also been targeted with vandalism and death threats, and had a dead rat nailed to its door (Hickman 2019).
9. In full: 'gender identity means a person's gender-related identity, which may or may not correspond with their designated sex at birth, and includes the personal sense of the body (whether this involves medical intervention or not) and other expressions of gender, including dress, speech, mannerisms, names and personal preferences'. This definition was introduced in the Change or Suppression (Conversion) Practices Prohibition Act 2021 (VIC), amending the previous definition in the Equal Opportunity Act 2010 (VIC) which made reference to sex ('the identification…by a person of one sex as a member of the other sex…by assuming the characteristics of the other sex, whether by means of medical intervention, style of dressing or otherwise…'). The new definition is similar to that used in the Yogyakarta Principles.
10. Gender-critical feminists are routinely smeared as 'TERFs'. Feminist philosopher Jennifer Saul characterizes us in *The Conversation* as 'anti-trans activists', people who are 'committed to worsening the situation of some of the most marginalized women' (Saul 2020). Feminist philosopher Carol Hay wrote in *The New York Times* that gender-critical feminists are inspired by Janice Raymond's 1979 book *The Transsexual Empire* and comments 'for the record, many of us who are critics of TERFs consider Raymond's book to be hate speech' (Hay 2019). (For the record, it is a mistake to consider Raymond's book as the inspiration for gender-critical feminism, a mistake that comes from thinking of gender-critical feminism exclusively in terms of its position on trans/gender. Janice Raymond was a radical feminist, the author of many feminist books, and her position on the exclusion of transsexual women from women-only spaces was explained by her wider feminist commitments. As I have already argued in Chapters 2 and 3, gender-critical feminism is an evolution of radical feminism, not a new feminism 'about' trans/gender.) For other characterizations of gender-critical feminism as 'anti-trans', see also Burns (2019); Lewis (2019); and Dembroff (2021).
11. Different states protect trans people according to one or more of these attributes.

12. For further discussion of whether gender-critical speech, in particular, can plausibly be characterized as either hate speech or harmful speech, see Lawford-Smith, manuscript.
13. https://www.sofiehagen.com/newsletters/2020/2/26/also-im-not-a-woman-2019 accessed 19th May 2020.
14. Hacker (1951, p. 62).
15. Firestone (1970, p. 49).
16. Beauvoir (1949, Volume I, Part I, ch. 2).
17. Thompson (1943). See also Horney (1939, ch. 6) and Thompson (1941, 1942).
18. Raymond (1979).
19. Here I'm drawing on a description of sexual orientation, to deny that sexual orientation and gender non-conformity are relevantly similar: 'Homosexuality was removed from the World Health Organization (WHO) ICD-10 classification in 1992…Same-sex orientation is regarded as a normal, acceptable variation of human sexuality' (Griffin et al. 2021, p. 291).
20. The same is true for boys/men.
21. Doward (2019); Lane (2019); Evans (2020).
22. https://www.legislation.vic.gov.au/bills/change-or-suppression-conversion-practices-prohibition-bill-2020. See also my commentary in Lawford-Smith (2020*b*); Deves & Lawford-Smith (2020*a*, 2020*b*); and Lawford-Smith (2021).
23. Warrier et al. (2020); Griffin et al. (2021).
24. Thirteen per cent of the adolescents referred to a gender identity clinic in Finland in a two-year period were in foster homes (Griffin et al. 2021, p. 294, fig. 3).
25. Griffin et al. (2021, p. 296) cite testimony from female detransitioners as reasons for detransitioning, including 'realised the dysphoria was a result of abuse'. Abuse was present for more than 20 per cent of the female and more than 10 per cent of the male referrals to the Tavistock in 2012 (Griffin et al. 2021, p. 294, fig. 4, citing Holt et al. 2016).
26. A dataset of 641,860 individuals found that 'transgender and gender-diverse individuals have, on average, higher rates of autism, other neurodevelopmental and psychiatric diagnoses' (Warrier et al. 2020). At the Royal Children's Hospital in Melbourne, which is the busiest youth gender clinic in Australia, 45 per cent of patients showed mild to severe autism in screening (note further that 275 of the total 383 patients are female). Tony Attwood, a world expert on Asperger's, has called for an inquiry into the overrepresentation of autistic people in gender transition (Lane 2020). There is disagreement between researchers over the relation between being autistic and being transgender. Reubs Walsh and colleagues present two hypotheses about the relation (Walsh et al. 2018). One is that 'autistic traits may in some way cause, or create an illusion of, trans identity' (p. 4070). For example, rigid thinking might lead to a misinterpretation of gender-atypical interests as meaning one is trans, or hypersensitivity to touch

could lead to a preference for clothing that is gender-norm violating (p. 4071). One of the papers cited on the latter possibility includes case studies of two autistic boys preoccupied with 'feminine objects and interests', speculating that 'This preoccupation may relate to a need for sensory input that happens to be predominantly feminine in nature (silky objects, bright and shiny substances, movement of long hair, etc.' (Williams et al. 1996, p. 641). (It is worth noting that when I discussed this hypothesis with acquaintances who are autistic, parents of autistic kids, or work with autistic people, they all said they found this hypothesis implausible on the grounds that every autistic person is different, so any touch-hypersensitivity preferences are unlikely to track lines of sex, or provide a general explanation of autistic kids' disproportionate identification as trans). The other hypothesis is that 'individuals with autism are more prone to reject ideas they perceive as flawed or logically inconsistent, such as social conditioning and social norms, and this facilitates "coming out"' (Walsh et al. 2018, p. 4071; in-text references omitted). The authors themselves seem to favour this second hypothesis. They found elevated rates of nonbinary gender identities in a cohort of autistic people (100/675), and commented 'The finding that non-binary identities are most elevated seems to support hypotheses focused on autistic resistance to social conditioning' (p. 4074). On this picture, we all have gender identities, but 'typical' (i.e. not autistic) people suppress theirs as a result of sensitivity to social conditioning, while autistic people claim theirs, as a result of rejecting or resisting that social conditioning. Walsh et al. do not provide any evidence between these two main hypotheses. But their preferred hypothesis does not support autistic people *in fact being trans*. It predicts their being gender non-conforming. What that means depends on whether gender is norms (external) or identity (internal). If it is norms, then it is perfectly normal, and indeed desirable, to be gender non-conforming; it is not evidence of being trans. And if it is norms, then autistic women and girls are at particular risk, from a medical establishment and broader cultural messaging that will treat their gender non-conformity as evidence of being transgender, and potentially put them on a pathway to medical and surgical interventions. (The Australian comedian Hannah Gadsby, who is a gender non-conforming lesbian with an adult autism diagnosis, said in her stand-up show *Nanette* (2018) that she has been pressured by fans to 'come out as trans').

27. One group of authors providing information about a sample of 577 children and 243 adolescents referred to a gender identity service between 2008 and 2011 found that 76 per cent of the girls were lesbians, and commented '[a]nother parameter that has struck us as clinically important is that a number of youth comment that, in some ways, it is easier to be trans than to be gay or lesbian. One adolescent girl, for example, remarked "If I walk down the street with my girlfriend and I am perceived to be a girl, then people call us all kinds of names, like *lezzies* or *faggots*, but if I am perceived to be a guy, then they leave

us alone' (Wood et al. 2013, p. 5). Another group found that only 8.5 per cent of the females referred to the gender identity service in London were 'primarily attracted to boys', another way to say being that at least 91.5 per cent were lesbian or bisexual (Holt et al. 2016; cited in Griffin et al. 2021, p. 294). See also n. 39 to this chapter.

28. The Swedish documentary *Trans Train* has a good discussion of these issues. There is some discussion at (Gender Health Query 2019), and the documentary itself is available on YouTube. See https://www.youtube.com/watch?v=sJGAoNbHYzk and https://www.youtube.com/watch?v=73-mLwWIgwU
29. Quoted in Lane (2019). Lane's article is a lightly edited collection of excerpts from Moore & Brunskell-Evans (2019). The quote comes from their pp. 245–246. There are minor differences in grammar and capitalization from the original, and the word 'clinical' appears in the original: 'we are subjugating children's clinical needs to an ideological position' (p. 246).
30. Littman (2018). On trans identification as a social contagion, see also Marchiano (2017) and Shrier (2020). The Coalition for the Advancement and Application of Psychological Science released a position statement on 'rapid onset gender dysphoria' (ROGD) claiming that there is a 'lack of rigorous empirical support for its existence' (they seemed to assume that Littman intended it as a diagnosis). James Cantor (2021) provides an excellent response. He says 'The question has never been (and isn't supposed to be) whether ROGD exists: The question is whether the recent and explosive increase in trans referrals being reported across the world represents one of the previously well-characterized profiles (so we would know what to do) or something new (wherein we can't)' (Cantor 2021; in-text citations omitted).
31. Littman (2018, pp. 17–18). Littman's paper was re-reviewed by the journal *PLOS One* after activists complained, but the conclusions of the paper remained unchanged. As Littman herself put it in a later note, 'Other than the addition of a few missing values in Table 13, the Results section is unchanged in the updated version of the article' (Littman 2019). See also commentary in Bartlett (2019).
32. As reported in *The Telegraph:* 'There are concerns among some MPs that drug treatment is being offered too readily to children—some of them as young as 10—without fully understanding what lies behind their desire to change sex. In 2009/10 a total of 40 girls were referred by doctors for gender treatment. By 2017/18 that number had soared to 1,806. Referrals for boys have risen from 57 to 713 in the same period. Last year 45 children referred for NHS treatment were aged six or under, with the youngest being just four, though younger children are not given drugs' (Rayner 2018). The point about drug treatment being offered to children as young as 10 was confirmed in the High Court's *Bell v. Tavistock* judgement, which said 'Puberty blocking drugs can in theory be, and have in practice been, prescribed for gender dysphoria through the services provided by the defendant to children as young as 10' (point 5); and, 'As it is, for

the year 2019/2020, 161 children were referred by GIDS for puberty blockers (a further 10 were referred for other reasons). Of those 161, the age profile is as follows: 3 were 10 or 11 years old at the time of referral' (point 29).

33. Evans (2020).
34. Evans (2020).
35. Orange (2020).
36. See discussion in Vincent & Jane (forthcoming).
37. This tweet came from Law's account @mrbenjaminlaw, on the 12th of February 2020 at 7.58 a.m. It was part of a thread which he had started by accusing *The Australian* journalist Bernard Lane of 'attacking…transgender children and kids' hospitals', linking to an article at junkee.com whose headline was 'The Australian Has Compared Being Transgender to Having Coronavirus'. Online at https://twitter.com/mrbenjaminlaw/status/1227010643267444736 accessed 14th June 2020.
38. Shidlo & Schroeder (2002, pp. 249, 254–256).
39. Same-sex attraction is particularly significant given that the same marker—gender non-conformity—that might be used to infer or attribute trans status correlates strongly with non-heterosexual sexual orientation. One study of 2,428 girls and 2,169 boys 'found that the levels of gender-typed behaviour at ages 3.5 and 4.75 years…significantly and consistently predicted adolescents' sexual orientation at age 15 years' (Li et al. 2017, p. 764); another using data from a longitudinal study of 5,007 young people said 'Gender nonconformity was strongly associated with later male and female nonheterosexuality' (Xu et al. 2019, p. 1226); a paper discussing the relationship between the science of sexual orientation and the politics of it notes 'childhood gender nonconformity—behaving like the other sex—is a strong correlate of adult sexual orientation that has been consistently and repeatedly replicated', and explained further, 'In girls, gender nonconformity comprises dressing like and playing with boys, showing interest in competitive sports and rough play, lacking interest in conventionally female toys such as dolls and makeup, and desiring to be a boy' (Bailey et al. 2016, p. 57).
40. The term 'puberty blockers' refers to a Gonadotropin-Releasing Hormone agonist (GnRHa), originally developed to treat prostate cancer, and also used to delay abnormally early puberties. An endocrinologist in Amsterdam in 1994 used it 'to stop normal puberty altogether' (Biggs 2019, p. 1). A 2011 experimental study in the UK gave puberty blockers to forty-four children. University of Oxford sociologist Michael Biggs uses information obtained under the Freedom of Information Act to argue that the results of this 'experiment' were more negative than positive, and concludes that negative evidence has been ignored or suppressed (Biggs 2019). The NHS themselves admit that GnRHa 'was not licensed for use in addressing dysphoria in gender identity disorders', although they say that this is common (NHS 2019). The Society for Evidence-Based Gender

Medicine summarize a review—undertaken in 2020, published in 2021—by the UK's National Institute for Health and Care Excellence (NICE): 'The review of GnRH agonists (puberty blockers) makes for sobering reading. Its major finding is that GnRH agonists lead to little or no change in gender dysphoria, mental health, body image and psychosocial functioning. In the few studies that did report change, the results could be attributable to bias or chance, or were deemed unreliable. The landmark Dutch study by De Vries et al. (2011) was considered "at high risk of bias," and of "poor quality overall." The reviewers suggested that findings of no change may in practice be clinically significant, in view of the possibility that study subjects' distress might otherwise have increased. The reviewers cautioned that all the studies evaluated had results of "very low" certainty, and were subject to bias and confounding. The review of cross-sex hormones identified similar shortcomings in the quality of the evidence. The reviewers noted that "a fundamental limitation of all the uncontrolled studies in this review is that any changes in scores from baseline to follow-up could be attributed to a regression-to-the-mean," rather than the beneficial effects of hormone treatment. No study reported concomitant treatments in detail, meaning that it is unclear if positive changes were due to hormones or the other treatments participants may have received. The reviewers suggested that hormones may improve symptoms of gender dysphoria, mental health, and psychosocial functioning, but cautioned that potential benefits are of very low certainty and "must be weighed against the largely unknown long-term safety profile of these treatments"' (SEGM 2021).

41. Lyons (2016).
42. Vrouenraets et al. (2015).
43. Kirkup (2020).
44. de Vries et al. (2011); see also discussion in Kearns (2019).
45. de Vries et al. (2011).
46. *Bell v. Tavistock Judgement*, paragraph 56, p. 14 of PDF.
47. Their judgement acknowledged one expert saying that 'of the adolescents who started puberty suppression, only 1.9 per cent stopped the treatment and did not proceed to cross-sex hormones', but also cited another, saying that of forty-nine children and young people who had accessed endocrinology services 'only 55% (27 individuals) were subsequently approved for or accessed cross-sex hormones during their time with GIDS' (paragraph 26, p. 9 of PDF).
48. See discussion in Kearns (2019); and e.g. Wallien & Cohen-Kettenis (2008); Ristori & Steensma (2016); and Steensma & Cohen-Kettenis (2018). Studies on desistance tend to be based on people who experienced childhood gender dysphoria, so it's not clear whether the same findings will apply to the 'rapid onset gender dysphoria' that is more common in adolescents and young adults today, especially girls.

49. Quoted in Kearns (2019).
50. See further discussion in Moore & Brunskell-Evans (2019). The *Bell v. Tavistock* judgement also supports this point about pathway dependence: 'The evidence shows that the vast majority of children who take PBs [puberty blockers] move on to take cross-sex hormones, that Stages 1 and 2 are two stages of one clinical pathway and once on that pathway it is extremely rare for a child to get off it' (point 136). Although, cf. the Court of Appeals judgement, paragraph 26 (details in n. 47).
51. The judgement (*Bell v. Tavistock*) is online here: https://www.judiciary.uk/wp-content/uploads/2020/12/Bell-v-Tavistock-Judgment.pdf
52. They did question the empirical claims made in two of the points, namely whether there really is pathway dependence between puberty blockers and cross-sex hormones, and whether puberty blockers really are an 'experimental' treatment. Court of Appeals, paragraphs 63 and 64, pp. 18–19 of PDF.
53. Court of Appeals, paragraph 92, p. 25 of PDF.
54. Cohen & Barnes (2019); Ferguson & O'Connell (2019).
55. E.g. Schneider et al. (2017).
56. Pang et al. (2020).
57. According to 'The Report of the 2015 U.S. Transgender Survey 2015', 36 per cent of transgender men had had chest surgery reduction or reconstruction, 14 per cent had had a hysterectomy (removal of the uterus), 2 per cent had had metoidioplasty (creation of a 'neophallus' or new penis out of clitoral growth created by taking testosterone), 3 per cent had had phalloplasty (construction of a penis using skin grafts from the arm, leg, or torso), and 6 per cent had had another procedure not listed. Of those surveyed who hadn't had the procedures yet, 61 per cent wanted chest surgery reduction or reconstruction, 57 per cent wanted a hysterectomy, 49 per cent wanted metoidioplasty, and 43 per cent wanted phalloplasty. In comparison, among girls who identified as nonbinary, only 6 per cent had had chest surgery reduction or reconstruction and only 2 per cent had had hysterectomies, although 42 per cent wanted the former and 30 per cent wanted the latter (James et al. 2016).
58. According to 'The Report of the 2015 U.S. Transgender Survey 2015', 48 per cent of transgender women had had hair removal or electrolysis, 12 per cent had had vaginoplasty or labiaplasty (in trans cases this means the construction of a 'neovagina' or 'neolabia' and/or 'neoclitoris' from existing genital tissue), 11 per cent had had augmentation mammoplasty (breast construction or enhancement), 11 per cent had had an orchiectomy (removal of the testicles), 7 per cent had had facial feminization surgery, 5 per cent had had a tracheal shave (reduction of the Adam's apple), 3 per cent had had silicone injections, 1 per cent had had voice surgery, and 6 per cent had had other procedures not listed. 54 per cent of those surveyed who hadn't had the procedures yet wanted

to have vaginoplasty or labiaplasty, and over 40 per cent wanted to have hair removal or electrolysis, augmentation mammoplasty, orchiectomy, and facial feminization surgery (James et al. 2016). A 2016 study by the Williams Institute put the number of transgender people in the United States at 0.6 per cent of the population, most common in the 18–24-year-old age bracket.

59. For example, the Tasmanian Law Reform Institute considered thirty-five peer-reviewed studies, and concluded 'peer-reviewed empirical studies indicate that SOGI [sexual orientation and gender identity] conversion practices have significant and prolonged harmful effects on people subjected to them. These include depression, loneliness, alienation, increased risk of drug abuse, and suicidal ideation and suicide attempts' (Tasmanian Law Reform Institute 2020, p. 15). But only thirteen of the papers even mention gender identity. Conclusions about sexual orientation seem to have been generalized to gender identity; it is unclear whether this is simply because there has been a habit of pairing sexual orientation and gender identity as 'SOGI' since the Yogyakarta Principles were drafted, or because the structure of the two is assumed to be the same, or for some other reason.
60. Ehrensaft (2017).
61. It is unfortunate that the research report did not announce the sex breakdown of the nonbinary respondents, although they did collect the data. The report is linked here https://www.gov.uk/government/publications/national-lgbt-survey-summary-report see 'National LGBT Survey: Research Report', p. 19, fig. 3.3; and Annex 2, Question 3, p. 272.
62. An Australian study from 2018 reported on nonbinary identification by sex, finding that of 1,613 trans and gender diverse respondents, 53.5 per cent were nonbinary, with a ratio of 39.2 per cent female to only 14.3 per cent male (the study uses the phrases 'assigned female at birth' and 'assigned male at birth') (Callander et al. 2019, p. 6). A large American study from 2015 on 27,715 transgender respondents asked about the sex respondents were 'assigned at birth, on [their] original birth certificate', and found that of the 35 per cent non-binary respondents, 80 per cent were female, and only 20 per cent male (James et al. 2016, p. 45). So it seems fairly safe to assume that the UK data (see n. 61 above), had it been reported, would have also shown a skew towards female people being identified as nonbinary.
63. https://www.gov.uk/government/publications/national-lgbt-survey-summary-report/national-lgbt-survey-summary-report#the-results
64. A similar trend has been observed at a clinic in Wellington, New Zealand, with a 'particular increase in referrals for people under age 30, as well as an increasing proportion of people requesting female-to-male (FtM) therapy so that it is now approaching the number of people requesting male-to-female therapy (MtF)' (Delahunt et al. 2018, p. 33).

65. Callander et al. (2019, p. 10).
66. The study left it unclear whether these experiences happened *while* trans-identified or could be what *led* girls to identify out of girl-/womanhood.
67. Government Equalities Office (2018, p. 57).
68. Winer (2015). Note that homosexuality is illegal in Iran, and the state subsidizes sex reassignment surgery. This means it is likely that at least some of the people who have had sex reassignment surgery in Iran are in fact gay men, *not* transwomen (and so my description of the soccer team's players may be incorrect). See discussion in *The Economist* (2019): 'Gay Iranians face pressure to change their sex regardless of whether they want to, say activists and psychologists in Iran.'
69. Bannerman (2017).
70. Rodgers (2019).
71. Pulver (2018).
72. Strudwick (2015); Bartosch (2018).
73. Darbyshire (2018); Bannerman (2018).
74. Ekman (2018); Sutton (2019); Hunter (2020).
75. Brean (2018).
76. Lorde (1984, p. 78).
77. Lorde (1984, p. 78).
78. Finlayson et al. (2018).
79. Finlayson et al. (2018).
80. Kathleen Stock dates this as starting around 1990, with Judith Butler's influential book *Gender Trouble* (which directed people to 'trouble' the existing binary gender categories), but really taking off in the 2000s, getting a big boost in 2007 with Julia Serano's *Whipping Girl* (which proclaimed that gender identity is what makes a person a woman or man). Stock says the word 'transgender' got its contemporary meaning in 1992, 'trans' in 1998. Before that it was 'transsexual' and this meant specifically a person who had had sex reassignment surgery. See discussion in Stock's book *Material Girls*, ch. 1 (Stock 2021).
81. To quote them more fully: 'from an academic standpoint the medical field is suffering from a paucity of published data on the care of transgender patients and outcomes related to this care, especially in core medical journals. This is likely a result of a dearth of submissions from physician-researchers, lack of original research, and an overall lack of high-quality research. Our review demonstrates that most of the published work that exists is not primary research, and there are very few studies that look at long-term outcomes. Even fewer studies are prospective in nature, and only 11 were randomized controlled trials. While we acknowledge that such research design may not always be feasible or ethical, carefully designed studies will ultimately be the driving factor in moving the field towards a more evidence-based model of medicine. This, combined with longer patient follow-up and more prospective trials, will

improve our overall quality of research and allow us to better care for our patients' (Wanta & Unger 2017). The authors also noted that there were only forty-six articles on the epidemiology of transgenderism, the most robust of which came from only six European countries, and no comprehensive epidemiological studies done in the United States (Wanta & Unger 2017, p. 122).

82. For a more detailed discussion of the idea of 'gender identity', told in 'eight key moments', see discussion in Stock's *Material Girls*, chs. 1 and 4 (2021).
83. McCook (2018); Wadman (2018); Marcus (2020).
84. See n. 58 to this chapter.
85. For the considerable expansion of the community considered 'trans' today, see the 'Transgender Umbrella' image from *The Gender Book*, online at www.thegenderbook.com and reproduced in Griffin et al. 2021, p. 292).
86. 'Queer' arguably is such a concept, so imagine that all the people doing empirical research into sexual orientation could now *only* work with cohorts of people who self-identify as 'queer', which might mean that they are heterosexual but polyamorous; heterosexual but claim a cross-sex or no-sex gender identity; or heterosexual but in some other way feel the label 'queer' is appropriate to them.
87. Blanchard (1989, p. 324).
88. Blanchard (1989, p. 325).
89. Blanchard (1989, p. 327).
90. Lawrence (2017, p. 41).
91. Lawrence (2017, p. 41).
92. Bailey (2003); Lawrence (2013). Lawrence reports on some of the personal narratives she collected from autogynephilic males over thirteen years. Here are just a few, to illustrate: 'My sexual fantasies all include myself in female form, either being forced to become female or voluntarily. Frequently they involve a submissive element on my part: I am either forced to be a woman or forced to behave in a particularly submissive manner' (Lawrence 2013, p. 47). 'I know that I don't simply have a cross-dressing fetish, because my greatest sexual fantasy is going through puberty again as a girl and experiencing breast development, as well as being in pillow fights and bubble-gum blowing contests with other girls' (p. 48). Lawrence summarizes the major themes of the 249 informants' personal narratives as follows: 'Usually concede that they were not overtly effeminate during childhood but instead displayed many male-typical interests and behaviours'; 'Often report that autogynephilic erotic arousal has continued throughout their lives, including after sex reassignment'; 'Usually give a history of erotic arousal associated with the fantasy or act of wearing particular items of women's clothing'; 'Almost always report a history of erotic arousal associated with the fantasy or reality of having female breasts or genitalia'; 'Sometimes give a history of erotic arousal associated with fantasies of menstruating, breast-feeding, or being pregnant'; and 'Often report a history of erotic arousal associated with

the fantasy or act of engaging in behaviours considered typical or characteristic of females' (Lawrence 2013, pp. 53; for the full summary see pp. 53–54).

93. Documented in detail in Dreger (2008).
94. See e.g. Joel (2015); Fine (2017).
95. Bailey & Triea (2007, p. 527).
96. Blanchard (1985); Serano (2010); Lawrence (2017, p. 42).
97. Serano (2010, p. 177).
98. Blanchard (2005, p. 444).
99. Serano (2010) claims that it's natural for gender dysphoric people to fantasize about their sex lives 'inhabiting the "right" body', and even suggests that doing so is a 'coping mechanism' (Serano 2010, p. 184). But it's hard to square this sanitized version of autogynephilia (which she calls 'cross-gender arousal') with what autogynephilic people actually say, for examples of which see (Lawrence 2013) and n. 92 above.
100. Blanchard et al. (1987, p. 143). Compare this to the women: out of seventy-two, seventy-one were homosexual and one was heterosexual. It seems there is no sexual excitement to be found in dressing like a man or being treated like a man, perhaps because maleness is not subordinated and therefore not culturally taboo.
101. See n. 88 to this chapter.
102. There's an excellent discussion between counsellor Sasha Ayad and psychotherapist Stella O'Malley about boys who identify as transgender in the podcast *Gender: A Wider Lens*, episodes 'Gender Dysphoria in Boys: Part 1' and 'Gender Dysphoria in Boys: Part 2' (episode 20, 23rd April 2021; and episode 21, 30th April 2021). Both agree that there is a category of boys today that don't fit the older typology. As Ayad puts it 'there's something else going on here' (episode 20, 00:01:46). Online at https://gender-a-wider-lens.captivate.fm/episode/20-gender-dysphoria-in-boys-part-1
103. Stone (2006); Feinberg (2006). For a more recent version, see Dembroff (2018).
104. Dhejne et al. (2011, p. 3).
105. In full: 'regarding any crime, males-to-females had a significantly increased risk for crime compared to female controls...but not compared to males...This indicates that they retained a male pattern regarding criminality' (Dhejne et al. 2011, p. 6).
106. The adjustment for psychiatric morbidity was thought necessary because 'transsexual individuals had been hospitalized for psychiatric comorbidity other than gender identity disorder prior to sex reassignment about four times more often than controls' (Dhejne et al. 2011, p. 4). It's not clear that women should be interested in what the risk of violent crime by transsexual women would be *if four times as many transsexual women as other males didn't have psychiatric comorbidities*. Arguably, we should be interested in the actual risk, given the comorbidities. The data comparing rates of violent crime in transsexual women relative to 'birth sex' (i.e. male) controls is available in table S1, and

relative to 'final sex' controls (i.e. female) is available in table S2 in the section 'Supporting Information' for the paper online: https://journals.plos.org/plosone/article?id=10.1371/journal.pone.0016885#s5

107. If we consider only the data for *all transsexual subjects* in the study, rather than considering transsexual men and transsexual women separately, then this mixed-sex cohort is more likely to have been convicted for any crime or violent crime than non-transsexual controls (Dhejne et al. 2011, p. 6). This finding was significant in the time-divided cohort 1973–88, but there was inadequate data to reach a conclusion for the 1989–2003 cohort. (Some commentators have slipped into claiming that the finding was *not significant* in the later cohort, or was *only significant* in the earlier cohort, both of which are strictly true, but misleading.) Emphasizing this point allows the speculative explanation that it was the social conditions pre-1989 that explained the findings. Dhejne et al. comment on the improved survival of transsexual subjects in the later cohort that it 'might be explained by improved health care for transsexual persons during 1990s, along with altered social attitudes towards persons with different gender expressions' (Dhejne et al. 2011, p. 6). But even if that speculative explanation were correct, in considering whether we could expect it to generalize we would need to consider that (i) most transwomen today are not transsexual; and (ii) most live in countries that are not Sweden, and so may not have Sweden's post-1990 social conditions.

108. Let me be absolutely clear that the issue here is sex (being male or female), not gender identity or transgender status (specifically, being a transwoman). Dhejne et al. are also clear on this point, noting that their male-pattern crime finding had nothing to do with sex reassignment and everything to do with being male. They said 'Criminal activity, particularly violent crime, is much more common among men than women in the general population...In this study, male-to-female individuals had a higher risk for criminal convictions compared to female controls but not compared to male controls. This suggests that the sex reassignment procedure neither increased nor decreased the risk for criminal offending in male-to-females' (Dhejne et al. 2011, p. 6). There is no claim being made, either by them or by me, that being trans in general, or being a transwoman in particular, involves specific traits that make that group dangerous to women. (For an example of this misunderstanding, see e.g. Rebecca Solnit (2020), who wrote 'One of the really weird fears about trans women is that they're men pretending to be women to do nefarious things to other women'.) The issue is maleness. Gender-critical feminists do not need to take a stand on whether it is male biology, testosterone, male socialization, sex-differentiated evolved psychology, or any other of a range of competing hypotheses that account for observed differences between the sexes, particularly when it comes to physical and sexual violence. None of these hypotheses plausibly rule in non-trans men and rule out transwomen.

109. See e.g. Weale (2017); McCook (2018); Marcus (2020); and Gliske (2020).
110. See also Bailey (2003).
111. Bicchieri (2017).
112. Kuran (1990).
113. I am wary of discussing being gay and being trans together, given their recent pairing in conversion therapy legislation around the world, which applies data about attempts to change or suppress sexual orientations over to gender identities in order to mandate strict affirmation policies. They are not the same. But many gender non-conforming boys will turn out to be gay, so it is relevant to discuss them together here. On feminine boys, see Bailey (2003).
114. How trans people are protected at the moment is complicated and differs between countries. In Victoria, Australia, any transwoman who has secured a legal change of sex (which is just a matter of a statutory declaration) is legally female. All other transwomen are protected via 'gender identity', which is a protected attribute. In all cases where there are exceptions to anti-discrimination legislation on the basis of sex, e.g. to permit some single-sex activities or spaces, gender identity *trumps* sex (so such spaces could exclude a non-trans man, but not a transwoman). The only exception is elite sports, where it is permissible to exclude on the basis of *both* sex and gender identity. So when I say 'protected as the sex they identify as', I mean either by being classed as legally that sex, or by their status as a person with a gender identity trumping sex as a protected attribute and so effectively securing the same thing as if they had the legal sex.
115. Frye's essay 'Lesbian Feminism and the Gay Rights Movement: Another View of Male Supremacy, Another Separatism' makes a persuasive case against thinking that gay men and lesbian women have anything much in common—she says that their 'femininity' is 'a casual and cynical mockery of women, for whom femininity is the trappings of oppression' and a 'serious sport' (Frye 1983, pp. 128–151).
116. Legislation passed recently in Victoria, Australia, for example makes it a criminal offence to engage in a 'change or suppression' practice (defined as a failure to 'support or affirm' a person's gender identity, with limited exceptions) where that practice results in injury or serious injury. The original target of such legislation, a version of which already exists in Queensland and the Australian Capital Territory, was to prohibit the 'conversion' of homosexual sexual orientations by faith groups. Gender identity has simply been added in alongside sexual orientation, as though it has the same status and history. See references in nn. 22 and 59 to this chapter.
117. An employment tribunal in the UK awarded £20,000 to Sonia Appleby, the child safeguarding lead for an NHS gender identity clinic, who was subjected to hostile treatment in the workplace after raising concerns about the clinic's practices (Griffiths & Das 2021). There is testimony throughout Michelle Moore & Heather Brunskell-Evans' book *Inventing Transgender Children and*

Young People from clinicians and other practitioners about the 'affirmation-only' culture inside gender medicine (Moore & Brunskell-Evans 2019). The Society for Evidence-Based Gender Medicine were not allowed to have a stand at the recent American Academy of Paediatrics conference (SEGM 2021). Endocrinologist Will Malone said, on the podcast *Gender: A Wider Lens*, that at the conference where affirmative-care standards were introduced, there was no counterpoint presented (unlike every other session, where one expert argues for a new medical intervention and another expert argues the counterpoint) (Ayad & O'Malley 2021, 00:20:24–00:23:47). The Care Quality Commission Report (January 2021) of the Tavistock and Portman NHS Foundation Trust's Gender Identity Services (GIDS) rated the service 'inadequate', and noted that 'Staff did not always feel respected, supported, and valued. Some said they felt unable to raise concerns without fear of retribution' (p. 4).

118. See e.g. Chambers (2008, ch. 5); Jeffreys (2014, ch. 8).
119. As discussed in Littman (2018).
120. See also Vincent & Jane (forthcoming).
121. For more on gender abolitionism versus gender revisionism, see Lawford-Smith (2020*a*).

Chapter 6

1. She tweeted 'If sex isn't real, there's no same-sex attraction. If sex isn't real, the lived reality of women globally is erased. I know and love trans people, but erasing the concept of sex removes the ability of many to meaningfully discuss their lives. It isn't hate to speak the truth' (J. K. Rowling @jk_rowling, 6th June 2020 at 8.02 a.m., online at https://twitter.com/jk_rowling/status/1269389298664701952). Some of the abusive responses to her have been collated here:https://medium.com/@rebeccarc/j-k-rowling-and-the-trans-activists-a-story-in-screenshots-78e01dca68d posted 9th June 2020 accessed 13th June 2020.
2. A fourth explanation, which I don't have space to develop here, is that such antagonism is tribal, less about the gender-critical feminists who are the targets of the animosity and more about what *expressions* of animosity signal socially. For more on this theme, in connection with the use of slurs, see Nunberg (2017).
3. Murphy (2020*a*).
4. Sundar (2020).
5. Sundar (2020).
6. Murphy (2020*a*).
7. Sundar (2020).
8. 'Desi' means something like 'ex-pat'; Indian, Pakistani, or Bangladeshi people who live abroad.
9. Sundar (2020).

10. Murphy says she thinks those who most frequently oppose her tend to be leftist men, anarchists, and college student activists, as well as women who are sex worker rights activists and trans rights activists. Those who petitioned to have her fired from *Rabble* in 2015 describe themselves as 'feminists, grassroots community groups and organizations that support intersectional feminism'—see nn. 13 and 14.
11. In 1793 the feminist Olympe de Gouges was executed by guillotine in Paris, one of roughly 370 women to be killed this way during the French Revolution. Historian Oliver Blanc told *Haaretz* 'She [Gouges] is much more than the first feminist in the modern era. She is one of the first women who entered political life. She was a model for other women, and for that she also paid with her life' (Bar 2017). In 1943, Marie-Louise Giraud was executed by guillotine for performing illegal abortions—one of the last five women to be executed this way in France (Conerly 2017).
12. Acosta (2019).
13. https://www.change.org/p/rabble-ca-we-demand-that-rabble-ca-end-your-association-with-meghan-murphy-as-editor-and-columnist
14. https://rabble.ca/blogs/bloggers/rabble-staff/2015/05/statement-on-review-meghan-murphy-petitions
15. Murphy, p.c.
16. Ekman ([2010] 2013, p. 116).
17. Ekman ([2010] 2013, p. 116).
18. Lewis (2019).
19. The Heritage Foundation hosted an event called 'The Inequality of the Equality Act: Concerns from the Left', featuring speakers Julia Beck, Jennifer Chavez, Kara Dansky, and Hasci Horvath (a full video is available on their website). The event was initiated by Katherine Cave of the Kelsey Coalition, which is non-partisan. In an interview with Meghan Murphy for *Feminist Current*, Julia Beck explains that 'Cave spent four years searching for anyone willing to speak publicly about how "gender identity" impacts children and their parents. She asked every left-leaning think tank she could find, but they either flatly refused with accusations of "transphobia", or simply did not reply. Eventually, Cave and WoLF [radical feminist organization Women's Liberation Front] worked together to plan a panel of left-leaning people to speak at The Heritage Foundation. At the beginning of 2019, no other platform with half as much political influence as Heritage even dared to challenge the status quo, and that remains the same today' (Murphy 2019*c*).
20. Hay (2019). Murphy (2019*b*) is a useful reply to Hay.
21. Burns (2019).
22. See e.g. https://www.nature.com/articles/d41586-018-07238-8 and https://www.nature.com/news/sex-redefined-1.16943

23. To give some examples: laws in Australia, Canada, the UK, the United States, and a number of other countries have been rapidly changed to introduce gender identity ideology, in sex self-identification bills, conversion therapy bills, and vilification/hate speech bills. In my own state, Victoria, Australia, since 2019, we have had the Births, Deaths and Marriages Registration Amendment Bill (sex self-identification), the Change or Suppression (Conversion) Practices Prohibition Bill (conversion therapy), and Racial and Religious Tolerance Amendment Bill (vilification). The first makes change of legal sex obtainable by statutory declaration, the second prohibits the change or suppression of gender identities, and the third will prohibit vilification on the grounds of gender identity. Major lesbian, gay, bisexual, and transgender (LGBT) charities have become preoccupied by gender identity activism (for example, Stonewall in the UK—see discussion in Siddique 2021). University policies are entrenching the ideology through diversity and inclusion policy. My own university, the University of Melbourne, in 2021 issued a draft 'Gender Affirmation Policy' for consultation, which would give gender identity activist groups on campus veto power over events on campus (at my time of writing this, a revised draft was due to be released). Oxford sociologist Michael Biggs has collated data on the words 'lesbian', 'gay', 'bisexual', and 'transgender' appearing in annual reports over the years for Stonewall, the Equality Network, LGBT Youth Scotland, and the Human Rights Commission, most showing a radical increase for (and contemporary disproportionate focus on) 'transgender' over time; as well as funding from Big Lottery Fund, BBC Children in Need, and academic grants, to trans-related projects; and increases in funding over time to Mermaids, a UK trans-focused charity. See https://users.ox.ac.uk/~sfos0060/LGBT_figures.shtml#GLAAD
24. Byrne (2020).
25. Dembroff (2021, pp. 1 (abstract) and 11). Page numbers correspond to the pre-print of paper, archived at https://philpapers.org/rec/DEMETN 20th April 2020.
26. To be even more precise, the slogan as it appears on billboards and pamphlets (as Dembroff described) is 'woman [line break] wʊmən [line break] *noun* [line break] adult human female'. There is an image of a billboard put up by the campaign group Speak Up For Women New Zealand in 2021 in Wells (2021).
27. Some women have gotten so fed up of leftist identity politics and its failure to take adequate action on issues that affect women that they've given up memberships in left-wing parties, and in some cases given up identifying with 'the left' at all. This happened recently in the UK, when members of the UK Labour party signed a pledge to expel members who had expressed 'transphobic' views. See discussion in Parker (2020). Needless to say, this doesn't make those who left the party 'conservative'.
28. Ekman ([2010] 2013, p. 22).

29. This comes under the heading 'Repeated and/or non-consensual slurs, epithets, racist and sexist tropes, or other content that degrades someone'. The policy reads 'We prohibit targeting others with repeated slurs, tropes or other content that intends to dehumanize, degrade or reinforce negative or harmful stereotypes about a protected category. *This includes targeted misgendering or deadnaming of transgender individuals*' (my emphasis). Online at https://help.twitter.com/en/rules-and-policies/hateful-conduct-policy
30. See further discussion in Lawford-Smith & Megarry (forthcoming).
31. Macandrew et al. (2019).
32. I say 'uses the name' rather than is named, as does Libby Brooks writing for *The Guardian* (Brooks 2019), because bizarrely, this transwoman seems to have taken the name 'Cathy Brennan' from a prominent radical feminist activist in the United States.
33. Davidson (2019*a*).
34. Brooks (2019).
35. Davidson (2019*a*).
36. Davidson (2019*a*).
37. Twitter, @TownTattle, Replying to @fem_dr, 8th May 2019, 12.09 a.m. (my emphasis).
38. Baynes (2019).
39. Davidson (2019*b*).
40. Izaakson (2018).
41. Vonow (2017). *The Sun* reports the Hyde Park event as a talk titled 'What is Gender? The Gender Recognition Act and Beyond' (Vonow 2017). But seeing as the *Sun* reporter describes MacLachlan as 'a member of TERF'—and describes the altercation in the rather colourful terms, 'Fists went flying at Speakers' Corner, London, when the Trans-Exclusionary Radical Feminists (TERFs) and their enemies Trans Activists clashed in the bust-up about 7pm on September 3' (Vonow 2017)—I'm going to assume that *Feminist Current* has the more accurate information.
42. Pearson-Jones (2018).
43. Izaakson (2018).
44. Izaakson (2018).
45. Sommers (1994, p. 29).
46. Stoljar (1995, p. 265).
47. In the first book-length indictment of this kind of feminism—arguing for the conclusion that there is no such thing as 'women as a class' and denying that white middle-class women are oppressed—the antagonists identified as deserving a chapter of their own were the following rather curious bunch: *Plato, Aristotle* (neither generally considered a feminist), Simone de Beauvoir (writing more than a decade before the second wave began), and Nancy Chodorow (Spelman 1988). A few other culprits have been named elsewhere,

most notably Betty Friedan, named by bell hooks ([1984] 2000, pp. 1–3), and Mary Daly, named by Audre Lorde in 'An Open Letter to Mary Daly' (Lorde 1984). Friedan's mistake was writing about the predicament of a majority of American women (roughly two-thirds, according to hooks) without acknowledging that they were *only* a majority, rather than 'women' in general (hooks [1984] 2000, p. 2). Friedan's mistake may have been less in failing to acknowledge that some women were black, as in failing to acknowledge that half of all black people were women. Daly's mistake was in writing about ancient goddesses from the European tradition, and failing to mention the African goddesses (Lorde 1984, pp. 66–71).

48. Frye ([1981] 1983, pp. 110–127).
49. Peoples (2016).
50. hooks (1982, ch. 4).
51. hooks ([1984] 2000, ch. 5, esp. pp. 69–70).
52. For example, the Human Rights Campaign resource, '5 Things to Know to Make Your Feminism Trans-Inclusive', is focused on transwomen and includes the section 'Centering the Most Marginalized Is Key' (https://www.hrc.org/resources/5-things-to-know-to-make-your-feminism-trans-inclusive). See also Saul (2020), who describes transwomen as 'some of the most marginalised women'. Obviously, which social groups come out as 'the most marginalized' will depend on what we consider to be marginalization, and how we conceptualize the social group (consider the difference between lesbians, on the one hand, and the LGBTQIA+ (lesbian, gay, bisexual, trans, queer, intersex, and asexual plus), on the other; or transsexuals, on the one hand, and anyone with an atypical gender identity (relative to their sex), on the other). But there is evidence that some of the claims about marginalization frequently repeated across the media, for example about murder and suicide rates, are false. See discussion in Biggs (2015) and Reilly (2019).
53. Wittgenstein (1969).
54. See discussion in Pritchard (2011, pp. 524–532).
55. Pritchard (2011, p. 528).
56. See discussion in Cohen (2003).
57. Rowland (2017, p. 812).
58. See overview in Gosepath (2007).
59. Flynn (2000).
60. See e.g. Sunstein (1999).
61. Judith Butler has said, for example, 'every person should have the right to determine the legal and linguistic terms of their embodied lives' (Williams n.d.).
62. Another might be, 'if a social group has high rates of suicide ideation we should give them whatever they're asking for'. (Suicide ideation is thoughts about suicide, including thinking about, considering, or planning it.) Suicide ideation tends to be weaponized by trans activists—a mother threatening the Tavistock

gender clinic in the UK with litigation to stop her autistic daughter being medicalized says that suicide is used as 'emotional blackmail to show why we should capitulate with every single demand around trans rights' (Lane 2019). A problem with this 'value' is that suicide is a problem for adolescent males *in general*, not just those who identify as transgender. Suicide is the third most common cause of death for adolescent males globally, and in Australia the leading cause of death for males aged 15–25 years old (King et al. 2020, p. 1). One group of researchers have argued that norms of 'ideal' masculinity contribute to this, finding that 'greater conformity to heterosexual norms was associated with reduced odds of reporting suicide ideation' (p. 5). In other words, less masculine-conforming males were more likely to have thought about suicide. This may be because conformity to gender norms has a 'protective effect' (p. 6) (conformity is rewarded while violation is sanctioned). This is likely to implicate transgirls and transwomen, but it is significant that it is *not limited to* them. The result persisted even when sexual minorities were removed from the sample.

63. Most recently, gender identity activist Peter Tatchell pulled out of a podcast debate with gender-critical feminist Kathleen Stock, after pressure from other gender identity activists (Kelleher 2021). See also discussion in (Turner 2018).
64. Dembroff et al. (2019).
65. Stock et al. (2019); see also discussion in Lawford-Smith (2019).
66. Stanley (2015).
67. Stanley (2015, p. 53).
68. Stanley (2015, p. 58).
69. Stanley (2015, p. 57).
70. Stanley (2015, p. 60).
71. Stanley (2015, p. xiv).
72. Lance (2019).
73. Lance (2019).
74. Lance (2019; my emphasis).
75. To be fair, some of the radical feminists were guilty of these tactics. Janice Raymond wrote that 'all transsexuals *rape* women's bodies by reducing the real female form to an artifact, appropriating this body for themselves' (Raymond 1979, p. 104; my emphasis). Jo Freeman does the same thing, writing that '[t]rashing is a particularly vicious form of character assassination which amounts to psychological *rape*' (Freeman 1976; my emphasis). Shulamith Firestone, herself Jewish, wrote in *The Dialectic of Sex* that love—specifically men's love of women—was a *holocaust* (Firestone 1970, p. 119).
76. Stanley (2015, pp. 3–8).
77. Sheila Jeffreys, p.c.
78. Ekman ([2010] 2013, pp. 15–30).
79. Ekman ([2010] 2013, p. 104).

80. Ekman ([2010] 2013, pp. 104–105).
81. Ekman ([2010] 2013, pp. 94–100).
82. Ross et al. (2004) see also discussion in Ekman ([2010] 2013, pp. 102–103).
83. For six of the countries in the study (Canada, Colombia, Germany, Mexico, Turkey, and Zambia—a majority), data is gathered on 'women', but for three (South Africa, Thailand, and the USA), it's 'people' (allowing for the men, children, and trans people who work in prostitution) (see Farley et al. 2004, p. 48).
84. Farley et al. (2004).
85. Farley et al. (2004, pp. 33–34, 56); see also discussion in Ekman ([2010] 2013, p. 102).
86. 'Listen to sex workers' (deference) (Scarlet Alliance 2011); 'The Convention on the Rights of the Child (CRC) takes a similar approach, promoting measures that curb and punish the activities of those who sexually exploit children, without any reference to the emerging sexual rights and agency of children and young people' (agency) (Otto 2007, p. 269, in-text references removed); 'I want people to engage in educated conversations and disagreements so we can get to the best possible place to protect surrogates and the intended parents' right to make the choice that works for them' (choice) (Rosen 2020. See also Rudrappa (2010) and Riggs (2016) for extensive commentary on narratives about 'choice' in contract pregnancy.
87. McKinnon's contribution was not peer-reviewed. This is standard practice for book symposiums at the journal.
88. McKinnon (2018, p. 484).
89. Allen et al. (2018*a* and 2018*b*). See also https://terfisaslur.com/and https://www.reddit.com/r/terfisaslur/ for examples of its use.
90. See e.g. the empirical evidence collected in Fine (2010).
91. Dembroff (2018). The full paragraph is: 'I consider nonbinary identity to be an unabashedly political identity. It is for anyone who wishes to wield self-understanding in service of dismantling a mandatory, self-reproducing gender system that strictly controls what we can do and be'.
92. https://adfmedialegalfiles.blob.core.windows.net/files/SouleDisqualifyMotionAndMemo.pdf p. 36 (page numbers correspond to the PDF, not to page headers or document page numbers). In response to a follow-up question by the Plaintiff's council, the court allowed that the transwomen athletes could be referred to as 'transgender athletes', and that it was acceptable to refer to their having 'male bodies', and having gone through 'male puberty'. The bright line was that they not be referred to as simply 'male'. In their later motion to disqualify, arguing that the court's request with respect to language showed bias, the Plaintiff's council wrote 'The use of the word "male" to describe individuals who have been genetically male since conception and possess male bodies is accurate, consistent with timeless use as well as formal definitions of "male", and follows widespread usage in legal contexts in which accuracy is required' (p. 8).

93. https://assets.publishing.service.gov.uk/media/5e15e7f8e5274a06b555b8b0/Maya_Forstater__vs_CGD_Europe__Centre_for_Global_Development_and_Masood_Ahmed_-_Judgment.pdf It's worth noting that in reaching judgements like this, courts seem to be relying on outdated understandings of who is 'trans' (as discussed above). It's clearly not a violation of human decency or human dignity to call a politically motivated nonbinary person, or a person who has transitioned because of social contagion, by their sex-corresponding pronouns.
94. Posie Parker makes a similar point in an interview for Triggernometry in 2019: https://www.youtube.com/watch?v=Pdpc2r4cBxQ&t=2220s
95. Ekman (2018).
96. 'Punching down' refers to targeting people who are positioned lower than you in the social hierarchy, while 'punching up' refers to targeting people who are positioned higher than you. This is possibly best-known as a rule in progressive stand-up comedy circles: don't punch down, only punch up.
97. Saul (2020).
98. A similar point is also made, albeit with a needlessly incendiary analogy to a date rape drug, in Kerr (2019).
99. It is noteworthy that a lot of the vitriol coming from journalists and academics is coming out of the United States, which has substantially worse protections in place for transgender people, and being directed at women speaking out in countries like the United Kingdom, Australia, and New Zealand, which have substantially better protections in place for transgender people. It's not clear whether this is strategic. If it is—a contribution to a global political debate designed to make domestic political gains—then it belongs under the umbrella of this section (it is political propaganda). The alternative explanation is less charitable, namely that the Americans making these interventions are simply ignorant about the significant differences in context between themselves and those they are arguing against, and they are 'universalizing' the American context.

Chapter 7

1. Chesler (2018, p. 227).
2. @UN_Women, Twitter, Jan 5th 2019. Online at https://twitter.com/UN_Women/status/1081469111975272448?s=20
3. I'll use the term 'intersectionality' to cover all of the discussion within black feminism about incorporating multiple axes of oppression within a single movement. This may be idiosyncratic relative to the contemporary discussion, in which intersectionality is most often associated with Kimberlé Crenshaw, who coined the term. But I think the intellectual history is continuous, that many women were getting at the same or a similar idea, and that Crenshaw simply proposed one refinement of it. Because that idea is most closely associated with the term 'intersectionality' today, that's the term I'll use. So when I go on to

argue that gender-critical feminism need not be intersectional, what I mean is *both* that it need not be about multiple axes of oppression (it can be about sex alone) and that it need not be about the intersections between sex and other axes that create novel forms of oppression (it can be about non-intersectional oppression alone, in this refined sense).

4. Wong (2010).
5. I say 'refocusing' rather than 'focusing' because this is an old idea that has gotten lost in contemporary feminism, not a new idea. Janet Radcliffe Richards, for example, wrote in 1980 'If, for instance, there are men and women in slavery, it is not the business of feminism to start freeing the women. Feminism is not concerned with a group of people it wants to benefit, but with a type of injustice it wants to eliminate' (Radcliffe Richards 1980, p. 24).
6. Nash (2019, p. 36).
7. See discussion in Nash (2019).
8. Cooper (1892).
9. Kate Phelan and I argue that it is possible to distinguish at least six understandings of intersectionality across the black feminist literature. There are experiential claims (about what it is like to be multiply oppressed), epistemic claims (about what a multiply oppressed person knows), legal claims (about ways in which a multiply oppressed person lacks legal protection), explanatory claims (about what ultimately explains people's oppression), political claims (about what is best in eliminating oppression), and metaphysical claims (about what oppression ultimately is) Lawford-Smith & Phelan 2021*)*.
10. https://iwda.org.au/learn/what-is-feminism/
11. Cooper (1892).
12. Combahee River Collective (1977; my emphasis).
13. Beal (1969); King (1988).
14. Crenshaw (1989; my emphasis).
15. UN Women (2017, pp. 5, 8, 9, 13).
16. hooks ([1984] 2000, p. 37).
17. Jeffreys (2009*a*, p. 9).
18. E.g. Morton et al. (2009).
19. hooks ([1984] 2000, p. 40).
20. hooks ([1984] 2000, p. 40).
21. hooks ([1984] 2000, p. 118–120); following Hodge (1975).
22. hooks ([1984] 2000, p. 118).
23. https://www.ancient.eu/article/1136/women-in-ancient-china/
24. https://www.ancient.eu/article/1152/caste-system-in-ancient-india/
25. For those who are curious, the philosopher is John Hodge. See discussion in hooks ([1984] 2000, pp. 36–39).
26. https://www.wgea.gov.au/data/fact-sheets/gender-workplace-statistics-at-a-glance
27. hooks (2000, pp. xiv–xv).

28. http://womensliberationfront.org/document-statement-of-principles/ accessed 18th May 2020.
29. Jefferson (1980).
30. hooks ([1984] 2000). In later work, bell hooks added class to her previous focus on race/sex, and claimed that these must be addressed together. She said 'class structure in American society has been shaped by the racial politic of white supremacy; it is only by analysing racism and its function in a capitalist society that a thorough understanding of class relationships can emerge. Class struggle is inextricably bound to the struggle to end racism' (hooks 2000, p. 3).
31. Crenshaw (1989, 1991).
32. Cooper (1892).
33. Combahee River Collective (1977).
34. Spelman (1988).
35. See discussion in Phelan, manuscript.
36. hooks ([1984] 2000, p. 2).
37. Nothing important hangs on the word 'disadvantage' here, I mean to include all/any of disadvantage, discrimination, marginalization, exploitation, oppression.
38. It's worth noting that in Rawls's case, prioritarianism came after equality. Departures from an equal distribution of material resources were justified only if they were to the benefit of the least well off. It's not clear what this would mean for feminism. Perhaps: we should focus on issues that affect all women (baseline of equality) unless focusing on issues that affect some women would mean that the worst-off women became better-off than they were in the baseline. If there are 'trickle-down' benefits, this could justify focusing on the *best-off* women. For example, imagine that closing the pay gap between actors and actresses in Hollywood would actually improve the situation of the worst-off women. This is likely to strike many feminists as deeply unintuitive.
39. See e.g. Cox (2016).
40. Uta Johansdottir @UtaJohansdottir in reply to Kirsten Gillibrand @SenGillibrand, 5th December 2018 at 3.49 p.m. Online at https://twitter.com/UtaJohansdottir/status/1070178335051915264
41. To the extent that intersectionality has caught on in the leftist popular imagination, *all* movements will be urged to be intersectional, and what I am describing for feminism will happen elsewhere too. Maybe this will be a good thing—instead of many specialized movements with a narrow focus, there will eventually just be one big movement supporting all the social justice projects. The worry remains though that a movement that tries to do everything will end up being able to do virtually nothing.
42. Criado-Perez (2019).
43. Criado-Perez (2019).
44. Topping (2020).
45. Frye (1983, p. 16).

46. Frye (1983, p. 16).
47. Dworkin (1974, p. 23).
48. Dworkin (1974, pp. 23–24).
49. Woman's Place UK @Womans_Place_UK, 28th September 2019 at 7.05 p.m. Online at https://twitter.com/Womans_Place_UK/status/117787189455032320 1?s=20.Seealsohttps://womansplaceuk.org/2020/02/03/50-years-of-womens-liberation-in-the-uk-pragna-patel/
50. Jefferson (1980).
51. Crenshaw (1989, pp. 158–159).
52. See e.g. testimony from women in the documentary *On The Record* (Dick & Ziering 2020), or Phyllis Chesler's discussion of this issue (Chesler 2018, pp. 197–286). Kate Phelan and I discuss these issues in Lawford-Smith & Phelan (2021).
53. See discussion in Jacobs (2017–2018).
54. Scotland (2020).
55. Cf. Natalie Stoljar, who writes 'Consider a white, able-bodied, heterosexual woman who is privileged along the first three dimensions of her identity, yet disadvantaged by virtue of being a woman. Can this woman be said to suffer discrimination when her overall individual situation is one of privilege?' (Stoljar 2017, p. 69). For the antidote, see MacKinnon (1991*a*).
56. Those who associate intersectionality with Crenshaw are likely to find this remark odd. For a fuller explanation, see n. 3 to this chapter.
57. Crenshaw (1989, pp. 139–140).
58. Crenshaw (1989, p. 142; case in n. 8).
59. Freeman (2005).
60. Lorde (1984, p. 52).
61. Lorde (1984, p. 60).
62. Lorde (1984, p. 52).
63. As Shirley Chisholm experienced in the 1970s; and as Rose McGowan, who would surely be described as 'privileged' if anyone is, experienced in the 1990s, and as was revealed as part of the global #metoo movement revealing women's experiences of sexual abuse and sexual harassment (Levin & Solon 2017).

Chapter 8

1. Firestone (1970, p. 203).
2. Salk, Hyde, & Abramson (2017).
3. Bodily autonomy will still be important (this is something all types of feminists agree about), and it's possible that as surgeons become more proficient—currently they are much more proficient in transforming male bodies than in transforming female bodies—demand for 'designed' bodies, including bodies designed to

look as the opposite sex, will increase. This interacts with increased interest in 'transhumanism' too, the improvement of human life using technological advancements, including integration of the physical body with technology. There are interesting treatments of this issue in the British television series *Years and Years* (BBC & HBO 2019), and the novel *Inappropriation* by Lexi Freiman (2018). On the philosophy of transhumanism, see e.g. More (2013).

4. Sargent (2010, p. 21).
5. Alderman (2016).
6. Vonnegut (1961).
7. More ([1516] 2000).
8. Anderson (2014, p. 16).
9. Abbott (1903).
10. See discussion in Williams (2013).
11. As Nicholas Southwood and David Wiens (2016) have pointed out, it's not always the case that something's becoming actual establishes that it was feasible, because some actual things were fluky. If something comes about by fluke, then it may not count as feasible in the sense that moral and political philosophers, and policy-makers and activists besides, are interested in. I'll proceed on the assumption that the success of the major social justice movements I'm using as examples wasn't fluky.
12. I'm aware that asymmetric criminalization is normally considered a model for prostitution *not including* pornography, but because I don't see any meaningful difference between the two industries, I also don't see any meaningful difference in how they should be dealt with. See also Chapter 6.
13. Southwood (2017).
14. Mac & Smith (2018).
15. Ekman ([2010] 2013).
16. Jeffreys (2009*b*, pp. 124–125).
17. See further discussion in Lawford-Smith (2020*a*).
18. So long as, as I said earlier, they aren't actual *and* the result of a fluke. See n. 11.
19. See discussion in Cox (2017).
20. Some argue against particular alliances, e.g. between radical feminists and conservatives, on symbolic grounds—almost as though there is a moral taint involved in working with people who we disagree with on other issues. Others argue against it on more pragmatic grounds, e.g. that it may damage the progressive credentials of the radical feminists, or that it may lead to backsliding on feminist issues because it ultimately empowers conservatives. The former is ideological puritanism because it can mean refusing to make alliances that would actually be successful in securing gains for women. The latter is not (so long as the pragmatic concerns are well-founded).

21. Mac & Smith (2018).
22. See discussion in Aroney & Crofts (2019).
23. For simplicity here I'm just talking about pornography simpliciter rather than specific kinds of pornography. Some might think that this is too broad, because there can be 'feminist pornography'. Women working from their bedrooms via webcams, solo porn, lesbian porn filmed by women, and porn designed from a woman's perspective for a woman's enjoyment are all candidates for morally acceptable pornography. The counter-argument, inspired by MacKinnon (1989) is that the most entrenched gender expectation for women is sexual availability to men, which is behind both women's sexual objectification and sexual violence against women and girls. If this is right—and I agree with MacKinnon that it's a big part of the story even if it's not the whole story—then even solo porn, lesbian porn, and porn by women for women will still be viewed by men as confirming their stereotypes and prejudices about 'what women are for', and in that sense 'feminist pornography' is an oxymoron. So I will proceed on the assumption that the gender-critical feminist is committed to full abolition. This doesn't mean that *in the utopia* some form of pornography couldn't re-emerge, from a novel starting point and with none of the baggage of porn under patriarchy.
24. See the original petition here https://www.change.org/p/shut-down-pornhub-and-hold-its-executives-accountable-for-aiding-trafficking and the current version of the petition here https://www.traffickinghubpetition.com/
25. https://www.similarweb.com/website/pornhub.com
26. https://traffickinghub.com/
27. Bicchieri (2017, pp. 147–153).
28. Hudson (2012).
29. For an overview of alternatives, see Southwood (2018).
30. Some think these two ideas go together: something can be judged to be infeasible *because* it's immoral. This is one version of *implicit constraints*, discussed in Section 8.3. For criticism of this idea, see Lindauer & Southwood (forthcoming).
31. Hill (2019).
32. Gilabert & Lawford-Smith (2012, pp. 813–814, 2013, p. 255).
33. It *is* an objection to a general theory of political feasibility, which would ideally apply to both individuals and legal/political reforms. For alternative approaches to feasibility, see discussion in (Southwood 2018), who has work in progress defending a novel approach likely to come out in the next couple of years.
34. Lawford-Smith (2013).
35. For debate over this idea of 'remit', see discussion in Collins & Lawford-Smith (2016); cf. Berkey (2019).
36. See discussion in Anderson (2014).
37. See discussion in Stamp (2013).

Chapter 9

1. Sundar (2020).
2. Mehat (2015).
3. Sanchez (2017).
4. An alternative way to make sense of the radical/liberal distinction is in terms of whether the feminist takes a revolutionary or an incremental/gradualist approach to reform. This does seem to describe the difference between activist groups, e.g. The Feminists (radical) breaking away from the National Organization for Women (liberal) in the United States, and the Women's Electoral Lobby (liberal) breaking away from the Women's Liberationists (radical) in Australia. It's not clear whether it also describes the theoretical disagreement. Aside from some dismissive talk about 'reformers' (as opposed to e.g. revolutionaries) by the radical feminists, there's not much explicit discussion about this difference as being a key or relevant distinction between radical and liberal feminism. So I won't say more about it here.
5. Blackford (2018, p. 16).
6. Blackford (2018, p. 16).
7. Locke (1689, p. 6). Page numbers correspond to the PDF here: https://socialsciences.mcmaster.ca/econ/ugcm/3ll3/locke/toleration.pdf
8. Locke (1689, p. 6).
9. Locke (1689, p. 7).
10. Locke (1689, p. 6).
11. Locke (1689, p. 12).
12. Rawls (1971, p. 14), cited in Gibson (1977, p. 194); see also Jaggar (1983, ch. 3).
13. Mill (1859, p. 73).
14. Mill (1859, pp. 74–75).
15. Mill (1859, p. 74).
16. Mill (1859, p. 81).
17. Mill (1859, ch. IV).
18. Berlin (1969).
19. Jean-Paul Sartre talked in *Being and Nothingness* (1956, p. 553) about this kind of freedom. Wherever there was the alternative of 'suicide or…desertion', there was free choice. He applies the same reasoning to rape in marriage, arguing that women are merely 'self-deceived' and attempting to distract themselves from the 'pleasure'; she had the choice of suicide instead of sex and chose sex, so she is free (see discussion in Frye 1983, p. 55). Frye's description of this is enjoyable: 'Sartre took this economical route to freedom and embraced the absurd condition as profundity…It should not be surprising that the same small mind, embracing a foolish consistency, cannot recognize rape when he sees it and employs a magical theory of "bad faith" to account for its evidence' (Frye 1983, pp. 54–55).
20. Taylor (1979).

21. Gaus (2000, ch. 5).
22. Pettit (1996, 1997).
23. Pettit (1993).
24. Cf. Burgess-Jackson (1995), who argues that Mill was a radical feminist.
25. Also Elizabeth Holtzman, Bella Abzug, Eleanor Smeal, Pat Schroeder, and Patsy Mink, although these names are likely to be less familiar (Tong 1989, p. 13).
26. Tong (1989, p. 28); following Eisenstein (1986, p. 176).
27. Tong (1989, p. 28).
28. Gloria Steinem had a higher public profile than Friedan, but there is controversy about how to classify her, with many classifying her as liberal and her classifying herself as radical.
29. Radcliffe Richards ([1980] 1994, p. 94–95).
30. Radcliffe Richards ([1980] 1994, p. 97).
31. Radcliffe Richards ([1980] 1994, p. 98).
32. Radcliffe Richards ([1980] 1994, pp. 104–105).
33. Radcliffe Richards ([1980] 1994, p. 108; her emphasis). It might seem that radical and gender-critical feminists want to do exactly what Radcliffe Richards is describing when they advocate for the Nordic Model (which criminalizes the purchase of sex). But the Nordic Model is justified in terms of taking away *men's right to buy sex*, not taking away women's right to sell it in order to 'liberate' them (even though abolishing the sex industry is one key component of ending up in a future in which women are, in fact, liberated from male domination). (See also Chapter 6.)
34. Radcliffe Richards ([1980] 1994, p. 120).
35. Radcliffe Richards ([1980] 1994, pp. 120–121).
36. In an essay titled 'The Great Gulf of Feminism', published in an updated edition of *The Sceptical Feminist* in 1994, Radcliffe Richards distinguishes 'egalitarian feminism' from 'liberal feminism', saying that there is a difference between a feminism that wants to get rid of a sexual double standard and see men and women treated the same *no matter the background political theory*, liberal or otherwise (this she called 'egalitarian feminism'), and a feminism specifically committed to liberalism that wanted to see liberal values realized equally in the cases of women and men. She thought the 'great gulf' was actually between egalitarian feminists, who worked for equality within the status quo whatever it was, and 'radical' feminists, who challenged the status quo. (I use quote marks for 'radical' because she seems to be referring to *difference feminism* in the examples of thinkers and ideas that she gives, rather than the broader range of views I'm talking about as radical feminism in this book.) Given how much work would actually have to be done to achieve equality, she thinks 'egalitarian feminism' is actually 'radical' (here she seems to mean *more ambitious than its critics give it credit for*): '[t]he feminism that seeks equality within the status quo, properly understood, is as radical as any movement there has ever been'

(Radcliffe Richards [1980] 1994, p. 395). In Chapter 4, I suggested we should leave much of difference feminism behind, so her criticism of what she's calling 'radical' feminism does not apply to the radical, and then gender-critical, feminism that I've been defending throughout this book.

37. Gibson (1977, pp. 200–208).
38. Gibson (1977, pp. 208–209).
39. Gibson (1977, p. 200).
40. Gibson (1977, p. 193).
41. Chambers (2008, pp. 162–164).
42. Chambers criticizes a prominent liberal feminist, Martha Nussbaum, for focusing on autonomy over big decisions but not the more everyday ones. This was not an oversight: 'Nussbaum argues that her position ... allows people to live nonautonomous lives, for autonomy may be counter to their conception of the good, particularly if that conception is religious' (Chambers 2008, p. 164). Chambers argues that Nussbaum's view is inconsistent, based on Nussbaum's *feminist* commitment against female genital mutilation (FGM). If it were only a matter of choosing at the level of big decisions, then a girl could in principle decide that she wants to lead a life where she has FGM and so can marry within her community. This would be a sacrifice of everyday autonomy, especially in decisions about sexual pleasure which would be entirely foregone. But it doesn't look structurally different from the case of choosing to enter the army or the convent. But Nussbaum thinks FGM is wrong. Chambers thinks Nussbaum is right about FGM, and that her reasoning about it extends to other kinds of cases, like the social practice of women undergoing cosmetic breast implant surgeries.
43. Chambers (2008, p. 194).
44. Chambers (2008, p. 194).
45. Chambers (2008, p. 196).
46. Jeffreys (2009*a*).
47. Frye (1983).
48. MacKinnon (1982).
49. MacKinnon (1982).
50. Jeffreys (2009*a*).
51. Miriam (2005).
52. Brownmiller (1976).
53. Ginsberg in Jaschick (2009).
54. Atkinson (1974*c*; Frye (1983)).
55. Atkinson (1974*c*, p. 110). [Sic.]
56. *Channel 4 News* (2018).
57. Lerner (1986, p. 12).
58. Lerner (1986, p. 13).
59. Firestone wrote in 1968 that the abolitionists had sold out women: 'The Abolitionists, who had been glad to accept the alliance with women all along,

suddenly decided that now it was "the Negro's hour,"—that the cause of women was too unimportant to delay for a minute any advances in the liberation of the blacks. Needless to say they had forgotten that HALF of the black race was female, so they sold out their own cause as well' (p. 5). This might sound 'intersectional', like she's making the point that it doesn't make sense to put black liberation before women's liberation when some black people are women. But I read her as making a point about alliances. She goes on to say, 'Once again the principle was proved that unless oppressed groups stick together, *and on alliances of self-interest rather than do-goodism*, nothing can be accomplished in the long run to dismantle the apparatus of oppression' (Firestone 1968, p. 5; my emphasis). Indeed, she says a little later in the same article 'we should keep in mind that revolutions anywhere are always glad to use any help they can get, even from women. But unless women also use the Revolution to further their own interests as well as everyone else's, unless they make it consistently clear that all help given now is expected to be returned, both now and after the Revolution, they will be sold out again and again' (p. 5).

60. Lerner (1986, p. 226). Although Lerner is not the only person to attribute these words ('existential nothingness') to Daly, I have not been able to find them in Daly's work. Another source provides a reference to *The Church and the Second Sex*, p. 70—but at least in my copy, they are not there; Google Books turns up the same source, p. 68—but again, in my copy, they are not there.
61. Friedan ([1963] 2013), p. 83).
62. Atkinson (1974*c*, p. 111).

Chapter 10

1. See also an alternative list of demands put together by Woman's Place UK with feedback from the gender-critical feminist community at https://womanspla-ceuk.org/wpuk-manifesto-2019/ and the global Declaration on Women's Sex-Based Rights at https://www.womensdeclaration.com/en/declaration-womens-sex-based-rights-full-text/
2. The Victorian Parliament's Change or Suppression (Conversion) Practices Prohibition Act 2021, which was passed in February 2021, redefines sexual orientation as a protected attribute under the Equal Opportunity Act 2010 (p. 15), from 'homosexuality (including lesbianism), bisexuality or heterosexuality' to 'a person's emotional, affectional and sexual attraction to, or intimate or sexual relations with, persons of a different gender or the same gender or more than one gender' (pp. 39–40).
3. The first ten items are derived from a thread by Alessandra Asteriti—@AlessandraAster—on Twitter, 29th March 2019. The thread is here: https://twitter.com/AlessandraAster/status/1111709720258203648?s=20 The full list that

appears here was published to Medium on the 7th of June 2019. That post is archived here: https://hollylawford-smith.org/radical-feminist-wish-list-2019/

4. John Schwenkler challenged me on this demand, on the grounds that some women are pushed into *having* abortions they don't wish to have by partners, and noting that state support can skew women's incentives in either direction (free and accessible abortions might signal a preference for abortion in cases of uncertainty, whereas a strong programme of support for pregnancy and maternal health might signal the opposite. I think these are fair points. 'Full reproductive rights' should be taken to include rights to abortion *if* that is what is wanted, and rights not to have abortions if *that* is what is wanted. In either case, control should not rest with male partners (although cf. Mathison & Davis 2017, esp. p. 318, whose discussion of 'ectogenesis'—the development of a foetus entirely outside the womb—has interesting implications for how much say prospective fathers should get in decisions about abortion). On the issue of state policy, I have less to say, because as Cass Sunstein has observed, there's a 'nudge' either way (see e.g. Sunstein 2019). That's just how it goes with policy—we have to choose which nudge is worse. I think restricted access to abortion is a worse nudge in terms of social outcomes for women.

Afterword

1. Hochschild (2005).
2. On this point, see also Phelan (forthcoming); and see n. 29 to Chapter 2.

References

á Campo, J., Nijman, H., Merckelbach, H., & Evers, C. 'Psychiatric Comorbidity of Gender Identity Disorders: A Survey among Dutch Psychiatrists', *The American Journal of Psychiatry* 160 (2003), pp. 1332–1336.

Abbott, Lyman. 'Why Women Do Not Wish the Suffrage', *The Atlantic*, September 1903.

Acosta, Katherine. 'Vancouver Panel on Gender Identity and Media Bias Encapsulated Conflict between Women and Trans Activists', *Feminist Current*, 6th November 2019.

Alarcón, Rubén, de la Iglesia, Javier, Casado, Nerea, & Montejo, Angel. 'Online Porn Addiction: What We Know and What We Don't—A Systematic Review', *Journal of Clinical Medicine* 8/1 (2019), pp. 1–20.

Alderman, Naomi. *The Power* (London: Viking, 2016).

Allen, Jeffner. *Lesbian Philosophy* (Palo Alto, CA: Institute of Lesbian Studies, [1986] 2001).

Allen, Sophie, Finneron-Burns, Elizabeth, Jones, Jane Clare, Lawford-Smith, Holly, Leng, Mary, Reilly-Cooper, Rebecca, & Simpson, Rebecca. 'Derogatory Language in Philosophy Journal Risks Increased Hostility and Diminished Discussion (Guest Post)', *Daily Nous*, 27th August 2018*a*.

Allen, Sophie, Finneron-Burns, Elizabeth, Jones, Jane Clare, Lawford-Smith, Holly, Leng, Mary, Reilly-Cooper, Rebecca, & Simpson, Rebecca. 'On An Alleged Case of Propaganda: Reply to McKinnon'. Manuscript, 9th September 2018*b*.

Ananthaswamy, Anil, & Douglas, Kate. 'The Origins of Sexism: How Men Came to Rule 12,000 Years Ago', *New Scientist*, 18th April 2018.

Anderson, Craig. 'Violent Video Games: Myths, Facts, and Unanswered Questions', *Psychological Science Agenda*, October 2003.

Anderson, Elizabeth. 'Social Movements, Experiments in Living, and Moral Progress: Case Studies from Britain's Abolition of Slavery', *The Lindley Lecture, The University of Kansas*, 11th February 2014.

Andrews, Travis. 'She Gained Fame as an Early Transgender Advocate. Now, She's Charged with Triple Homocide', *The Washington Post*, 18th November 2016.

Appiah, Anthony. *The Honour Code: How Moral Revolutions Happen* (New York: W.W. Norton & Co., 2010).

Aroney, Euridice, & Crofts, Penny. 'How Sex Worker Activism Influenced the Decriminalisation of Sex Work in NSW, Australia', *Crime Justice Journal* 8/2 (2019), pp. 50–67.

Ásta. *Categories We Live By* (Oxford: Oxford University Press, 2018).

Atkinson, Ti-Grace. 'Radical Feminism' (The Feminists, New York, 1969).

Atkinson, Ti-Grace. *Amazon Odyssey* (New York: Links Books, 1974*a*).

Atkinson, Ti-Grace. 'Radical Feminism and Love', in *Amazon Odyssey* (New York: Links Books, 1974*b*).

Atkinson, Ti-Grace. 'Some Notes Toward a Theory of Identity', in *Amazon Odyssey* (New York: Links Books, 1974*c*).

Atkinson, Ti-Grace. 'Declaration of War', in *Amazon Odyssey* (New York: Links Books, 1974*d*).

Aubusson, Kate. 'The question female doctors never want to hear again', *The Sydney Morning Herald*', 18th November 2019.

Ayad, Sasha, & O'Malley, Stella. 'Hormonal Interventions—From Fringe to Mainstream: A Conversation with Dr. Will Malone', *Gender: A Wider Lens Podcast*, 8th January 2021. Online at https://gender-a-wider-lens.captivate.fm/episode/hormonal-interventions-from-fringe-to-mainstream-a-conversation-with-dr-will-malone

Bailey, J. Michael. *The Man Who Would Be Queen: The Science of Gender-Bending and Transsexualism* (Washington, DC: Joseph Henry Press, 2003).

Bailey, J. Michael, & Triea, Kiira. 'What Many Transgender Activists Don't Want You to Know: And Why You Should Know It Anyway', *Perspectives in Biology and Medicine* 50/4 (2007), pp. 521–534.

Bailey, Michael, Vasey, Paul, Diamond, Lisa, Breedlove, Marc, Vilain, Eric, & Epprecht, Marc. 'Sexual Orientation, Controversy, and Science', *Psychological Science in the Public Interest* 17/2 (2016), pp. 45–101.

Bannerman, Lucy. 'Trans Teenager Lily Madigan Voted in as a Labour Women's Officer', *The Times*, 20th November 2017.

Bannerman, Lucy. 'Anger Over Women's Business Honour for Cross-dressing Banker', *The Times*, 22nd September 2018.

Bar, Roni. 'Olympe De Gouges, the Radical French Feminist Who Was Murdered Twice', *Haaretz*, 3rd November 2017.

Barker, Victoria. 'Definition and the Question of "Woman"', *Hypatia* 12/2 (1997), pp. 185–215.

Bartlett, Tom. 'Journal Issues Revised Version of Controversial Paper that Questioned Why Some Teens Identify as Transgender', *The Chronicle of Higher Education*, 19th March 2019.

Bartosch, Josephine. 'The Limits of Stonewall's Tolerance', *The Spectator*, 31st July 2018.

Baynes, Chris. 'Julie Bindel: Feminist Writer Claims She Was "Physically Attacked" by Trans Activist after University Talk on Violence against Women', *Independent*, 6th June 2019.

BBC. 'Germany "Cannibal" Trial: Former Policeman Is Sentenced', *BBC News*, 1st April 2015.

BBC. 'Woman Billboard Removed After Transphobia Row', *BBC News*, 26th September 2018. Online at https://www.bbc.com/news/uk-45650462 accessed 30th June 2020.

BBC & HBO. *Years and Years* (2019).

Beal, Frances. 'Double Jeopardy: To Be Black and Female', *Meridians* 8/2 [1969] (2008), pp. 166–176.

Beauvoir, Simone de. *The Second Sex*. Trans. Constance Borde & Sheila Malovany-Chevallier (Paris: Vintage [1949] 2011).

Ben-Yehuda, Nachman. 'The European Witch Craze of the 14th to 17th Centuries: A Sociologist's Perspective', *American Journal of Sociology* 86/1 (1980), pp. 1–31.
Berkey, Brian. 'Collective Obligations and Demandingness Complaints', *Moral Philosophy and Politics* 6/1 (2019), pp. 113–132.
Berlin, Isaiah. 'Two Concepts of Liberty', in *Four Essays on Liberty* (Oxford: Oxford University Press, 1969), pp. 118–172.
Berns, Magdalen. 'RE: "Are Genital Preferences Transphobic?" Give It Up, Riley!' YouTube, 31st March 2017. Online at https://www.youtube.com/watch?v=F_5FFGrGzJw
Bettcher, Talia Mae. 'Trans Identities and First-Person Authority', in Laurie Shrage (Ed.), *You've Changed: Sex Reassignment and Personal Identity* (Oxford: Oxford University Press, 2009).
Bicchieri, Cristina. *Norms in the Wild* (Oxford: Oxford University Press, 2017).
Biggs, Michael. 'The 41% Trans Suicide Attempt Rate: A Tale of Flawed Data and Lazy Journalists', *4thWaveNow*, 3rd August 2015.
Biggs, Michael. 'The Tavistock's Experiment with Puberty Blockers'. Manuscript, 29th July 2019.
Bindel, Julie. 'My Sexual Revolution', *The Guardian*, 30th January 2009.
Bindel, Julie. *The Pimping of Prostitution* (Melbourne: Spinifex, 2017).
Bindel, Julie. 'The Left Has Forgotten What Feminism Looks Like', *UnHerd*, 10th September 2018.
Bindel, Julie, & Kelly, Liz. 'A Critical Examination of Responses to Prostitution in Four Countries: Victoria, Australia; Ireland; the Netherlands; and Sweden', Routes Out Partnership Board, 2003.
Bisch, Kevin. 'The Gang's All Here', *Salon*, 31st August 1999.
Blackford, Russell. *The Tyranny of Opinion* (New York: Bloomsbury, 2018).
Blackless, Melanie, Charuvastra, Anthony, Derryck, Amanda, Fausto-Sterling, Anne, Lauzanne, Karl, & Lee, Ellen. 'How Sexually Dimorphic Are We? Review and Synthesis', *American Journal of Human Biology* 12/1 (2000), pp. 151–166.
Blanchard, Ray. 'Typology of Male-to-Female Transsexualism', *Archives of Sexual Behaviour* 14 (1985), pp. 247–261.
Blanchard, Ray. 'The Concept of Autogynephilia and the Typology of Male Gender Dysphoria', *Journal of Nervous and Mental Disease* 177 (1989), pp. 616–623.
Blanchard, Ray. 'Early History of The Concept of Autogynephilia', *Archives of Sexual Behaviour* 34/4 (2005), pp. 439–446.
Blanchard, Ray, Clemmensen, Leonard, & Steiner, Betty. 'Heterosexual and Homosexual Gender Dysphoria', in *Archives of Sexual Behaviour* 16/2 (1987), pp. 139–152.
Bolinger, Renee. 'Moral Risk and Communicating Consent', *Philosophy and Public Affairs* 47/2 (2019), pp. 179–207.
Borissenko, Sasha. 'How to Spot a Brocialist: The Guys With Righteous Politics but a Dodgy Attitude to Girls', *Vice*, 11th April 2016.
Brean, Joseph. 'Forced to Share a Room with Transgender Woman in Toronto Shelter, Sex Abuse Victim Files Human Rights Complaint', *National Post*, 2nd August 2018.
Brennan, Geoffrey., Eriksson, Lina., Goodin, Robert., & Southwood, Nicholas. *Explaining Norms* (Oxford: Oxford University Press, 2013).

Brooks, Libby. 'Edinburgh LGBT+ Committee Resigns in Row over Speakers at Feminist Meeting', *The Guardian*, 7th June 2019.

Brown, G. R., & Jones, K. T. 'Mental Health and Medical Health Disparities in 5135 Transgender Veterans Receiving Healthcare in the Veterans Health Administration: A Case-control Study', *LGBT Health* 3 (2016), pp. 122–131.

Brownmiller, Susan. *Against Our Will: Men, Women and Rape* (New York: Bantam, 1976).

Budapest, Zsuzsanna. *The Holy Book of Women's Mysteries* (Berkeley, CA: Wingbow Press, [1980] 1989).

Burgess-Jackson, Keith. 'John Stuart Mill, Radical Feminist', *Social Theory and Practice* 21/3 (1995), pp. 369–396.

Burns, Katelyn. 'The Rise of Anti-trans "Radical" Feminists, Explained', *Vox*, 5th September 2019.

Butler, Judith. 'Sex and Gender in Simone de Beauvoir's Second Sex', *Yale French Studies* 72 (1986), pp. 35–49.

Butler, Judith. *Gender Trouble* (Abingdon: Routledge, 1990).

Byrne, Alex. 'Is Sex Binary?' *ARC Digital*, 2nd November 2018.

Byrne, Alex. 'Are Women Adult Human Females?' *Philosophical Studies* 177 (2020), pp. 3783–3803.

Callander, D., Wiggins, J., Rosenberg, S. Cornellisse, V. J., Duck-Chong, E., Holt, M., Pony, M., Vlahakis, E., MacGibbon, J., & Cook, T. *The 2018 Australian Trans and Gender Diverse Sexual Health Survey: Report of Findings* (Sydney, NSW: The Kirby Institute, University of New South Wales, 2019).

Cameron, Deborah. *Feminism: A Brief Introduction to the Ideas, Debates, & Politics of the Movement* (Chicago, IL: University of Chicago Press, 2019).

Cameron, Jessica Joy. *Reconsidering Radical Feminism* (Vancouver: UBC Press, 2018).

Campbell, Alastair. 'Why a Market in Organs is Inevitably Unethical', *Asian Bioethics Review* 8/3 (2016), pp. 164–176.

Cantor, James. 'CAAPS, ROGD, and the Science Neglected', *Sexology Today*, 9th August 2021. Online at http://www.sexologytoday.org/2021/08/caaps-rogd-and-science-neglected.html

Chambers, Clare. *Sex, Culture, and Justice: The Limits of Choice* (University Park, PA: Penn State University Press, 2008).

Channel 4 News. 'Germaine Greer on Women's Liberation, the Trans Community and Her Rape', YouTube, 23rd May 2018.

Chatterjee, Rhitu. 'Where Did Agriculture Begin? Oh Boy, It's Complicated', *NPR*, 15th July 2016.

Chesler, Phyllis. *A Politically Incorrect Feminist* (New York: St. Martin's Press, 2018).

Cho, Seo-Young. 'An Analysis of Sexual Violence—The Relationship between Sex Crimes and Prostitution in South Korea', *Asian Development Perspectives* 9/1 (2018), pp. 12–34.

Cohen, Deborah, & Barnes, Hannah. 'Gender Dysphoria in Children: Puberty Blockers Study Draws Further Criticism', *British Medical Journal* 366 (2019), pp. 1–4.

Cohen, G. A. 'Facts and Principles', *Philosophy & Public Affairs* 31/3 (2003), pp. 211–245.

Collins, Stephanie. *The Core of Care Ethics* (London: Palgrave Macmillan, 2015).

Collins, Stephanie, & Lawford-Smith, Holly. 'Collectives' and Individuals' Obligations: A Parity Argument', *Canadian Journal of Philosophy* 46/1 (2016), pp. 38–58.
Combahee River Collective, The. 'A Black Feminist Statement', in Akasha (Gloria T.) Hull, Patricia Bell Scott, & Barbara Smith (Eds.), *All the Women Are White, All the Blacks Are Men, But Some of Us Are Brave*, 2nd Ed. (New York: Feminist Press, [1977] 1982).
Conerly, Jennifer. 'The Last Woman Guillotined in WWII France Risked Her Life Over Abortion Rights', *History Collection*, 8th July 2017.
Cooper, Anna Julia. *A Voice From The South* (1892).
Cox, Susan. 'Why Do Women Fail to Vote as a Class?' *Feminist Current*, 18th November 2016.
Cox, Susan. 'Prostitution Legislation Must Include Women in the Porn Industry', *Feminist Current*, 23rd March 2017.
Crenshaw, Kimberlé. 'Demarginalizing the Intersections of Race and Sex: A Black Feminist Critique of Antidiscrimination Doctrine, Feminist Theory, and Antiracist Politics', *University of Chicago Legal Forum* (1989), pp. 139–167.
Crenshaw, Kimberlé. 'Mapping the Margins: Intersectionality, Identity Politics, and Violence against Women of Colour', *Stanford Law Review* 43/6 (1991), pp. 1241–1279.
Criado-Perez, Caroline. *Invisible Women* (London: Chatto & Windus, 2019).
Daisley, Stephen. 'Labour's Trans Rights Problem', *The Spectator*, 24th February 2020.
Daly, Mary. *Beyond God The Father: Toward a Philosophy of Women's Liberation* (Boston, MA: Beacon Press, 1973).
Daly, Mary. 'The Qualitative Leap beyond Patriarchal Religion', *Quest* 1/4 (1975), pp. 20–40.
Daly, Mary. *Gyn/Ecology* (Boston, MA: Beacon Press, 1978).
Daly, Mary, & Caputi, Jane. *Webster's First New Intergalactic Wickedary of the English Language* (Boston: Beacon Press, 1987).
Danaher, John. 'A Defence of Sexual Inclusion', *Social Theory and Practice* (forthcoming).
Darbyshire, Madison. 'HERoes: Champions of Women in Business', *Financial Times*, 20th September 2018.
Davidson, Gina. 'Feminist Speaker Julie Bindel "Attacked by Transgender Person" at Edinburgh University after Talk', *The Scotsman*, 6th June 2019*a*.
Davidson, Gina. 'Protester Charged for "Abusing" Feminist', *The Scotsman*, 22nd June 2019*b*.
Dehghan, Saeed Kamali. 'Kidney for Sale: Poor Iranians Compete to Sell Their Organs', *The Guardian*, 27th May 2012.
Delahunt, John, Denison, Hayley, Sim, Dalice, Bullock, Jemima, & Krebs, Jeremy. 'Increasing Rates of People Identifying as Transgender Presenting to Endocrine Services in the Wellington Region', *New Zealand Medical Journal* 131/1468 (2018), pp. 33–42.
Dembroff, Robin. 'Why Be Nonbinary?' *Aeon*, 30th October 2018.
Dembroff, Robin. 'Escaping the Natural Attitude About Gender', *Philosophical Studies* 178/3 (2021), pp. 983–1003.
Dembroff, Robin. & Wodak, Daniel. 'He/She/They/Ze', *Ergo* 5 (2018*a*).

Dembroff, Robin. & Wodak, Daniel. 'If Someone Wants to Be Called "They" and Not "He" or "She", Why Say No?' *The Guardian*, 4th June 2018*b*.

Dembroff, Robin, Kukla, Rebecca, & Stryker, Susan. 'Retraction Statement by Robin Dembroff, Rebecca Kukla and Susan Stryker', *IAI News*, 26th August 2019.

Dennis, Riley J. 'Can Having Genital Preferences for Dating Mean You're Anti-Trans?' *Everyday Feminism*, 21st April 2017.

Denton, Fatma. 'Climate Change Vulnerability, Impacts, and Adaptation: Why Does Gender Matter?', *Gender and Development* 10/2 (2002), pp. 10–20.

Destro-Bisol, Giovanni, Donati, Francesco, Coia, Valentina, Boschi, Ilaria, Verginelli, Fabio, Caglia, Alessandra, Tofanelli, Sergio, Spedini, Gabriella, & Capelli, Cristian. 'Variation of Female and Male Lineages in Sub-Saharan Populations: The Importance of Sociocultural Factors', *Molecular Biology and Evolution* 21/9 (2004), pp. 1673–1682.

Deves, Katherine, & Lawford-Smith, Holly. 'What is Victoria's bBan on "Conversion Therapy" Actually Trying to Achieve?' *Crikey*, 22nd December 2020*a*.

Deves, Katherine, & Lawford-Smith, Holly. 'Gender Bill Risks Too Great', *Herald Sun*, 28th December 2020*b*.

Dhejne, Cecilia, Lichtenstein, Paul, Boman, Marcus, Johansson, Anna, Langstrom, Niklas, & Landen, Mikael. 'Long-Term Follow-Up of Transsexual Persons Undergoing Sex Reassignment Surgery: Cohort Study in Sweden', *PLOS One* 6/2 (2011), e16885.

Dick, Kirby, & Ziering, Amy. *On The Record* (California: HBO Max, 2020).

Dickinson, Helen., & Bismark, Marie. 'Female doctors in Australia are hitting glass ceilings—why?' *The Conversation*, 6th January 2016.

Dickson, Sandra. 'Sex in the City: Mapping Commercial Sex across London', The POPPY Project, Eaves Housing for Women, 2004.

Dines, Gail. *Pornland: How Porn Has Hijacked Our Sexuality* (Boston, MA: Beacon Press, 2010).

Dinour, Lauren. 'Speaking Out on "Breastfeeding" Terminology: Recommendations for Gender-Inclusive Language in Research and Reporting', *Breastfeeding Medicine* 14/8 (2019), pp. 523–532.

Donnelly, Laura. 'Don't Call Pregnant Women "Expectant Mothers" as It Might Offend Transgender People, BMA Says', *The Telegraph*, 29th January 2017.

Doward, Jamie. 'Politicised Trans Groups Put Children at Risk, Says Expert', *The Guardian*, 28th July 2019.

Dreger, Alice. 'The Controversy Surrounding *The Man Who Would Be Queen:* A Case History of the Politics of Science, Identity, and Sex in the Internet Age', *Archives of Sexual Behaviour* 37 (2008), pp. 366–421.

Dreger, Alice. 'Is Anatomy Destiny?' *TED Talk*, 10th June 2011. Online at https://youtu.be/59-Rn1_kWAA

Dretske, Fred. 'Epistemic Operators', *The Journal of Philosophy* 67/24 (1970), pp. 1007–1023.

Dworkin, Andrea. *Woman Hating* (New York: E.P. Dutton, 1974).

Economist, The. 'Why Are So Many Teenage Girls Appearing in Gender Clinics?' *The Economist*, 1st September 2018.

Economist, The. 'Why Iran Is a Hub for Sex-reassignment Surgery', *The Economist*, 6th April 2019.

Ehrensaft, Diane. 'Gender Nonconforming Youth: Current Perspectives', *Adolescent Health, Medicine, and Therapeutics* 8 (2017), pp. 57–67.

Eisenstein, Zillah. *The Radical Future of Liberal Feminism* (Boston, MA: Northeastern University Press, 1986).

Ekman, Kajsa Ekis. *Being and Being Bought: Prostitution, Surrogacy and the Split Self* (Melbourne: Spinifex Press, [2010] 2013).

Ekman, Kajsa Ekis. 'The Modern John Got Himself a Queer Nanny', *Feminist Current*, 24th August 2016.

Ekman, Kajsa Ekis. 'En man som styckar kvinnor ska inte sitta i kvinnofängelse', *Debatt*, 21st September 2018.

Engels, Friedrich. *The Origin of the Family, Private Property, and the State*, 4th Ed. (Foreign Languages Publishing House, 1891).

Evans, Marcus. 'Why I Resigned from Tavistock: Trans-identified Children Need Therapy, Not Just "Affirmation" and Drugs', *Quillette*, 17th January 2020.

Faludi, Susan. 'Death of a Revolutionary', *The New Yorker*, 8th April 2013.

Farley, Melissa, Cotton, Ann, Lynne, Jacqueline, Zumbeck, Sybille, Spiwak, Frida, Reyes, Maria, Alvarez, Dinorah, & Sezgin, Ufuk. 'Prostitution and Trafficking in Nine Countries: An Update on Violence and Posttraumatic Stress Disorder', *Journal of Trauma Practice* 2/3–4 (2004), pp. 33–74.

Farley, Melissa, Bindel, Julie, & Golding, Jacqueline. 'Men Who Buy Sex: Who They Buy and What They Know', *Research Report for Eaves*, December 2009.

Fausto-Sterling, Anne. 'The Five Sexes: Why Male and Female Are Not Enough', *The Sciences*, March/April 1993, pp. 20–25.

Fausto-Sterling, Anne. 'Why Sex Is Not Binary', *The New York Times*, 25th October 2018.

Fausto-Sterling, Anne. 'The Five Sexes, Revisited', *The Sciences*, July/August 2000, pp. 18–23.

Feinberg, Leslie. *Stone Butch Blues* (Michigan: Firebrand Books, 1993).

Feinberg, Leslie. 'Transgender Liberation: A Movement Whose Time Has Come' (1992), in Susan Stryker & Stephen Whittle (Eds.), *The Transgender Studies Reader* (New York: Routledge, 2006), pp. 205–220.

Feminists, The. 'The Feminists: A Political Organization to Annihilate Sex Roles' (1970), in Anne Koedt, Ellen Levine, & Anita Rapone (Eds.), *Radical Feminism* (New York: Quadrangle Books, 1973), pp. 368–378.

Ferguson, Grant, & O'Connell, Michele. 'Gender Dysphoria: Puberty Blockers and Loss of Bone Mineral Density', *British Medical Journal* 367 (2019), p. 1.

Fickling, David. 'Cannibal Killer Gets Life Sentence', *The Guardian*, 9th May 2006.

Fine, Cordelia. *Delusions of Gender* (New York: Norton, 2010).

Fine, Cordelia. *Testosterone Rex—Myths of Sex, Science, and Society* (New York: W.W. Norton & Co., 2017).

Fine, Cordelia, Sojo, Victor, & Lawford-Smith, Holly. 'Why Does Workplace Gender Diversity Matter? Justice, Organizational Benefits, and Policy', *Social Issues and Policy Review* 14/1 (2020), pp. 36–72.

Finlay, Karen. 'After Thousands of Women Object, Male Student Withdraws from Women-only University', *Women Are Human*, 14th February 2020.

Finlayson, Lorna, Jenkins, Katharine, & Worsdale, Rosie. '"I'm Not Transphobic, but…": A Feminist Case against the Feminist Case against Trans Inclusivity', *Verso*, 17th October 2018.

Finn, Suki. 'The Metaphysics of Surrogacy', in David Boonin (Ed.), *The Palgrave Handbook of Philosophy and Public Policy* (Cham: Springer, 2018), pp. 649–659.

Firestone, Shulamith. 'The Women's Rights Movement in the U.S.: A New View', in *Notes from the First Year: Women's Liberation Movement* (New York: 1968).

Firestone, Shulamith. *The Dialectic of Sex* (New York: William Morrow, 1970).

Fisher, Anna. 'A Critical Review of "Revolting Prostitutes: The Fight for Sex Workers' Rights" by Juno Mac and Molly Smith', nordicmodelnow.org, 7th February 2019.

Flynn, James. *How To Defend Humane Ideals* (Nebraska: University of Nebraska Press, 2000).

Frederick, David, St. John, Kate, Garcia, Justin, & Lloyd, Elisabeth. 'Differences in Orgasm Frequency Among Gay, Lesbian, Bisexual, and Heterosexual Men and Women in a U.S. National Sample', *Archives of Sexual Behavior* 47 (2018), pp. 273–288.

Freeman, Jo. 'Trashing: The Dark Side of Sisterhood', *Ms. Magazine*, April 1976, pp. 49–51, 92–98.

Freeman, Jo. 'Shirley Chisholm's 1972 Presidential Campaign', jofreeman.com, February 2005.

Freiman, Lexi. *Inappropriation* (Sydney: Allen & Unwin, 2018).

Friedan, Betty. *The Feminine Mystique* (New York: W. W. Norton & Company Inc., [1963] 1997).

Friedan, Betty. *The Feminine Mystique* (New York: W. W. Norton & Company, [1963] 2013).

Frye, Marilyn. 'On Being White: Toward a Feminist Understanding of Race and Race Supremacy', *The Politics of Reality* (New York: Crossing Press, [1981] 1983).

Frye, Marilyn. *The Politics of Reality* (New York: Crossing Press, 1983).

Fuss, Diana. *Essentially Speaking: Feminism, Nature, and Difference* (New York: Routledge, 1989).

Gaus, Gerald. Political Concepts and Political Theories (Boulder: Westview Press, 2000).

Gavey, Nicola. *Just Sex? The Cultural Scaffolding of Rape*, 2nd Ed. (Abingdon: Routledge, 2019).

Gender Health Query. 'Swedish Documentary Highlights Mental Health Issues and Transgender Transition Regret', genderhq.org, 1st May 2019.

Gibson, Mary. 'Rationality', *Philosophy & Public Affairs* 6/3 (1977), pp. 193–225.

Gilabert, Pablo, & Lawford-Smith, Holly. 'Political Feasibility: A Conceptual Exploration', *Political Studies* 60 (2012), pp. 809–825.

Gilligan, Carol. *In A Different Voice* (Cambridge, MA: Harvard University Press, 1982).

Gilligan, Carol. 'Revisiting "In a Different Voice"', *LEARNing Landscapes* 11/2 (2018), pp. 25–30.

Gleeson, Hayley. 'What Happens When an Abused Woman Fights Back?' *ABC News*, 30th July 2019.

Gliske, Stephen. 'Response to Retraction of My Paper on Gender Dysphoria', *Medium*, 30th April 2020.

Glosswitch. 'Sex-positive Feminism Is Doing Patriarchy's Work for It', *New Statesman*, 7th March 2014.

Goldberg, Michelle. 'The Trans Women Who Say That Trans Women Aren't Women', *Slate*, 9th December 2015.

Goldstein, Deborah, Sarkodie, Eleanor, & Hardy, David. 'Transgender and Nontrans Patients Do Not Receive Statistically Different Quality Primary Care at Whitman-Walker Health, 2008–2016', *Transgender Health* 4/1 (2019), pp. 200–208.

Goodin, Robert, & Barry, Christian. 'Benefiting from the Wrongdoing of Others', *Journal of Applied Philosophy* 31/2 (2014), pp. 363–376.

Gosepath, Stefan. 'Equality', *Stanford Encyclopedia of Philosophy* (Standford, CA: Standford University Press, [27th March 2001] 27th June 2007).

Gouges, Olympe de. *Declaration of the Rights of Woman and of the Female Citizen* (1791).

Government Equalities Office. 'National LGBT Survey: Research Report', July 2018. Online at https://www.gov.uk/government/publications/national-lgbt-survey-summary-report

Grant, Melissa Gira. 'Let's Call Sex Work What It Is: Work', *The Nation*, 5th March 2014.

Grant, Melissa Gira. 'Liberal Feminism Has a Sex Work Problem', *The New Republic*, 24th October 2019.

Greer, Germaine. *The Female Eunuch* (London: Fourth Estate, 1970).

Greer, Germaine. *On Rape* (Melbourne: Melbourne University Press, 2018).

Griffin, Lucy, Clyde, Katie, Byng, Richard, & Bewley, Susan. 'Sex, Gender and Gender Identity: A Re-evaluation of the Evidence', *BJPsych Bulletin* 45/5 (2021), pp. 291–299.

Griffin, Susan. *Woman and Nature: The Roaring Inside Her* (New York: Harper Colophon, 1980).

Griffiths, Sian, & Das, Shanti. 'Gender Identity Clinic Whistleblower Wins Damages for "Vilification"', *The Times*, 4th September 2021. Online at https://www.thetimes.co.uk/article/gender-identity-clinic-whistleblower-wins-damages-for-vilification-cwj2m3t0s

Guillamon, A., Junque, C., & Gómez-Gil, E. 'A Review of the Status of Brain Structure Research in Transsexualism', *Archives of Sexual Behaviour* 45 (2016), pp. 1615–1648.

Hacker, Helen Mayer. 'Women as a Minority Group', *Social Forces* 30/1 (1951), pp. 60–69.

Hald, Gert, Malamuth, Neil, & Yuen, Carlin. 'Pornography and Attitudes Supporting Violence against Women: Revisiting the Relationship in Nonexperimental Studies', *Aggressive Behaviour* 36 (2010), pp. 14–20.

Harvard Health Publishing. 'Mars vs. Venus: The Gender Gap in Health', *Harvard Men's Health Watch*, August 26th 2019.

Haslanger, Sally. 'Gender and Race: (What) Are They? (What) Do We Want Them To Be?' *Nous* 34.1 (2000), pp. 31–55.

Hay, Carol. 'Who Counts as a Woman?' *The New York Times*, 1st April 2019.

Heilburn, Carolyn. *Toward a Recognition of Androgyny* (New York: Alfred Knopf, 1973).

Hickman, Mary. 'What's Current: Vancouver Rape Relief Targeted with Vandalism and Death Threats', *Feminist Current*, 27th August 2019.

Hill, Jess. *See What You Made Me Do* (Melbourne: Black Inc. Books, 2019).

Hindriks, Frank. 'But Where Is the University?' *Dialectica* 66/1 (2012), pp. 93–113.

Hochschild, Adam. *Bury the Chains* (London: Macmillan Publishers, 2005).

Hodge, John. *The Cultural Basis of Racism and Group Oppression* (Berkeley, CA: Time Readers Press, 1975).

Holmes, Bob. 'The First Real Farmers: How Agriculture Was a Global Invention', *New Scientist*, 28th October 2015.

Holt, Vicky, Skagerberg, Elin, & Dunsford, Michael. 'Young People with Features of Gender Dysphoria: Demographics and Associated Difficulties', *Clinical Child Psychology and Psychiatry* 21 (2016), pp. 108–118.

hooks, bell. *Feminism Is for Everybody* (London: Pluto Press, 2000).

hooks, bell. *Feminist Theory: From Margin to Centre*, 2nd Ed. (London: Pluto Press, [1984] 2000).

hooks, bell. *Ain't I A Woman* (London: Pluto Press, 1982).

Horney, Karen. *New Ways in Psychoanalysis* (New York: Norton, 1939).

Hudson, John. 'How Brazilian Soap Operas Can Save the World', *The Atlantic*, 28th June 2012.

Hull, Carrie. 'Letter to the Editor', *American Journal of Human Biology* 15/1 (2003), pp. 112–116.

Hungerford, Elizabeth. 'Sex and Gender: The Law in the USA', Woman's Place UK, 19th October 2019.

Hunter, Brad. 'HUNTER: "Psychopathic" Child Sex Killer Uses Trans Card', *Toronto Sun*, 1st February 2020.

Izaakson, Jen. 'Trans-identified Male, Tara Wolf, Convicted of Assault after Hyde Park Attack', *Feminist Current*, 27th April 2018.

Jacobs, Michelle S. 'The Violent State: Black Women's Invisible Struggle against Police Violence', *William & Mary Journal of Race, Gender, and Social Justice* 24/1 (2017–2018), pp. 39–100.

Jaggar, Alison. *Feminist Politics and Human Nature* (Maryland: Rowman & Littlefield, 1983).

James, S. E., Herman, J. L., Rankin, S., Keisling, M., Mottet, L., & Anafi, M. *The Report of the 2015 U.S Transgender Survey* (Washington, DC: National Center for Transgender Equality, 2016).

Jaschick, Scott. 'The Evolution of American Women's Studies', *Inside Higher Ed*, 27th March 2009.

Jefferson, Margaret. [Interviewed in] 'Some American Feminists' (1980), YouTube, from 10.45.

Jeffreys, Sheila. 'The Need for Radical Feminism', *Scarlet Woman* 5 (1977). Online at https://finnmackay.wordpress.com/articles-i-like/the-need-for-revolutionary-feminism-by-sheila-jeffreys-1977/

Jeffreys, Sheila. *The Industrial Vagina* (Abingdon: Routledge, 2009*a*).

Jeffreys, Sheila. 'Military Prostitution', *The Industrial Vagina* (Abingdon: Routledge, 2009*b*).

Jeffreys, Sheila. *Beauty and Misogyny: Harmful Cultural Practices in the West* (Abingdon: Routledge, 2014).

Jenkins, Katharine. 'Toward an Account of Gender Identity', *Ergo* 5/21 (2018), pp. 713–744.

Jensen, Robert. *The End of Patriarchy* (Melbourne: Spinifex, 2017).

Joel, Daphna. 'Sex beyond the Genitalia: The Human Brain Mosaic', *Proceedings of the National Academy of Sciences* 112/50 (2015), pp. 15468–15473.

Joel, Daphna, & Vikhanski, Luba. *Gender Mosaic* (London: Octopus, 2019).

Jones, Jane Clare. 'On Feminist Genealogy: Reading the Reading of "Rereading the Second Wave"', janeclarejones.com, 16th May 2014.

Jones, Jane Clare. '"You Are Killing Me": On Hate Speech and Feminist Silencing', troubleandstrife.org, 16th May 2015.

Jones, Owen. 'Simon Danczuk MP Has Watched Porn—Why Should We Care?' *The Guardian*, 31st March 2015.

Joyce, Helen. *Trans: When Ideology Meets Reality* (London: Oneworld, 2021).

Kaplan, Gisela, Bottomley, Gill, & Rogers, Lesley. 'Ardent Warrior for Women's Rights', *The Sydney Morning Herald*, 31st July 2003.

Kaufmann, Eric. 'How the Trans Pledge Damaged the Labour Party', *Quillette*, 27th February 2020.

Kaufman, Eric. 'The Threat to Academic Freedom: From Anecdotes to Data', *Quillette*, 12th March 2021.

Kearns, Madeleine. 'The Tragedy of the "Trans" Child', *National Review*, 21st November 2019.

Keen-Minshull, Kellie-Jay. 'Posie Above the Parapet—Changes to the GRA 2004', 3rd July 2018. Online at https://www.youtube.com/watch?v=f6DLhFiLqds

Kelleher, Patrick. 'Peter Tatchell Pulls Out of Debate with Trans-exclusionary Professor Kathleen Stock after Backlash', *Pink News*, 26th August 2021.

Kelly, Liz. 'The Wrong Debate: Reflections on Why Force Is Not the Key Issue with Respect to Trafficking in Women for Sexual Exploitation', *Feminist Review* 73 (2003), pp. 135–139.

Kelly, Raymond. *Warless Societies and the Origins of War* (Michigan: University of Michigan Press, 2000).

Kerr, Barra. 'Pronouns Are Rohypnol', *Fair Play for Women*, 4th June 2019.

King, Deborah. 'Multiple Jeopardy, Multiple Consciousness: The Context of a Black Feminist Ideology', *Signs* 14/1 (1988), pp. 42–72.

King, Tania, Shields, Marissa, Sojo, Victor, Daraganova, Galina, Currier, Dianne, O'Neil, Adrienne, King, Kylie, & Milner, Allison. 'Expressions of Masculinity and Associations with Suicidal Ideation among Young Males' *BMC Psychiatry* 20/288 (2020), pp. 1–10.

Kipnis, Laura. *Unwanted Advances* (New York: Harper, 2017).

Kirkup, James. 'The NHS Has Quietly Changed Its Trans Guidance to Reflect Reality', *The Spectator*, 4th June 2020.

Koedt, Anne,Levine, Ellen,& Rapone, Anita(Eds.), *Radical Feminism* (New York: Quadrangle, 1973).

Koslowski, Max. 'Is This Why There Are So Few Women in Politics?' *The Sydney Morning Herald*, 25th June 2019.

Kreps, Bonnie. 'Radical Feminism 1', in Anne Koedt, Ellen Levine, & Anita Rapone (Eds.), *Radical Feminism* (New York: Quadrangle, 1973).

Kuran, Timur. 'Private and Public Preferences', *Economics and Philosophy* 6 (1990), pp. 1–26.

Lance, Mark. 'Taking Trans Lives Seriously', *Inside Higher Ed*, 30th July 2019.

Landrine, Hope. 'Race x Class Stereotypes of Women', *Sex Roles* 13/1–2 (1985), pp. 65–75.

Lane, Bernard. 'Cookie-cutter Gender Clinics for Troubled Teens', *The Australian*, 25th November 2019*a*.

Lane, Bernard. 'Reason Lost to Suicide in Trans Debate', *The Australian*, 1st November 2019*b*.

Lane, Bernard. 'Gender Change Is "No Fix for Autism"', *The Australian*, 3rd June 2020.

Lane, Bernard. 'Mothers Group in Turmoil Over "Chestfeeding" Pressure', *The Australian*, 9th May 2021.

Langton, Rae. 'Speech Acts and Unspeakable Acts', *Philosophy & Public Affairs* 22/4 (1993), pp. 293–330.

Lawford-Smith, Holly. 'Understanding Political Feasibility', *The Journal of Political Philosophy* 21/3 (2013), pp. 243–259.

Lawford-Smith, Holly. 'How the Trans-Rights Movement Is Turning Philosophers into Activists', *Quillette*, 20th September 2019.

Lawford-Smith, Holly. 'Ending Sex-based Oppression: Transitional Pathways', *Philosophia* (2020*a*), pp. 1–21 [early view].

Lawford-Smith, Holly. 'An Australian Bill Criminalizing "Conversion Therapy" May Harm Kids Deemed "Trans" as well as Those Who Treat Them', *Feminist Current*, 18th December 2020*b*.

Lawford-Smith, Holly. 'A Warning from Australia on the Transgender Debate', *The Spectator*, 13th February 2021.

Lawford-Smith, Holly. 'Tribalism & Trashing in the Gender Wars', in Mark Alfano (Ed.), *Moral Psychology of Hate*, Volume 14 (Maryland: Rowman & Littlefield International, forthcoming).

Lawford-Smith, Holly. *Sex Matters: Essays in Gender Critical Feminism*. Manuscript.

Lawford-Smith, Holly, & Megarry, Jessica. 'Is There Collective Responsibility For Misogyny Perpetrated On Social Media?' in Carissa Veliz (Ed.), *Oxford Handbook of Digital Ethics* (Oxford: Oxford University Press, forthcoming).

Lawford-Smith, Holly, & Phelan, Kate. 'The Metaphysics of Intersectionality Revisited', *The Journal of Political Philosophy* (2021), [early view].

Lawrence, Anne. *Men Trapped In Men's Bodies: Narratives of Autogynephilic Transsexualism* (New York: Springer 2013).

Lawrence, Anne. 'Autogynephilia and the Typology of Male-to-Female Transsexualism', *European Psychologist* 22/1 (2017), pp. 39–54.

Leeds Revolutionary Feminist Group. 'Love Your Enemy? The Debate between Heterosexual Feminism and Political Lesbianism' (London: Onlywomen Press, 1981).

Leeson, Peter, & Russ, Jacob. 'Witch Trials', *The Economic Journal* 128 (2018), pp. 2066–2105.

Lerner, Gerda. *The Creation of Patriarchy* (Oxford: Oxford University Press, 1986).

Levin, Sam, & Solon, Olivia. 'Rose McGowan Alleges Rape by Harvey Weinstein—and Amazon Ignored Claim', *The Guardian*, 13th October 2017.

Lewis, Helen. 'Rereading the Second Wave: Why Feminism Needs to Respect Its Elders', *New Statesman*, 12th May 2014.

Lewis, Sophie. 'How British Feminism Became Anti-trans', *The New York Times*, 7th February 2019.

Li, Gu, Kung, Karson, & Hines, Melissa. 'Childhood Gender-typed Behaviour and Adolescent Sexual Orientation: A Longitudinal Population-based Study', *Developmental Psychology* 53/4 (2017), pp. 764–777.

Lindauer, Matthew, & Southwood, Nicholas. 'How to Cancel the Knobe Effect: The Role of Sufficiently Strong Moral Censure', *American Philosophical Quarterly* (forthcoming).

Littman, Lisa. 'Parent Reports of Adolescents and Young Adults Perceived to Show Signs of a Rapid Onset of Gender Dysphoria', *PLoS ONE* 13/8 (2018), pp. 1–44.

Littman, Lisa. 'Correction: Parent Reports of Adolescents and Young Adults Perceived to Show Signs of a Rapid Onset of Gender Dysphoria', *PLOS One* 14/3 (2019).

Littman, Lisa. 'Individuals Treated for Gender Dysphoria with Medical and/or Surgical Transition Who Subsequently Detransitioned: A Survey of 100 Detransitioners', *Archives of Sexual Behaviour* 2021 [early view].

Locke, John. *A Letter Concerning Toleration*. Trans. William Popple (1689).

Lorde, Audre. *Sister Outsider: Essays and Speeches by Audre Lorde* (Berkeley, CA: Crossing Press, [1984] 2007).

Lowrey, Kathleen. 'From South American Anthropology to Gender-crit Cancel Culture: My Strange Feminist Journey', *Quillette*, 12th June 2020.

Lyons, Kate. 'UK Doctor Prescribing Cross-sex Hormones to Children as Young as 12', *The Guardian*, 11th July 2016.

Mac, Juno, & Smith, Molly. *Revolting Prostitutes* (London: Verso, 2018).

Macandrew, Ruby, Long, Jessica, & Deguara, Brittney. 'Banned from Twitter but Welcome at Massey: Radical Feminist Group to Host Event', stuff.co.nz, 28th September 2019.

Mackay, Finn. *Radical Feminism: Feminist Activism in Movement* (London: Palgrave MacMillan, 2015).

Mackay, Fiona. 'Jane Mansbridge—a Quietly Dangerous Woman', *Dangerous Women Project*, 8th March 2017.

MacKinnon, Catharine. 'Feminism, Marxism, Method, and the State: An Agenda for Theory', *Signs* 7/3 (1982), pp. 515–544.

MacKinnon, Catharine. 'Feminism, Marxism, Method, and the State: Toward Feminist Jurisprudence', *Signs* 8/4 (1983), pp. 635–658).

MacKinnon, Catharine. 'Difference and Dominance', in *Feminism Unmodified* (Cambridge, MA: Harvard University Press, 1987), pp. 32–45.

MacKinnon, Catharine. *Toward a Feminist Theory of the State* (Cambridge, MA: Harvard University Press, 1989).

MacKinnon, Catharine. 'From Practice to Theory, or What Is a White Woman Anyway?' *Yale Journal of Law and Feminism* 4/1 (1991*a*), pp. 13–22.

MacKinnon, Catharine. 'Pornography as Defamation and Discrimination', *Boston University Law Review* 71/5 (1991*b*), pp. 793–818.

MacKinnon, Catharine. *Only Words* (Cambridge, MA: Harvard University Press, [1993] 1996).

MacLennan, Cat. 'Why the New Strangulation Law Matters', *The Spinoff*, 7th December 2018.

Malik, Kenan. 'If Identity Politics Is a Force for Good, How Does White Nationalism Fit In?' *The Guardian*, 7th April 2019.

Mandler, C. 'Please Stop Wearing Those Pussy Hats to Women's Marches', *Seventeen*, 18th January 2019.

Marchiano, Lisa. 'Outbreak: On Transgender Teens and Psychic Epidemics', *Psychological Perspectives* 60/3 (2017), pp. 345–366.

Marcus, Adam. 'Journal Retracts Paper on Gender Dysphoria after 900 Critics Petition', *Retraction Watch*, 30th April 2020.

Marlowe, Frank. *The Hadza: Hunter-Gatherers of Tanzania* (California: University of California Press, 2010).

Mathison, Eric., & Davis, Jeremy. 'Is There A Right To The Death Of The Foetus?' *Bioethics* 31/4 (2017), pp. 313-320.

McConnell, Elizabeth, Odahl-Ruan, Charlynn, Kozlowski, Christins, Shattell, Mona, & Todd, Nathan. 'Trans Women and Michfest: An Ethnophenomenology of Attendees' Experiences', *Journal of Lesbian Studies* 20/1 (2016), pp. 8–28.

McCook, Alison. 'Reader Outcry Prompts Brown to Retract Press Release on Trans Teens', *Retraction Watch*, 29th August 2018.

McCulloch, Craig. 'Sophie Elliot's Mum Backs Law Criminalising Strangulation', *Radio New Zealand*, 3rd December 2018.

McKinnon, Rachel. 'The Epistemology of Propaganda', *Philosophy and Phenomenological Research* XCVI/2 (2018), pp. 483–489.

McLaughlin, Kelly. 'Here's Why Lori Loughlin Will Likely Spend 2 Months in Prison for the College Admissions Scandal while Felicity Huffman Was Sentenced to 14 Days', *Insider*, 22nd May 2020.

Mehat, Jindi. 'Shit Liberal Feminists Say: Choice', *Feminist Current*, 14th December 2015.

Mill, John Stuart. 'The Subjection of Women', in Alice Rossi (Ed.), *Essays on Sex Equality* (Chicago, IL: University of Chicago Press, [1869] 1970), chapter 4.

Mill, John Stuart. *On Liberty*. Ed. Elizabeth Rapaport. (Indianapolis: Hackett Publishing Company, [1859] 1978).

Millett, Kate. 'Sexual Politics: A Manifesto for Revolution', in Anne Koedt, Ellen Levine, & Anita Rapone (Eds.), *Radical Feminism* (New York: Quadrangle, [1968] 1973), pp. 365–367.

Millett, Kate. *Sexual Politics* (Champaign, IL: University of Illinois Press, [1970] 2000).

Minefield, The. 'International Women's Day—Cause for Celebration, or Commiseration?' *ABC*, 4th March 2020.

Miriam, Kathy. 'Stopping the Traffic in Women: Power, Agency and Abolition in Feminist Debates over Sex-Trafficking', *Journal of Social Philosophy* 36/1 (2005), pp. 1–17.

Mofokeng, Tlaleng. 'Why Sex Work Is Real Work', *Teen Vogue*, 26th April 2019.

Moore, Michele, & Brunskell-Evans, Heather. *Inventing Transgender Children and Young People* (Newcastle Upon Tyne: Cambridge Scholars Publishing, 2019).

Moran, Rachel. *Paid For: My Journey Through Prostitution* (Dublin: Gill & Macmillan, 2013).

More, Max. 'The Philosophy of Transhumanism', in Max More & Natasha Vita-More (Eds.), *The Transhumanist Reader: Classical and Contemporary Essays on the Science, Technology, and Philosophy of the Human Future*, 1st Ed. (Oxford: John Wiley & Sons, Inc., 2013).

More, Thomas. *Utopia* (London: Bibliolis, [1516] 2000).

Morgenroth, Thekla, & Ryan, Michelle. 'Gender Trouble in Social Psychology: How Can Butler's Work Inform Experimental Social Psychologists' Conceptualization of Gender?' *Frontiers in Psychology* 9/1320 (2018), pp. 239–247.

Morley, Louise. 'Feminist Academics: Disruption, Development and Disciplines', *Organizing Feminisms*, Women's Studies at York Series (London: Palgrave Macmillan, 1999).

Morton, Thomas, Postmes, Tom, Haslam, S., & Hornsey M. 'Theorizing Gender in the Face of Social Change: Is There Anything Essential about Essentialism?' *Journal of Personality and Social Psychology* 96/3 (2009), pp. 653–664.

Murphy, Meghan. 'PODCAST: What Happens When Your Husband Decides He's a Woman?' *Feminist Current*, 12th January 2018.

Murphy, Meghan. 'Discontinuation of Grant to Vancouver Rape Relief Shows Trans Activism Is an Attack on Women', *Feminist Current*, 20th March 2019*a*.

Murphy, Meghan. '"TERF": A Handy Guide for Irresponsible Journalists, Shady Academics, and Irate Men', *Feminist Current*, 1st April 2019*b*.

Murphy, Meghan. 'INTERVIEW: Julia Beck on the Equality Act, Sex Self-identification, and Why She Persevered in the Face of Controversy', *Feminist Current*, 24th September 2019*c*.

Murphy, Meghan. 'PODCAST: Indian Filmmaker Vaishnavi Sundar Made a Film about Sexual Harassment, Then Got Cancelled by Liberal Feminists', *Feminist Current*, 24th March 2020*a*.

Murphy, Meghan. 'PODCAST: Michelle Mara on the Truth about the Decriminalized Sex Trade in New Zealand', *Feminist Current*, 13th April 2020*b*. Online at https://www.feministcurrent.com/2020/04/13/podcast-michelle-mara-on-the-truth-about-the-decriminalized-sex-trade-in-new-zealand/ accessed 15th April 2020.

Nash, Jennifer. *Black Feminism Reimagined: After Intersectionality* (Croydon: Duke University Press, 2019).

National Health Service. 'Investigation into the Study "Early Pubertal Suppression in a Carefully Selected Group of Adolescents with Gender Identity Disorders"', NHS Health Research Authority, 14th October 2019.

New York Radical Feminists. 'Politics of the Ego: A Manifesto for New York Radical Feminists' (1969), in Anne Koedt, Ellen Levine, & Anita Rapone (Eds.), *Radical Feminism* (New York: Quadrangle Books, 1973), pp. 379–383.

Noddings, Nel. *Caring: A Feminine Approach to Ethics and Moral Education* (Berkeley, CA : University of California Press, 1984).

nordicmodelnow.org. 'FACT: Buying Sex Makes Men More Prone to Violence against Women', n.d. Online at https://nordicmodelnow.org/facts-about-prostitution/fact-buying-sex-makes-men-more-prone-to-violence-against-women/ accessed 24th May 2020.

Norma, Caroline. 'Transgenderism: The Latest Anti-Feminist Wedge of the Left' *ABC*, 28th October 2015.

Norma, Caroline. 'The Australian Left Gives away its anti-feminist game', *Feminist Current*, 28th December 2018.
O'Connor, Cailin. 'The Evolution of Gender', *The Origins of Unfairness* (Oxford: Oxford University Press, 2019), pp. 84–102.
Orange, Richard. 'Teenage transgender row splits Sweden as dysphoria diagnoses soar by 1,500%', *The Guardian*, 23rd February 2020.
Otto, Dianne. 'Making sense of zero tolerance policies in peacekeeping sexual economies', in Vanessa Munro & Carl Stychin (Eds.), *Sexuality and the Law: Feminist Engagements* (London: Taylor & Francis, 2007).
Pang, Ken, Notini, Lauren, McDougall, Rosalind, Gillam, Lynn, Savulescu, Julian, Wilkinson, Dominic, Clark, Beth, Olson-Kennedy, Johanna, Telfer, Michelle, & Lantos, John. 'Long-term Puberty Suppression for a Nonbinary Teenager', *Pediatrics* 145/2 (2020), pp. 1–6.
Parker, Jessica. 'Labour leadership: Long-Bailey backs calls to expel "transphobic" members', *BBC News*, 12th February 2020.
Parsons, Vic. '13 Troubling Problems with White Feminism, According to a White Feminist Who's Seen Them Firsthand', *Pink News*, 22nd May 2020.
Pateman, Carole. *The Sexual Contract* (Stanford, CA: Stanford University Press, 1988).
Pateman, Carole. 'Self-ownership and Property in the Person: Democratization and a Tale of Two Concepts', *The Journal of Political Philosophy* 10/1 (2002), pp. 20–53.
Pearson-Jones, Bridie. 'Transgender Model Who Punched Feminist and Smashed Her £120 Camera in Violent Brawl at Hyde Park Speakers' Corner Protest Walks Free from Court' *Daily Mail Australia*, 14th April 2018.
Pease, Bob. *Facing Patriarchy* (London: Zed Books, 2019).
Penna, Dominic. 'University Speakers with Gender-critical Views Are Most Likely to be Banned from Addressing Students', *The Telegraph*, 20th February 2021.
Pennyworth, Humphrey. 'Cyberstar Aiming for Sabrina's Gangbang Record', *AVN*, 29th May 2003.
Perhach, Paulette. 'A Story of a Fuck Off Fund', *The Billfold*, 20th January 2016.
Perry, Louise. 'How a Feminist Prophet Became an Apostate—An Interview with Dr Phyllis Chesler', *Quillette*, 20th June 2019.
Peoples, Lindsay. 'Bridging the Gap between Black and White Feminism', *The Cut*, 22nd January 2016.
Pettit, Philip. 'Liberalism and Republicanism', *Australian Journal of Political Science* 28/4 (1993), pp. 162–189.
Pettit, Philip. 'Freedom as Antipower', *Ethics* 106/3 (1996), pp. 576–604.
Pettit, Philip. *Republicanism* (Oxford: Clarendon Press, 1997).
Phelan, Kate. 'Feminism as Epic Theory', *British Journal of Political Science* (forthcoming).
Pinker, Stephen. *The Blank Slate* (New York: Viking, 2002).
Pizan, Christine de. *The Book of the City of Ladies*. Trans. Rosalind Brown-Grant (London: Penguin, [1405] 1999), Part I, pp. 5–11, 78–80.
Pratz, Clair de. *France From Within* (London: Hodder & Stoughton, 1912).
Pritchard, Duncan. 'Wittgenstein on Scepticism', in Oskari Kuusela & Marie McGinn (Eds.), *The Oxford Handbook of Wittgenstein* (Oxford: Oxford University Press, 2011).
Pulver, Andrew. 'BFI Criticized for Naming Trans Activist Munroe Bergdorf as Speaker at Women's Summit', *The Guardian*, 15th June 2018.

Rachelle, Vivian. 'Japan's #KuToo movement is fighting back against regressive dress codes for women', *Quartz*, 30th August 2019.

Radcliffe Richards, Janet. *The Sceptical Feminist* (Harmondsworth: Penguin Books, [1980] 1994).

Rawls, John. *A Theory of Justice* (Cambridge, MA: Harvard University Press, 1971).

Raymond, Janice. 'The Illusion of Androgyny', *Quest* 11/1 (1975), pp. 57–66.

Raymond, Janice. *Women as Wombs: Reproductive Technologies and the Battle Over Women's Freedom* (San Francisco, CA: Harper, 1993).

Raymond, Janice. *The Transsexual Empire: The Making of the She-Male* (New York: Teachers College Press [1979] 1994).

Raymond, Janice. *A Passion For Friends: Toward a Philosophy of Female Affection* (Boston, MA: Beacon Press, 1996).

Rayner, Gordon. 'Minister Orders Inquiry into 4,000 Per Cent Rise in Children Wanting to Change Sex', *The Telegraph*, 16th September 2018.

Redstockings. 'Redstockings Manifesto', 1969.

Rees, Yves. 'Reading the Mess Backwards', *Australian Book Review* 422/June-July (2020).

Reeve, Kesia, Casey, Rionach, Batty, Elaine, & Green, Stephen. 'The Housing Needs and Experiences of Homeless Women Involved in Street Sex Work in Stoke-on-Trent', Centre for Regional Economic and Social Research, Sheffield Hallam University, December 2009.

Reilly, Peter. 'Lesbians Want a Church of Their Own and IRS Approves', *Forbes*, 3rd August 2018.

Reilly, Wilfred. 'Are We in the Midst of a Transgender Murder Epidemic?' *Quillette* 7th December 2019.

Reilly-Cooper, Rebecca. 'Comment: The Attack on Germaine Greer Shows Identity Politics Has Become a Cult', politics.co.uk, 28th October 2015.

Reilly-Cooper, Rebecca. 'Gender Is Not a Spectrum', *Aeon*, 28th June 2016*a*. Online at https://aeon.co/essays/the-idea-that-gender-is-a-spectrum-is-a-new-gender-prison accessed 23rd May 2020.

Reilly-Cooper, Rebecca. 'Equality for Trans People Must Not Come at the Expense of Women's Safety', politics.co.uk, 26th January 2016b.

Rich, Adrienne. 'Compulsory Heterosexuality and Lesbian Existence', *Signs* 5/4 (1980), pp. 631–660.

Ridley, Matt. *Nature Via Nurture* (New York: Harper Collins, 2003).

Riggs, Damien. 'Narratives of Choice amongst White Australians Who Undertake Surrogacy Arrangements in India', *Journal of Medical Humanities* 37 (2016), pp. 313–325.

Ristori, Jiska, & Steensma, Thomas. 'Gender Dysphoria in Childhood', *International Review of Psychiatry* 28/1 (2016), pp. 13–20.

Robillard, Michael. & Strawser, Bradley J. 'The Moral Exploitation of Soldiers', *Public Affairs Quarterly* 30/2 (2016), pp. 171–195.

Rodgers, Sienna. 'Rania Ramli Elected Labour Students Chair as Corbynsceptics Sweep to Victory', *Labour List*, 7th March 2019.

Rosen, Ali. 'Surrogacy Is Misunderstood and Unfairly Maligned: We Need to Change the Narrative', *The Washington Post*, 24th January 2020.

Rosewarne, Lauren. 'Radical Feminists' Objection to Sex Work Is Profoundly Un-feminist', *The Conversation*, 9th August 2017.

Ross, Colin., Farley, Melissa., & Schwartz, Harvey. 'Dissociation Among Women in Prostitution', Journal of Trauma Practice 2/3-4 (2004), pp. 199-212.

Roszak, Betty. 'The Human Continuum', in Betty Roszak & Theodore Roszak (Eds.), *Masculine/Feminine* (New York: Harper & Row, 1969).

Rowland, Richard. 'The Significance of Significant Fundamental Moral Disagreement', *Nous* 51/4 (2017), pp. 802–831.

Rowling, J. K. [Writing under the pseudonym Robert Galbriath]. *Troubled Blood* (London: Sphere, 2020).

Rudrappa, Sharmila. 'Making India the "Mother Destination": Outsourcing Labour to Indian Surrogates', *Research in the Sociology of Work* 20 (2010), pp. 253–285.

Salk, Rachel, Hyde, Janet, & Abramson, Lyn. 'Gender Differences in Depression in Representative National Samples: Meta-Analyses of Diagnoses and Symptoms', *Psychological Bulletin* 143/8 (2017), pp. 783–822.

Sanchez, Raquel Rosario. 'Liberal Feminists Ushered Ivanka Trump into the White House', *Feminist Current*, 20th January 2017.

Sankaran, Kirun. 'What's New in the New Ideology Critique?' *Philosophical Studies* 177 (2020), pp. 1441–1462.

Sargent, Lyman Tower. *Utopianism: A Very Short Introduction* (Oxford: Oxford University Press, 2010).

SaAUrtre, Jean-Paul. *Being and Nothingness*. Trans. Hazel E. Barnes (New York: Philosophical Library, 1956).

Satz, Debra. 'Markets in Women's Reproductive Labour', *Philosophy & Public Affairs* 21/2 (1992), pp. 107–131.

Satz, Debra. *Why Some Things Should Not Be For Sale: The Moral Limits of Markets* (Oxford: Oxford University Press, 2010).

Saul, Jennifer. 'Why the Words We Use Matter When Describing Anti-trans Activists', *The Conversation*, 6th March 2020.

Savic, I., & Arver, S. 'Sex Dimorphism of the Brain in Male-to-Female Transsexuals', *Cerebral Cortex* 21 (2011), pp. 2525–2533.

Sax, Leonard. 'How Common is Intersex? A Tesponse to Anne Fausto-Sterling', *The Journal of Sex Research* 39/3 (2002), pp. 174–178.

Scarlet Alliance. 'Listen to Sex Workers: Support Decriminalisation and Anti-discrimination Protections', *Interface* 3/2 (2011), pp. 271–287.

Schneider, Maiko, Spritzer, Poli, Soll, Bianca, Fontanari, Anna, Carneiro, Marina, Tovar-Moll, Fernanda, Costa, Angelo, da Silva, Dhiordan, Schwarz, Karine, Anes, Mauricio, Tramontina, Silza, & Lobato, Maria. 'Brain Maturation, Cognition and Voice Pattern in a Gender Dysphoria Case Under Pubertal Suppression', *Frontiers in Human Neuroscience* 11/528 (2017), pp. 1–9.

Schor, Naomi. 'This Essentialism which Is Not One: Coming to Grips with Irigaray', in Naomi Schor & Elizabeth Weed (Eds.), *The Essential Difference* (Bloomington, IN: Indiana University Press, 1994).

Schulze, Erika, Novo Canto, Sandra Isabel, Mason, Peter, & Skalin, Maria. 'Sexual Exploitation and Prostitution and Its Impact on Gender Equality', European

Parliament, Directorate-General for Internal Policies, Citizens' Rights and Constitutional Affairs, 2014.

Scotland, Patricia. 'Women Shouldering the Burden of Climate Crisis Need Action, Not Speeches', *The Guardian*, 13th March 2020.

Searle, John. *The Construction of Social Reality* (New York: The Free Press, 1995).

Searle, John. 'What Is an Institution?' *Journal of Institutional Economics* 1 (2005), pp. 1–22.

Serano, Julia. *Whipping Girl* (Berkeley, CA: Seal Press, 2007).

Serano, Julia. 'The Case against Autogynephilia', *International Journal of Transgenderism* 12/3 (2010), pp. 176–187.

Shamsian, Jacob, & McLaughlin, Kelly. 'Here's the Full List of People Charged in the College Admissions Cheating Scandal, and Who Has Pleaded Guilty So Far', *Insider*, 22nd May 2020.

Sherfey, Mary Jane. 'A Theory on Female Sexuality', in Robin Morgan (Ed.), *Sisterhood is Powerful* (New York: Vintage Books, 1970), Part II.

Shidlo, Ariel, & Schroeder, Michael. 'Changing Sexual Orientation: A Consumers' Report', *Professional Psychology: Research and Practice* 33/3 (2002), pp. 249–259.

Shiffrin, Seana. 'Wrongful Life, Procreative Responsibility, and the Significance of Harm', *Legal Theory* 5 (1999), pp. 117–148.

Shrier, Abigail. *Irreversible Damage* (Washington, DC: Regnery Publishing, 2020).

Siddique, Haroon. 'Stonewall Is at Centre of a Toxic Debate on Trans Rights and Gender Identity', *The Guardian*, 5th June 2021.

Society for Evidence Based Gender Medicine (SEGM). 'New Systematic Reviews of Puberty Blockers and Cross-Sex Hormones Published by NICE', 31st March 2021*a*. Online at https://segm.org/NICE_gender_medicine_systematic_review_finds_poor_quality_evidence

Society for Evidence-Based Gender Medicine (SEGM). 'The AAP Silences the Debate on How to Best Care for Gender-Diverse Kids', 9th August 2021*b*. Online at https://segm.org/AAP_silences_debate_on_gender_diverse_youth_treatments

Solnit, Rebecca. 'Trans Women Pose No Threat to Cis Women, but We Pose a Threat to Them If We Make Them Outcasts', *The Guardian*, 10th August 2020.

Sommers, Christina Hoff. *Who Stole Feminism?* (New York: Touchstone, 1994).

Southwood, Nicholas. 'That's Just Not Feasible!', *TEDx Fullbright Canberra*, 28th July 2017. Online at https://www.youtube.com/watch?v=1wXtex5EtWQ

Southwood, Nicholas. 'The Feasibility Issue', *Philosophy Compass* 13/8 (2018), pp. 1–13.

Southwood, Nicholas, & Wiens, David. '"Actual" Does Not Imply "Feasible"', *Philosophical Studies* 173 (2016), pp. 3,037–3,060.

Spelman, Elizabeth. *Inessential Woman: Problems of Exclusion in Feminist Thought* (Boston, MA: Beacon Press, 1988).

Srinivasan, Amia. 'Does Anyone Have the Right to Sex?' *London Review of Books*, 22nd March 2018.

Srinivasan, Amia. *The Right to Sex* (London, Bloomsbury, 2021).

Stamp, Jimmy. 'Fact [or] Fiction? The Legend of the QWERTY Keyboard', *Smithsonian Magazine*, 3rd May 2013.

Stanley, Jason. *How Propaganda Works* (Princeton, NJ: Princeton University Press, 2015).

Steensma, Thomas, & Cohen-Kettenis, Peggy. 'A Critical Commentary on "A Critical Commentary on Follow-Up Studies and "Desistence" Theories about Transgender and Gender Non-conforming Children', *International Journal of Transgenderism* 19/2 (2018), pp. 225–230.

Stock, Kathleen. 'Academic Philosophy and the UK Gender Recognition Act', *Medium*, 8th May 2018.

Stock, Kathleen. *Material Girls* (London: Fleet, 2021).

Stock, Kathleen, Bindel, Julie, & Lawford-Smith, Holly. 'How Can Philosophy Help Us Understand Transgender Experiences?' *Institute of Art and Ideas*, 26th July 2019.

Stoljar, Natalie. 'Essence, Identity, and the Concept of Woman', *Philosophical Topics* 23/2 (Fall 1995), pp. 261–293.

Stojlar, Natalie. 'Discrimination and Intersectionality', in *The Routledge Handbook of the Ethics of Discrimination* (Abingdon: Routledge, 2017), pp. 68–79.

Stone, Sandy. 'The Empire Strikes Back: A Posttranssexual Manifesto' (1991), in Susan Stryker & Stephen Whittle (Eds.), *The Transgender Studies Reader* (New York: Routledge, 2006), pp. 221–235.

Strudwick, Patrick. 'This Trans Woman Kept Her Beard and Couldn't Be Happier', *Buzzfeed*, 17th July 2015.

Sundar, Vaishnavi. 'I Was Cancelled for My Tweets on Transgenderism', *Spiked*, 4th March 2020.

Sunstein, Cass. 'The Law of Group Polarization', University of Chicago Law School, John M. Olin Law & Economics Working Paper No. 91 (1999), pp. 1–38.

Sunstein, Cass. How Change Happens (Massachusetts: MIT Press, 2019).

Sutton, Candace. '7-Eleven Axe Attacker Evie Amati Involved in Jail Fight', news.com.au, 30th July 2019.

Taddeo, Lisa. *Three Women* (London: Bloomsbury, 2019).

Tasmanian Law Reform Institute. 'Sexual Orientation and Gender Identity Conversion Practices', Issues Paper No. 31, 2020.

Taylor, Charles. 'What's Wrong with Negative Liberty', in A. Ryan (Ed.), *The Idea of Freedom* (Oxford: Oxford University Press, 1979), pp. 175–193.

Taylor Mill, Harriet. 'Enfranchisement of Women' (1851), in Alice Rossi (Ed.), *Essays on Sex Equality* (Chicago, IL: University of Chicago Press, 1970), chapter 3.

Thompson, Clara. 'The Role of Women in This Culture', *Psychiatry: Interpersonal and Biological Processes* 4 (1941), pp. 1–8.

Thompson, Clara. 'Cultural Pressures in the Psychology of Women', *Psychiatry: Interpersonal and Biological Processes* 5 (1942), pp. 331–339.

Thompson, Clara. '"Penis Envy" in Women', *Psychiatry: Interpersonal and Biological Processes* 6/2 (1943), pp. 123–125.

Thornton, Mark. 'Alcohol Prohibition Was a Failure', *Cato Institute*, 17th July 1991.

Tong, Rosemary. 'Feminism, Pornography and Censorship', *Social Theory and Practice* 8/1 (1982), pp. 1–17.

Tong, Rosemary. *Feminist Thought* (Colorado: Westview Press, 1989).

Topping, Alexandra. 'Sexism on the Covid-19 Frontline: "PPE Is Made for a 6ft 3in Rugby Player"', *The Guardian*, 24th April 2020.

Turner, Janice. 'Trans Activists Think Debate Is Hate Speech', *The Times*, 14th April 2018.

Two to Tangle Productions.*Hot Girls Wanted*, Jill Bauer & Ronna Gradus (Directors), 2015.

Tyler, Meagan. *Selling Sex Short* (Newcastle upon Tyne: Cambridge Scholars Publishing, 2011).

Tyler, Meagan. 'Can Feminism Be Saved from Identity Politics?' *ABC Religion & Ethics*, 28th October 2019.

United Nations Women. 'Women's Economic Empowerment in the Changing World of Work: 2017 Commission on the Status of Women: Agreed Conclusions', March 2017.

UNODC (United Nations Office on Drugs and Crime). 'Global Report on Trafficking in Persons: Executive Summary', February 2009.

Vasquez, Tina. 'It's Time to End the Long History of Feminism Failing Transgender Women', *Bitch Media*, 17th February 2014.

Vincent, Nicole, & Jane, Emma. 'Interrogating Incongruence: Conceptual and Normative Problems with the ICD-11's and DSM-5's Diagnostic Categories for Transgender People', *Australasian Philosophical Review* (forthcoming).

Vonnegut, Kurt. 'Harrison Bergeron', *The Magazine of Fantasy and Science Fiction* (1961).

Vonow, Brittany. 'Rally Attack: Cops Release Pictures of Transgender Activists Wanted after 60-Year-Old Woman Was Attacked at Hyde Park Rally', *The Sun*, 26th October 2017.

Vries, Annelou de, Steensma, Thomas, Doreleijers, Theo, & Cohen-Kettenis, Peggy. 'Puberty Suppression in Adolescents with Gender Identity Disorder: A Prospective Follow-Up Study', *The Journal of Sexual Medicine* 8/8 (2011), pp. 2276–2283.

Vrouenraets, Lieke, Fredriks, Miranda, Hannema, Sabine, Cohen-Kettenis, Peggy, & de Vries, Martine. 'Early Medical Treatment of Children and Adolescents with Gender Dysphoria: An Empirical Ethical Study', *Journal of Adolescent Health* 57/4 (2015), pp. 367–373.

Wadman, Meredith. 'New Paper Ignites Storm Over Whether Teens Experience "Rapid Onset" of Transgender Identity', *Science*, 30th August 2018.

Wagoner, Bryce. (Director). *After Porn Ends* (Netflix: 2012).

Wallien, Madeleine, & Cohen-Kettenis, Peggy. 'Psychosexual Outcome of Gender-Dysphoric Children', *Journal of the American Academy of Child and Adolescent Psychiatry* 47/12 (2008), pp. 1413–1423.

Walsh, Reubs, Krabbendam, Lydia, Dewinter, Jeroen, & Begeer, Sander. 'Brief Report: Gender Identity Differences in Autistic Adults: Associations with Perceptual and Socio-cognitive Profiles', *Journal of Autism and Developmental Disorders* 48 (2018), pp. 4070–4078.

Wanta, Jonathon, & Unger, Cecile. 'Review of the Transgender Literature: Where Do We Go from Here?' *Transgender Health* 2/1 (2017), pp. 119–128.

Warrier, Varun, Greenberg, David, Weir, Elizabeth, Buckingham, Clara, Smith, Paula, Lai, Meng-Chuan, Allison, Carrie, & Baron-Cohen, Simon. 'Elevated Rates of Autism, Other Neurodevelopmental and Psychiatric Diagnoses, and Autistic Traits in Transgender and Gender-Diverse Individuals', *Nature Communications* 11/3959 (2020), pp. 1–12.

Watson, Christopher, Uberoi, Elise, & Kirk-Wade, Esme. 'Women in Parliament and Government', *House of Commons Library*, 25th February 2020.

Watson, Lori. 'The Woman Question', *Transgender Studies Quarterly* 3/1 (2016), pp. 248–255.

Watson, Lori, & Flanigan, Jessica. *Debating Sex Work* (Oxford: Oxford University Press, 2020).

Weale, Sally. 'University "Turned Down Politically Incorrect Transgender Research"', *The Guardian*, 26th September 2017.

Weisstein, Naomi. 'Psychology Constructs the Female' (1971), in Anne Koedt, Ellen Levine, & Anita Rapone (Eds.), *Radical Feminism* (New York: Quadrangle, 1973), pp. 178–197.

Wells, Imogen. 'Anti-trans' Billboard Removed from Wellington's CBD', *1 News*, 13th July 2021.

Wendell, Susan. 'A (Qualified) Defense of Liberal Feminism' *Hypatia* 2/2 (1987), pp. 65–93.

Widdows, Heather. *Perfect Me: Beauty as an Ethical Ideal* (Princeton, NJ: Princeton University Press, 2018).

Williams, Cristan. 'Gender Performance: The TransAdvocate Interviews Judith Butler', *The Trans Advocate*, n.d.

Williams, George. 'Gay Marriage Is Now Only a Matter of Political Will', *Newsroom*, 17th December 2013.

Williams, Patricia, Allard, Anna, & Sears, Lonnie. 'Case Study: Cross-gender Preoccupations in Two Male Children with Autism', *Journal of Autism and Developmental Disorders* 26/6 (1996), pp. 635–642.

Williams Institute, The. *How Many Adults Identify as Transgender in the United States?* June 2016.

Winer, Stuart. 'Iran Female Soccer Team Accused of Manning Up', *The Times of Israel*, 30th September 2015.

Witt, Charlotte. *The Metaphysics of Gender* (Oxford: Oxford University Press, 2011).

Wittgenstein, Ludwig. *On Certainty* (Oxford: Blackwell Publishing, 1969).

Wittig, Monique. 'One Is Not Born a Woman', *Proceedings of the Second Sex Conference, New York* (New York Institute for the Humanities, 1979).

Wittig, Monique. 'The Category of Sex', *Feminist Issues*, Fall ([1976] 1982), pp. 63–68.

Wollstonecraft, Mary. *A Vindication of the Rights of Woman* (London: Arcturus, [1792] 2017).

Wong, David. 'Christopher McMahon, Reasonable Disagreement: A Theory of Political Morality', *Notre Dame Philosophical Reviews*, 3rd November 2010.

Wood, Hayley, Sasaki, Shoko, Bradley, Susan, Singh, Devita, Fantus, Sophia, Owen-Anderson, Allison, Di Giacomo, Alexander, Bain, Jerald, & Zucker, Kenneth. 'Patterns of Referral to a Gender Identity Service for Children and Adolescents (1976–2011): Age, Sex Ratio, and Sexual Orientation', *Journal of Sex & Marital Therapy* 39/1 (2013), pp. 1–6.

Woolf, Virginia. *A Room of One's Own* (New York: Harcourt, Brace & World, Inc., 1929).

Workplace Gender Equality Agency. 'Gender Segregation in Australia's Workforce', 17th April 2019.

Wright, Paul J., & Tokunaga, Robert S. 'Men's Objectifying Media Consumption, Objectification of Women, and Attitudes Supportive of Violence against Women', *Archives of Sexual Behaviour* 45 (2016), pp. 955–964.

Wright, Paul J., Tokunaga, Robert S., & Kraus, Ashley. 'A Meta-analysis of Pornography Consumption and Actual Acts of Sexual Aggression in General Population Studies', *Journal of Communication*, 2015.

Wynn, Natalie. 'Autogynephilia | ContraPoints', YouTube, 2nd February 2018.

Xu, Yin, Norton, Sam, & Rahman, Qazi. 'Early Life Conditions and Adolescent Sexual Orientation: A Prospective Birth Cohort Study', *Developmental Psychology* 55/6 (2019), pp. 1226–1243.

Zeller, Tom. 'Defending Cruelty: It's Only a Game', *The New York Times*, 20th February 2006.

Index

For the benefit of digital users, indexed terms that span two pages (e.g., 52–53) may, on occasion, appear on only one of those pages.